What people are saying about *The World Peace Diet*

"Provocative and recommended."—*Library Journal*

"Use *The World Peace Diet* as a guide to empower yourself and others in making dietary choices that are powerful beyond what you can imagine."—**Julia Butterfly Hill,** environmental activist

"...one of the most provocative books I've ever read. I felt challenged and stimulated by its profound insights, and called to question ever more deeply what Will Tuttle calls 'the taboo against knowing what you eat.' This book . . . expose[s] the complacency of a culture." —**John Robbins,** author, *Diet For a New America* and *The Food Revolution*

"Profound, passionate—and ultimately hopeful and inspiring— Will Tuttle's *The World Peace Diet* should be required reading for students everywhere—and for all people with inquiring minds and open hearts. I recommend it most highly."—**Michael Klaper,** M.D.

"*The World Peace Diet* should be required reading for everyone regardless of their diet preferences."—**Harold Brown,** environmental activist and former rancher and dairy operator

"This is one of those 'necessary' books. It is a necessary catalyst for the transformation of human consciousness as it evolves from the domination and exploitation mindset to the paradigm of communion, cooperation, and reverence for all life." —**Judy Carman,** author, *Peace to All Beings*

"Will Tuttle, the author of this eloquently written book, challenges our thinking about our relationship to non-human animals with respect, sensitivity, and grace. His understanding of the human psyche is deep. His use of language is divine, and his compassion reaches out and jumps off each and every page. I highly recommend this book, and I dare you to not be moved by its gentle power." —**Colleen Patrick-Goudreau,** best-selling author and speaker

"A profoundly insightful and important book, *The World Peace Diet* is sure to be a catalyst and powerful tool in the evolution of human consciousness."—*Satya* **magazine**

"*The World Peace Diet* is outstanding. It has raised the bar in the understanding of diet's role in the order of all life on planet Earth. Reading this book will arm you with the information to become part of the solution and not part of the problem. Will Tuttle has struck a strong blow for the future of our children and grandchildren, and you can too by reading his book."
—**Howard F. Lyman** LL.D., author, *No More Bull!* and *Mad Cowboy*

"Will Tuttle has written a provocative book that provides much food for thought. His impassioned writing provides not only the moral framework for a peaceful diet, but also hope for a peaceful world."—**Zoe Weil**, President, International Institute for Humane Education; author, *Above All, Be Kind* and *The Power and Promise of Humane Education*

"As Gandhi observed, our fork can be a weapon of violence. Will Tuttle reminds us of this simple truth and invites us to keep violence off our plate by adopting a vegan way of being in the world. Everyone who works for peace will gain knowledge and draw inspiration from this fine book."—**Tom Regan**, author, *Empty Cages: Facing the Challenge of Animal Rights*

"Complete, compassionate, and profound. You'll never again take lightly the question 'What's for dinner?'"
—**Victoria Moran**, author, *Main Street Vegan*

"I believe *The World Peace Diet* is the most important book of the 21st century. If you read but one book in your life, make it *The World Peace Diet.*"—**James Macy**, M.D.

THE WORLD PEACE DIET

*Eating for Spiritual Health
and Social Harmony*

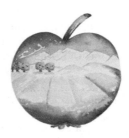

WILL TUTTLE, Ph.D.

Tenth Anniversary Edition

Lantern Books • New York
A Division of Booklight Inc.

2016 [2005]
Lantern Books
128 2nd Place
Brooklyn, NY 11231

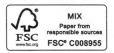

Cover painting by Madeleine W. Tuttle

Cover design by Josh Hooten. Tenth Anniversary design by Joe Lops.

Printed in the United States of America

Library of Congress Cataloging-in-Publication Data

Names: Tuttle, Will M., author.
Title: The world peace diet : eating for spiritual health and social harmony
   / Will Tuttle, Ph.D.
Description: Tenth anniversary edition. | New York : Lantern Books, A
   Division of Booklight Inc., 2016. | Includes bibliographical references.
Identifiers: LCCN 2016004453 | ISBN 9781590565278 (pbk.)
Subjects: LCSH: Food—Social aspects. | Food—Philosophy. | Diet—Moral
   and ethical aspects.
Classification: LCC RA601 .T88 2016 | DDC 613.2—dc23
LC record available at http://lccn.loc.gov/2016004453

ACKNOWLEDGMENTS

I am grateful to the many people who have helped along the way, contributing their insights and energy to the process of creating this book. My heartfelt appreciation to those who read the manuscript at some stage and offered helpful comments, particularly Judy Carman, Evelyn Casper, Reagan Forest, Lynn Gale, Cheryl Maietta, Laura Remmy, Veda Stram, Beverlie Tuttle, Ed Tuttle, and Madeleine Tuttle. Michael Greger, M.D., and John McDougall, M.D., provided valuable insights for chapter five and Michael Klaper, M.D., for chapters five through seven. Thanks also to Doug Davis, Joel and Michelle Levy, Howard Lyman, Norm Phelps, Zach Shatz, Jerry Simonelli, and Zoe Weil for their interest in the manuscript and helpful comments and to everyone above for their encouragement. I'm grateful to Sarah Gallogly and Martin Rowe for their skillful editing that clarified the manuscript.

Beyond these people, there are many more who have contributed to the book less directly through conversations, and through their writings, lectures, and creative efforts to uplift human consciousness. My deepest appreciation to all of you for your contributions! A big thank you to my dear wife Madeleine for sustaining me with loving-kindness, wonderful meals, and spirited discussion throughout the years this book was taking shape.

Finally, deep thanks to all the animals with whom we share this beautiful planet for their celebrative presence and their mysterious collaboration with the living forces that make everything possible here. May their suffering at our hands open our hearts to compassion.

TABLE OF CONTENTS

~~~

PREFACE TO THE TENTH
ANNIVERSARY EDITION

Aware that we are living in critical times, many of us feel called to contribute solutions to the problems that beset us. Because of this, when writing *The World Peace Diet*, I imagined a growing number of us making an effort to explore and share the most essential solution that is usually hidden from thought and discourse. This solution lies in understanding the connections that link our culture's routine abuse of animals for food and other products with the intractable problems of environmental destruction, world hunger, war, disease, and social injustice, as well as animal agriculture's unrecognized harm to the inner landscape of our consciousness. As *The World Peace Diet's* call to examine these deeper connections has gone forth over the past ten years, it has reached receptive hearts and minds, and this call has not just been heard but amplified through the countless efforts of inspired individuals. The book is now in many ways a movement—a bestseller published in fifteen languages—and its momentum continues to grow as the yearning for a more discerning understanding of compassion, health, spirituality, and justice gains traction worldwide.

Although a decade has passed since its first publication, the message of *The World Peace Diet* is as urgent and relevant today as ever. Certain facts and statistics have perhaps changed slightly, but the underlying patterns and truths still pertain. We heal our world and ourselves when we make an effort to understand the ramifications of our actions, especially those ramifications that are typically hidden and that resist being discussed or noticed. We can become a liberating influence in our world by questioning the official stories—particularly those that pertain to food and animals—and by making an effort to understand how to bring our daily lives into alignment with our values and contribute to a world where freedom, abundance, and peace are available for all.

This effort of moving both toward and within a more aware and nonviolent way of living is a continual adventure, and like any journey of awakening there is an evolution of understanding that moves through stages. *The World Peace Diet* is designed to speak to us wherever we are on this journey. For those of us in what could be called the pre-vegan stages of the adventure, the book offers a perspective to help us question the accepted narratives and understand the bigger picture of our society. For those of us in the beginning stages of veganism, it offers inspiration and practical information to support our ongoing quest for a better life for others and ourselves. For those of us who are more seasoned vegans and may find ourselves in what we may refer to as the angry vegan stage or the closet vegan stage, it offers a perspective that may help us become more peaceful, understanding, and assured, so that we thrive joyfully in our lives and become more effective in our advocacy for animals. And for those of us who are already opening to the further stages of vegan living that we can refer to as deep veganism, *The World Peace Diet* endeavors to help us access more doorways to embodying the timeless wisdom principles that are the foundation of living a life that fulfills our highest purpose—promoting harmony and liberation for all of us.

When *The World Peace Diet* was first released in 2005, Donald Watson, who coined the word vegan in 1944, was still alive, and a journalist friend traveled to England several times to interview him. He wrote articles describing how, at the age of 95, Watson was still spryly walking the hills surrounding his home. Then, in early 2006, this friend called us from England and said that the venerable old man was no longer walking through the hills, but was preparing to leave his body, and that every afternoon, he would sit in his bed while his son-in-law read him *The World Peace Diet*. Our friend told us that Donald Watson had expressed to those around him that this new book presented the message he'd had in mind when he created the word vegan. Over the ten years since then, it has become increasingly clear that *The World Peace Diet* is more than an individual's book. It is the articulation of a broad, timeless, and urgent vision that calls humanity to awaken to the unrecognized power of our food choices and heal our relationship with animals. Building on the efforts of Watson and others who have gone before, the intention of *The World Peace Diet* has been to receive the vision in all its extent and depth, and compose it as a foundational text for the next necessary stage in our collective adventure of evolving a way of living on this Earth that supports, rather than exploits, the web of life that includes all of us.

As the years have gone by, my partner Madeleine and I have heard from many people who've found this book to be a significant catalyst for transformation in their lives, and they've reported that reading it slowly and contemplatively, and multiple times, has been empowering and illuminating for them. Many have emphasized that they've found it's best to read straight through without skipping around, because later material builds on the earlier, although some have found it helpful to read Chapter 14 early on because it focuses on the author's personal background in writing the book.

Because of requests from readers, we began creating World Peace Diet training programs in order to help people integrate and embody the principles articulated in *The World Peace Diet* more deeply. This has led to the gradual creation of an international network of people who have completed this facilitator training, either through a live training or through our self-paced online training program. These people help support humanity's cultural progress through facilitating World Peace Diet study groups, as well as through coaching, writing, education, and advocacy efforts that take a variety of forms. Examples include people who have created vegan yoga studios, restaurants, meet-ups, and festivals, as well as a wide offering of music, art, books, blogs, radio shows, films, trainings, services, charitable foundations, sanctuaries, and public education campaigns that promote vegan living. To assist with this dimension of using *The World Peace Diet* as a source book for intensive study, we have included a brief section of study questions in this tenth anniversary edition.

In closing, I'm indebted to a vibrant web of caring people who have poured countless hours into organizing, translating, and helping to promote and embody the World Peace Diet solution and vision over the past decade. This perseverance and generosity of spirit are an inspiration, and we can give thanks knowing that as we make an effort to sow seeds of understanding in our brief sojourn on this beautiful Earth, we are helping all of us reap harmony and joy in our profoundly interconnected lives.

Will Tuttle
—*December 2015*

PREFACE TO THE ORIGINAL EDITION

~~~

Our Meals: The Hidden Key to Understanding
This book is an attempt to illuminate our culture's story and to present the outlines of a more empowering understanding of our world. The key to this understanding lies in comprehending the far-reaching implications of our food choices and the worldview they both reflect and mandate. At first glance it may seem unlikely that such a potent key could be found in the pedestrian place that food occupies in our culture, but if we look closely, we begin to realize that our shared cultural reality is profoundly affected by the attitudes, beliefs, and practices surrounding food. There are amazing unrecognized social, psychological, and spiritual consequences to our meals that ripple through all aspects of our lives.

Food is actually our most intimate and telling connection both with the natural order and with our living cultural heritage. Through eating the plants and animals of this earth we literally incorporate them, and it is also through this act of eating that we partake of our culture's values and paradigms at the most primal and unconscious levels. As children, through constant exposure to the complex patterns of belief surrounding our most elaborate group ritual, eating food, we ingested our culture's values and invisible assumptions. Like sponges, we learned, we noticed, we partook, and we became acculturated. Now, as adults, finding our lives beset with stress and a range of daunting problems of our own making, we rightly yearn to understand the source of our frustrating inability to live in harmony on this earth. When we look deeply enough, we discover a disturbing force that is fundamental in generating our dilemmas and crises, a force that is not actually hidden at all, but is staring up at us every day from our plates! It has been lying undiscovered all along in the most obvious of places: It is our food.

While debates rage over which diets are best in terms of health and longevity, this book is not about diet in this usual sense, but is an exploration of the profound cultural and spiritual ramifications of our food choices and the mentality underlying them. By placing humans at the top of the planet's food chain, our culture has historically perpetuated a particular worldview that requires from its members a reduction of essential feelings and awareness—and it is this process of desensitization that we must understand if we would comprehend the underlying causes of oppression, exploitation, and spiritual disconnectedness. When we practice eating for spiritual health and social harmony, we practice making certain essential connections that our culturally induced food rituals normally require us to block from awareness. This practice is an essential prerequisite for evolving to a state of consciousness where peace and freedom are possible.

We are in the midst of a profound cultural transformation. It is becoming increasingly obvious that the old mythos underlying our culture is collapsing. We are realizing that its core assumptions are obsolete and, if followed further, will result not only in the ecological devastation of our planet's intricate and delicate systems, but in our self-destruction as well. A new mythos, affirming cooperation, freedom, peace, life, and unity, is struggling to be born to replace the old mythos based on competition, separateness, war, exclusion, and the idea that might makes right. Food is a critical key to this birth, because our food habits condition our mentality profoundly—and because meals are the primary way our culture replicates and promulgates its value system through us. Whether this birth of a new mythos and more evolved spirituality and consciousness is successful will depend on whether we can transform our understanding and practice of food.

The Practice of Connecting

Our cultural predicament—the array of seemingly intractable problems that beset us, such as chronic war, terrorism, genocide, starvation, the proliferation of disease, environmental degradation, species extinction, animal abuse, consumerism, drug addiction, alienation, stress, racism, oppression of women, child abuse, corporate exploitation, materialism, poverty, injustice, and social malaise—is rooted in an essential cause that is so obvious that it has managed to remain almost completely overlooked. In trying to solve the social, environmental, and individual problems we face while ignoring the underlying cause that generates them, we are treating symptoms without addressing the root of the disease. Such efforts are ultimately doomed to failure. Instead, we need to build a web of understanding and awareness that helps us see the connections between our food choices, our individual and cultural health, our planetary ecology, our spirituality, our attitudes and beliefs, and the quality of our relationships. As we do this and act on this understanding, we contribute to the evolution of a more harmonious and liberated shared experience of life on this beautiful but misunderstood planet.

I believe that until we are willing and able to make the connections between what we are eating and what was required to get it on our plate, and how it affects us to buy, serve, and eat it, we will be unable to make the connections that will allow us to live wisely and harmoniously on this earth. When we cannot make connections, we cannot understand, and we are less free, less intelligent, less loving, and less happy. The most crucial task for our generation, our group mission on this earth, perhaps, is to make some essential connections that our parents and ancestors have been mostly unable to make, and thus to evolve a healthier human society to bequeath to our children. If we fail to make the connection between our daily meals and our cultural predicament, we will inevitably fail as a species to survive on this earth. By refusing to make this essential connection, we condemn others and ourselves to enormous suffering, without ever comprehending why.

The Call to Evolve

Though I spent the first twenty-two years of my life eating the large quantities of animal-based foods typical of our culture, I've spent the past thirty years or so exploring the fascinating connections and cause-effect relationships between our individual and cultural practice of using animals for food and the stress and difficulties we create for each other and ourselves. I've discovered that the violence we instigate for our plates boomerangs in remarkable ways.

It becomes immediately obvious, though, that our collective sense of guilt about our mistreatment of animals for food makes recognizing this basic connection enormously difficult. Eating animal foods is a fundamental cause of our dilemmas, but we will squirm every which way to avoid confronting this. It is our defining blind spot and is the essential missing piece to the puzzle of human peace and freedom. Because of our culturally inherited behavior of abusing the animals we use for food and ignoring this abuse, we are exceedingly hesitant to look behind the curtain of our denial, talk with each other about the consequences of our meals, and change our behavior to reflect what we see and know. This unwillingness is socially supported and continually reinforced.

Our behavior invariably reflects our understanding, and yet our behavior also determines what level of understanding we are able to attain.

The calling we hear today is the persistent call to evolve. It is part of a larger song to which we all contribute and that lives in our cells and in the essential nature of the universe that gives rise to our being. It is a song, ultimately, of healing, joy, and celebration because all of us, humans and non-humans alike, are expressions of a beautiful and benevolent universe. It is also a song of darkest pain and violation, due to our accepted practices of dominating, commodifying, and killing animals and people. In order to confine and kill animals for food, we must repress our natural compassion, warping us away from intuition and toward materialism, violence, and disconnectedness.

The song of the new mythos that yearns to be born through us requires our spirits to be loving and alive enough to hear and recognize the pain we are causing through our obsolete food orientation. We are called to allow our innate mercy and kindness to shine forth and to confront the indoctrinated assumptions that promote cruelty. While we are granted varying degrees of privilege depending on our species, race, class, and gender, we are all harmed when any is harmed; suffering is ultimately completely interconnected because we are all interconnected, and socially constructed privilege only serves to disconnect us from this truth of our interdependence.

This book is intended for readers of all religious traditions as well as those who do not identify with any particular tradition. Like the Golden Rule, which articulates a principle that is pronounced by all the world's religious traditions and is intuitively accepted by people of every culture and persuasion, the principles discussed in this book are universal and can be understood and practiced by all of us, whatever our religious affiliation or non-affiliation may happen to be. A moderately open mind and a willingness to make connections are all that are needed to apprehend these principles, and to see that they never contradict our deeper religious teachings or our spiritual yearnings, but always fulfill and illumine them.

The song of our necessary evolution and awakening is calling. Achieving the deeper understanding this song requires lies in uncovering connections and relationships that have been hidden or chronically ignored. A journey is required, and this is the adventure of discovery that beckons.

CHAPTER ONE

FOOD'S POWER

"The world is his who can see through its pretensions. What deafness,
what stone-blind custom, what overgrown error you behold, is there
only by sufferance—your sufferance. See it to be a lie, and you have
already dealt it a mortal blow."

—EMERSON

"The most violent weapon on earth is the table fork."

—MAHATMA GANDHI

Food as Metaphor

Since time immemorial—going back at least two and a half millennia to
Pythagoras in Greece, the Old Testament prophets in the ancient
Levant, and Mahavira and Gautama Buddha in India, as well as later
luminaries such as Plato, Plotinus, and the early Christian fathers—
social reformers and spiritual teachers have emphasized the importance
of attending to our attitudes and practices surrounding food. The fact
that these teachings have been aggressively ignored, discounted, and
covered up over the centuries is of paramount significance, and if we
look deeply into the wounds and attitudes responsible for this cover-up,
we will discover liberating truths about our culture and ourselves, and

about the way to positive personal and planetary transformation. What gives food such power, and why is this power still so unrecognized today? Answering this question requires us to pay attention in new ways and make connections we have been taught not to make.

Food is not only a fundamental necessity; it is also a primary symbol in the shared inner life of every human culture, including our own. It is not hard to see that food is a source and metaphor of life, love, generosity, celebration, pleasure, reassurance, acquisition, and consumption. And yet it is also, ironically, a source and metaphor of control, domination, cruelty, and death, for we often kill to eat. Every day, from the cradle to the grave, we all make food choices, or they are made for us. The quality of awareness from which these inevitable food choices arise—and whether we are making them ourselves or they are being made for us— greatly influences our ability to make connections. This ability to make meaningful connections determines whether we are and become lovers and protectors of life or unwitting perpetuators of cruelty and death.

I believe that at the deepest levels of our consciousness we all yearn to achieve authentic spiritual union with the source of being, to experience directly our true nature. It is this longing to experience wholeness, truth, and freedom from the painful illusion of fundamental separateness that urges us to explore and inquire into the mysteries surrounding us every day. We realize that looking deeply connects us with our spiritual roots and resources. Looking deeply into food, into what and how we eat, and into the attitudes, actions, and beliefs surrounding food, is an adventure of looking into the very heart of our culture and ourselves. As surprising as it may seem, as we shine the light of awareness onto this most ordinary and necessary aspect of our lives, we shine light onto unperceived chains of bondage attached to our bodies, minds, and hearts, onto the bars of cages we never could quite see, and onto a sparkling path that leads to transformation and the possibility of true love, freedom, and joy in our lives. We may want to laugh at such strong claims. Food? Our old friend, food? We have bigger projects and more pressing issues. Food is so pedestrian. We eat and run, or we eat to be comforted and sustained in our quests, or as background to fellowship or television. Food is just food, we might well protest. It's no big deal!

Sacred Feasts

As we look more deeply, we can see that food is a universal metaphor for intimacy. Many of us know the feeling of loving something or someone so deeply that we would like to become one with, and bring into ourselves, this apparent other. Perhaps it is a glorious sunrise that we drink in with our eyes, a melody that somehow opens our heart and melts something within us, or our beloved with whom we long to merge and become one. All the arts are conduits for the expression of this deep human longing for unity, but it is only in the art of food preparation and eating that this oneness is actually physically achieved. This is part of what makes eating such a powerful experience and metaphor: food art is eaten and *becomes* us. It enters as object and *becomes* subject; what is "not-me" is transformed into "me." What an alchemical miracle! It is the same as the miracle of spiritual illumination, and of forgiveness, and of love. What is not-me, the other, or even the potential enemy is somehow transmuted, by opening and embracing, into me, us. A healing occurs, an awakening to the larger wholeness in which the formerly separate "me" and "not-me" are united as co-elements, co-operators.

Partaking of food is thus a comprehensive metaphor for healing, spiritual transformation, forgiveness, and transcendent love. At a deep level, we all know this. Food preparation is the only art that allows us literally to incorporate what we create, and it is also the only art that fully involves all five senses. It also relies heavily on what is referred to in Buddhist teachings as the sixth sense: mentation, the mental activity that contextualizes what we perceive through our senses. We have incredibly intricate and complex layers of thinking and feeling attached to food that are an important part of our experience of eating. Our family and culture contribute enormously to these thoughts and feelings, and these memories and identifications give meaning to our meals.

Eating is thus the most intimate of all activities in which we actually accomplish the complex and longed-for union of self and other, subject and world. And so it has always been seen, cross-culturally, as the most sacred human activity, and the most culturally binding as well. We cannot become more intimate with someone or something than by eating them. They then literally become us. Such an intimate act must certainly be attended to with the greatest awareness, love, discrimination, and reverence. If it is not, then it is a clear indication that something is seriously awry.

Once we realize that preparing and eating food is humanity's fundamental symbol of intimacy and spiritual transformation, we can begin to understand why sacred feasts are essential to every culture's religious and social life. The metaphor of eating is central to spiritual communion with the divine presence. It is universally recognized that eating food is both a literally and symbolically sacred action: it is directly partaking of the infinite order that transcends our finite lives.

Though it appears that we are mere finite beings eating food, from another perspective we can see the infinite eternally feeding itself with itself. Through this act of partaking, we open, embrace, and actually embody the infinite order as a unique expression of itself, which is us, these human beings who are eating. This is an expression of the profoundest love. When we eat, we are loved by the eternal and mysterious force that births all life, that makes present all who ever preceded us, that manifests itself ceaselessly as us and experiences life through us, with a love that thoroughly gives of itself to us, to we who *are* this force. It is a love that our intuitive heart can sense and respond to and deeply, ecstatically appreciate, but that our rational mind can barely begin to comprehend.

Food, Life, and Death

What is so simple as eating an apple? And yet, what could be more sacred or profound? When we eat an apple we are not just eating an apple as a separate thing. The apple enters us, dissolves within us, contributes to us, and becomes us. And each apple is a manifestation of so much more! We are eating of the rain and the clouds and of all the trees that have gone before to bring this tree into manifestation, and of the tears, sweat, bodies, and breaths of countless generations of animals, plants, and people that have become the rain and soil and wind that feed the apple tree.

When we look into one apple, we see the entire universe. All the planets and stars, our sun and moon, the oceans, rivers, forests, fields, and creatures are in this apple. The apple tree is a manifestation of an infinite web of life, and for the tree to exist, every component of the web is vital. The apple is the gift of the tree and of the infinite universe propagating and celebrating itself through the apple. The seeds fall, in the apple, to become new trees, or are eaten by humans or bears or birds and thus distributed more widely, spreading and benefiting the tree and the whole system, unfolding in utter vastness, complexity, and perfection.

If we become aware of this when we eat an apple, we will know we are loved and nourished, and that we are part of something greater, a mystery so immense and benevolent and exciting that we can only be touched by the sense of sacredness. In virtually all societies, the times when we pause to remember the source of our life and to consciously connect with the great mystery are at death, with funerals, and at meals, with grace and prayers. Eating an apple with awareness can be a sacred feast, and yet it is usually done casually while we are preoccupied with something else.

We humans, eating apples, are in a true sense apples eating apples. The whole universe is not only in every apple but in every one of us. In eating, we see that there are no fundamentally separate things at all, but only processes. All things partake of each other, ever changing, and are eventually eaten by the process and by time, the great devourer. Food is the source and metaphor of the flow of life into death and of death into life.

We can see that the mythic and spiritual significance of eating food is profound and has been woven into the underlying mythos and religious traditions of many cultures, including our own. Besides the ongoing symbolic appeal of eating the sacramental Christian communion meal, transforming Jesus' death, there is the birth story. Jesus was born in a manger! What a potent symbol, to be born in someone's food bowl. He was born to be spiritual food for others, and the profound connections between the symbolism of the manger and of the Last Supper point to food's enduring power as a primary metaphor of the spiritual mystery that both embraces and transcends life and death.

As we evolve spiritually and awaken our potential, we can be food for others every day, sharing our love and understanding, our time and energy, nourishing others and ourselves in the process. It is not just our personal love, energy, or time that we share, for, like the apple, when we give of ourselves we are giving of the gifts we've received from our families, teachers, and friends, from the earth and her creatures, from the sun, moon, and stars, and from all our experiences. Ultimately, we are life itself giving to itself—feeding itself, exploring, satisfying, and rejuvenating itself. If we live well, we feed many with the most nourishing food: the fruits of compassion and wisdom. In the end, more than needing food for the journey, we can discover that we are the food for each other's journey, and that our deepest need and joy is not merely to consume but to be this nourishing food for others. We are all born in a symbolic manger, to be spiritual food for others, and we are called to discover our unique way of contributing.

Is it so surprising that something so mundane as eating appears to be could yet occupy the central place of power in our cultural and spiritual lives? In exploring this further, we must examine what we choose to eat. What lies behind our food choices?

The Origin of Our Food: Either Plants or Animals

In our culture, the distinction between food items that come from animals and those that come from plants is sometimes deliberately blurred and overlooked. In explicitly recognizing the obvious, though, we empower ourselves to understand more deeply.

Food of plant origin is most often the fruits and seeds that are freely released from certain plants. For example, grains such as wheat, oats, rice, corn, barley, quinoa, rye, and millet are the seeds and fruits of cereal grasses. Legumes such as soybeans, chickpeas, lentils, peas, beans, and peanuts are the seeds of leguminous plants. Fruit-vegetables like tomatoes, squashes, peppers, pumpkins, okra, eggplants, and cucumbers are the fruits and seeds of herbaceous plants. Fruits and seeds released from trees and other plants make up many of the other plant foods we eat, such as apples, oranges, bananas, papayas, avocados, breadfruit, melons, grapes, lemons, plums, peaches, cherries, apricots, olives, figs, dates, and other fruits; blackberries, strawberries, blueberries, cranberries, raspberries, and other berries; pecans, walnuts, hazelnuts, macadamias, cashews, almonds, coconuts, and other nuts; and sunflower seeds, sesame seeds, pumpkin seeds, cocoa, flax seeds, pine nuts, and other seeds. Some foods are seed-bearing flowers, like broccoli, cauliflower, brussels sprouts, and artichokes, or spore-bearing fruits of underground fungi, like mushrooms, or starchy tubers like potatoes and yams. A few are roots, like carrots and beets, or leaves, like chard, cabbage, and lettuce, or stalks, like asparagus, celery, and sugarcane.

Behind the plant foods on our plates, we see orchards and gardens, fields, forests, and seasons, and people nurturing and tending plants. If they are organically grown with sustainable and small-scale methods, we see the beauty and abundance of the earth yielding delicious and healthy foods to hands that practice caring and work in harmony with nature's rhythms.

Looking deeply, we see that there is very little suffering caused by eating these foods; most plant foods are fruits and seeds released from grasses, herbs, trees, vines, and other plants. In addition, unlike animals, which are mobile and thus need a nervous system with pain receptors to help them avoid self-damaging behaviors, plants have nothing analogous to a physical nervous system or pain receptors. Since they are rooted and stationary, there is no reason for nature to grant or evolve mechanisms that would help them by allowing them to feel pain.*

Food of animal origin is either the actual flesh and organs of dead animals, or animal excretions appropriated for food. In the former class of foods is the muscle flesh of a variety of animals who are killed to produce the foods that are the centerpieces of most of our culture's meals. The flesh of fish and shellfish is typically referred to by the animal's species, such as tuna, catfish, salmon, lobster, crab, and shrimp. Though amphibians and reptiles are less commonly eaten in the U.S. than in some countries, frogs, turtles, and alligators are nevertheless raised here to produce frog's legs and turtle and alligator meat for human consump-

---

* While some may argue that plants are nevertheless capable of suffering, this would be all the more reason not to consume animal-based foods, because it requires enormous amounts of grain to produce meat, eggs, dairy products, and farmed fish. It also requires the devastation of forests, prairies, and wildlife habitat for pasture and to grow these grains, and the destruction of marine ecosystems. See Chapter 11 for further details.

tion. The flesh of birds is also referred to by the animal's species, as when we eat chicken, turkey, duck, emu, and pheasant, and differentiation is often made between different types and colors of flesh, such as breast and leg, white meat and dark meat. In contrast to the above, the flesh of other mammals is rarely named by species but as a particular "cut" of flesh, such as loin, sirloin, flank, rump roast, shoulder roast, rib roast, T-bone, brisket, or as pork, bacon, ribs, veal, lamb chops, venison, mutton, ground beef, hamburger, hot dog, baloney, sausage, and ham. Certain internal organs are also eaten, particularly the kidneys and livers of young mammals, the fattened livers of ducks and geese (foie gras), and, less often, the stomach tissue (tripe) and the heart, tongue, brains, and feet of certain animals (sometimes referred to as head cheese). The milk of lactating mother cows, sheep, and goats is drunk and eaten as butter, yogurt, cream, and a variety of cheeses. The latter are formed using rennet, the stomach lining of slaughtered calves, to coagulate the milk. Birds' eggs are also appropriated for food, as is the honey excreted from the bodies of bees.

In contrast to plants, which naturally produce healthy and nourishing foods that involve little if any suffering, animals are routinely dominated and attacked in order to obtain the flesh, milk, and eggs we humans eat. This clearly involves suffering, for we all know with utter certainty that taking a knife and cutting into the skin of a dog, cow, cat, chicken, rabbit, or human is totally different from cutting into the skin of a tomato or grapefruit, that biting into the leg of a pig cannot be compared to biting into a fresh apple. The renowned ethologist Konrad Lorenz once remarked that anyone who couldn't see the difference between chopping up a dog and chopping up a lettuce should commit suicide for the benefit of society. We know today that all vertebrate animals are endowed with central nervous systems with proprioceptors that are sensitive to a variety of painful stimuli, including being cut, burned, crushed, confined, electrically shocked, and subjected to cold and heat, noxious smells, bruising, and chafing, and that they feel psychological pain as we would when they are physically confined, their babies are stolen from them, or their innate drives are systematically thwarted.

The Culture of Denial

The more forcefully we ignore something, the more power it has over us and the more strongly it influences us. Looking undistractedly into the animal-derived foods produced by modern methods, we inescapably find misery, cruelty, and exploitation. We therefore avoid looking deeply at our food if it is of animal origin, and this practice of avoidance and denial, applied to eating, our most basic activity and vital ritual, carries over automatically into our entire public and private life. We know, deep down, that we cannot look deeply anywhere, for if we do, we will have to look deeply into the enormous suffering our food choices directly cause. So we learn to stay shallow and to be willingly blind to the connections we could see. Otherwise, our remorse and guilt would be too painful to bear. The acknowledged truth would also conflict too strongly with our self-image, causing serious cognitive dissonance and emotional disturbance. We choose to ignore, and thus choose to be ignorant and inattentive.

Being unwilling and unable to see, confront, and take responsibility for the hidden ocean of horror that our most basic activity causes to those who are as sentient and vulnerable as we are, we have split ourselves into a schizophrenia of politeness and civility that lives uneasily with the remorseless cruelty that surfaces whenever we obtain or eat animal foods. I believe this split is *the* fundamental unrecognized wound we modern humans suffer, and from it many other wounds and divisions naturally and inevitably follow. It is so deep and terrible that it is taboo to discuss it publicly.

Choosing to be blind to what we are actually doing when we shop for, prepare, and eat food, we blind ourselves not only to the horror and suffering we are instigating and eating, but also to the beauty of the world around us. This acquired inability to actually see and appreciate the overwhelming loveliness of this earth allows us to ravage forests and oceans and systematically destroy the natural world. Becoming insensitive to the pain we cause daily to defenseless animals, we also become insensitive to the beauty and luminosity of the creation that we oppress and from which we disconnect at every meal.

The desensitizing of millions of children and adults—on the massive scale that consuming millions of tortured animals daily requires—sows countless seeds of human violence, war, poverty, and despair. These outcomes are unavoidable, for we can never reap joy, peace, and freedom for ourselves while sowing the seeds of harming and enslaving others. We may speak of love, kindness, freedom, and a gentler world, yet it is our actions, especially those that are habitually practiced, that determine what future outcomes we and others will experience. The cycles of violence that have terrorized people both historically and today are rooted in the violence of our daily meals. Though animals cannot retaliate like other people can, our violence toward them retaliates against us.

Inheriting Cruelty

By confining and killing animals for food, we have brought violence into our bodies and minds and disturbed the physical, emotional, mental, social, and spiritual dimensions of our selves in deep and intractable ways. Our meals require us to eat like predators and thus to see ourselves as such, cultivating and justifying predatory behaviors and institutions that are the antithesis of the inclusiveness and kindness that accompany spiritual growth. Because cruelty is inescapable in confining, mutilating, and slaughtering animals for food, we have been forced from childhood to be distracted and inattentive perpetrators of cruelty.

None of us ever consciously and freely chose to eat animals. We have all inherited this from our culture and upbringing. Going into the baby food department of any grocery store today, we see it immediately: beef-flavored baby food, chicken, veal, and lamb baby food, and even cheese lasagna baby food. Well-meaning parents, grandparents, friends, and neighbors have forced the flesh and secretions of animals upon us from before we can remember. As infants, we have no idea what "veal," "turkey," "egg," or "beef" actually are, or where they come from. We don't know what horror is visited upon helpless creatures in order to create the easily available concoctions being spooned into our little teething mouths. We find out slowly, and by the time we do, the cruelty and perversity involved seem natural and normal to us. We are never told that we humans are not designed to eat the large quantities of animal foods typical of our culture. We are never told of the extreme confinement, the routine unanesthetized castrations and other mutilations, and the brutal and often botched killings that stare up at us every day from our bowls and plates, and that we unthinkingly chew while watching television, reading, or conversing.

Thus, our deepest and most blessed connection with the earth and with the mystery of infinite spiritual consciousness—our daily meals—have become rituals of distraction and repressed sensitivity and guilt rather than rituals of heart-opening gratitude, connectedness, blessedness, and love. The price we pay for this is incalculable and includes, among other things, the dulling of our innate intelligence and compassion and a consequent loss of peace, freedom, and joy.

The Withering of Intelligence

Intelligence is the ability to make meaningful connections, and this is true for all living systems, such as humans, animals, communities, and societies. Participating in daily rituals that repress our ability to make connections severely impedes our intelligence, even amid our current glut of so-called information, and destroys our ability to deal effectively with the serious problems we generate. Because we are adept at disconnecting from the suffering we impose on animals, we naturally and inevitably become adept at disconnecting from the suffering we impose on hungry people, living biosystems, war-ravaged communities, and future generations. Our skills in forcefully blocking feedback also make us easily distracted and manipulated by corporate interests whose profits depend on our inability to make significant connections.

Compassion is ethical intelligence: it is the capacity to make connections and the consequent urge to act to relieve the suffering of others. Like cognitive intelligence, it is suppressed by the practice of eating animals. The ability to disconnect, practiced at every mealtime, is seen in perhaps more chilling guise in the modern scientist slowly freezing dogs to death to learn about human physiology, in modern soldiers looking straight into the eyes of helpless civilians and killing them, in hunters deceiving and chasing defenseless animals and killing them for sport, and in countless other legal and approved cultural activities.

As long as we remain, at core, a culture that sees animals merely as commodities and food, there is little hope for our survival. The systematic practice of ignoring, oppressing, and excluding that is fundamental to our daily meals disconnects us from our inner wisdom and from our sense of belonging to a benevolent and blessed universe. By actively ignoring the truth of our connectedness, we inescapably commit geocide and suicide, and forsake the innate intelligence and compassion that would guide us.

I-Thou vs. I-It

In the 1920s the philosopher Martin Buber introduced and articulated an essential distinction in our relations with others and in our consequent sense of self that is increasingly recognized for its importance. Proposing that we do not develop our sense of "I" in isolation, but rather through relationship with others, he went on to say that when we relate to others as being conscious, and as having feelings, experiences, desires, and purposes, we develop an "I-Thou" sense of self. When we relate to others as objects, as having no significant desires, purposes, or consciousness of their own, we develop an "I-It" sense of ourselves. Cultivating an I-Thou sense of self, we cultivate respect and sensitivity towards others and ourselves. Cultivating an I-It sense of self, we tend to relate to others as instruments to be used. This I-It sense of self leads to an increasingly deadened and depersonalized view of nature, animals, and other people, and to an inner hardening that shields us from feeling the pain of whomever and whatever we are using, consuming, and exploiting. According to Buber, the I-It sense of self requires and fosters an inner insensitivity that leads to an ever-increasing craving to consume more things. This ironic and impossible quest for happiness and fulfillment by an objectified, separate, anxious self that reduces others to instruments to be used for pleasure and gain is a primary driving force behind consumerism and the runaway industrialization, corporate capitalism, and environmental and social devastation that this mentality inevitably manifests.

While Buber's insights are certainly provocative and illuminating, it seems he failed to recognize the deeper dynamic responsible for the I-It sense of self: the food choices we learn from birth, in which mysterious, sensitive, and intelligent beings are continually and unquestioningly reduced to mere food objects to be used, killed, and eaten.

It's remarkable, we might think, that Buber couldn't make this rather obvious connection in over forty years of meditating and writing on the I-Thou and I-It mentalities. Yet what is far more remarkable is that out of the thousands of leading writers and researchers in the physical sciences, human sciences, and humanities over the last hundred years, virtually no one has produced a sentence on the subject! These great minds were among the most innovative and courageous of their time, willing to risk controversy and daring to offer the world many new ideas in sociology and social theory, psychology, philosophy, systems theory, science, economics, history, government, anthropology, theology, comparative religion, and spirituality.[1] How could something so central and obvious to our lives and thinking—our treatment of animals for food—go ignored by—and invisible to—so many for so long? It's eerie to contemplate the mountains of books, articles, essays, lectures, and documentaries produced by and about the great minds of modernity—and to realize how unmentionable this subject is. The idea that our routine violence against animals for food could be a primary driving force behind human suffering and war has managed to remain virtually completely unthinkable to this day.

Even the more radical and contemporary voices have been unwilling or unable to seriously address this subject, as have virtually all the current writers and leaders in the human potential, spiritual, environmental, social justice, holistic health, and peace movements.[2] This is not meant in any way as a criticism of any of these fine people and their contributions and ideas, but is intended rather to emphasize the amazing resistance our entire culture has to confronting its defining behavior, which is as pervasively obvious as cheeseburger ads and fried chicken but at the same time as invisible as air and uncannily unapproachable.

That is because we have all agreed that, at all costs, this truth *must* be ignored. One of Carl Jung's notable contributions was to articulate the character of the shadow archetype: it is what the self is and includes, but denies and represses. Though it is repressed, the shadow *will* be heard and is invariably projected in harmful and perhaps insidious

ways. Our mistreatment of animals for food is far and away our greatest cultural shadow. Our collective guilt drives us not only to hide the
violence we eat but also to act it out: in our aggressive lifestyle, in
movies, books, games, and other media, and in the violence we inflict
both directly and indirectly on each other.

We Are All Mysteries

Our ongoing practice of commodifying animals for food, besides violating the natural order in profound ways that cause enormous unrecognized suffering to us and to the other animals, also blinds us to what we
and the other animals actually are.* We err if we reduce ourselves to the
status of mere material entities that are born, live awhile, and die. Like
other animals, we are not fundamentally physical beings; we are essentially consciousness. We are all expressions of the infinite creative mystery force that births and sustains the universes of manifestation, and
our bodies and minds are sacred, as are the bodies and minds of all creatures. Like us, animals have feelings and yearnings; they nest, mate,
hunger, and are the conscious subjects of their lives. They make every
effort, as we do, to avoid pain and death and to do what brings them
happiness and fulfillment.

What we human beings are fundamentally is an enormous mystery.
The institutions of science, religion, education, and government have
done very little, ultimately, to reveal to us in any profound or transfor-
mational way what we humans essentially *are*. We remain perhaps as
mysterious to ourselves as we were in the days of Moses, Buddha,
Confucius, and Jesus. Some may argue that we know more and have
certainly evolved more; others may argue that we know less of what is
truly vital, and are more distracted and benighted than in earlier times.
No one, though, can argue that we are not mysteries to ourselves, for
all our scientific and theological investigations. And, just as we do not
actually know what a man or woman is, neither do we know what a

---

*It's important to say "other animals" here, because to set them apart from us is a tactic of
exclusion used to perpetuate exploitation and cruelty toward these beings. It also reinforces
the absurd notion that humans are not animals—mammals with bodies, brains, glands, reproductive systems, drives, and nervous systems. We feel pain and pleasure like other animals, and
we feel, dream, and relate socially to our species members as other animals do.

mare or stallion is, or a dog, an elephant, an eagle, a dolphin, a chicken, a swordfish, a lobster, an alligator, a mouse, a butterfly, an earthworm, a honeybee, or a housefly. They are all utterly mysterious to us, perhaps even more mysterious than we are to ourselves. They are truly *others*, and this essential understanding should create in us a sense of humility, wonder, and respect.

Unfortunately, though, we invent mental categories for the infinitely mysterious beings we encounter, such as "blacks," "slaves," and "pagans," or "food animals," "game," "pests," and "laboratory animals." These categories, and the violence with which we treat the magnificent beings thus categorized, do not fundamentally change or cheapen that sacred and enigmatic nature. They only cloud and enslave our minds with the distorted thinking born of our exclusionary and self-serving attitude. The light of the infinite spiritual source of all life shines in all creatures. By seeing and recognizing this light in others, we free both them and ourselves. This is love. Failing to see it, often because we never experienced others seeing it in us, we imprison ourselves, mistaking the confines of the shallows for the deep and free.

By seeing other animals merely as objects to be exploited for food, we have torn the fabric of essential harmony so deeply that we have created a culture that enslaves itself, often without realizing it. The domination of humans by humans is a necessary outgrowth of dominating other animals for food. As Jim Mason has demonstrated in *An Unnatural Order*, there is a strong historical link between the human enslavement of other humans and the human enslavement of animals for food. This enslaving mentality of domination and exclusion lies at the core of the spiritual malaise that allows us to wage war upon the earth and upon each other.

Love Is Understanding

When I was young, I often wondered if our culture really had to be like this. I've discovered that it does not. We can all make a most profound contribution to cultural transformation and world peace with our meals, which are our most vital connection to our culture and to the natural world.

Making the effort to cultivate our awareness and see beyond the powerful acculturation we endured brings understanding. Healing, grace and freedom come from understanding. Love understands. From understanding, we can embrace our responsibility and become a force for blessing the world with our lives, rather than perpetuating disconnectedness and cruelty by proxy. With awareness, our behavior naturally changes, and individual changes in behavior, rippling through the web of relationships, can lead to social transformation and bring new dimensions of freedom, joy, and creativity to everyone. It all begins with our most intimate and far-reaching connection with the natural order, our most primary spiritual symbol, and our most fundamental social ritual: eating.

CHAPTER TWO

OUR CULTURE'S ROOTS

" 'The multitude of your sacrifices—what are they to me?' says the Lord.
'I have more than enough of burnt offerings of rams and the fat of fattened animals; I have no pleasure in the blood of bulls and lambs and
goats. . . . Your hands are full of blood; wash and make yourselves
clean. Take your evil deeds out of my sight.' "
—ISAIAH 1:11, 15–16

"Cruelty to animals is as if man did not love God . . . there is something
so dreadful, so satanic, in tormenting those who have never harmed us,
and who cannot defend themselves, who are utterly in our power."
—CARDINAL JOHN HENRY NEWMAN

The Herding Culture

Most of us don't think of our culture as being a herding culture. Looking
around, we see mainly cars, roads, suburbs, cities, and factories, and
while there are enormous fields of grain, and cattle grazing in the countryside, we may not realize that almost all of the grain is grown as livestock feed, and that most of the untold billions of birds, mammals, and
fish we consume are confined out of sight in enormous concentration
camps called factory farms. Though it is not as obvious to us today as it

was to our forebears a few thousand years ago, our culture is, like theirs, essentially a herding culture, organized around owning and commodifying animals and eating them.

It was roughly ten thousand years ago that wandering tribes in the Kurdish hill country of northeastern Iraq began domesticating sheep and initiated a revolution with enormous consequences.[1] Anthropologists believe it was an outgrowth of the hunting practices of these tribes, who began attaching themselves to particular herds of wild sheep, culling them and increasingly controlling their mobility, food, and reproductive lives. They eventually learned to castrate and kill off male sheep so that the herd consisted primarily of females with a few rams; from this they learned selective breeding to create animals with more desirable characteristics. Goats were apparently domesticated soon after sheep, followed by cattle two thousand years later to the west and north, and subsequently by horses and camels another two to four thousand years after that.[2] Highly charged concepts of property ownership and of male bloodlines and bloodline purity gradually emerged, of which there is ample evidence by the time the historical period began about four thousand years ago.

Our Western culture can be seen as having two main roots: ancient Greece and the ancient Levant (the eastern Mediterranean basin and Middle East). Reading the earliest extant writings from these cultures from about three thousand years ago, like Homer's *Iliad* and *Odyssey*, and the Old Testament accounts of the ancient kings and their wars, we find that these cultures were oriented around meat eating, herding, slavery, violent conquest, male supremacy, and offering animal sacrifices to their mostly male gods.

For the old herding cultures, confined animals were not just food; they were also wealth, security, and power. The first money and form of capital were sheep, goats, and cattle, for only they were consumable property with tangible worth.[3] In fact, our word "capital" derives from *capita*, Latin for "head," as in head of cattle and sheep. The first capitalists were the herders who fought each other for land and capital and created the first kingdoms, complete with slavery, regular warfare, and power concentrated in the hands of a wealthy cattle-owning elite. Our word *pecuniary* comes from the Latin word *pecus,* meaning cattle, and the ancient Roman coin, the *denarius,* was so named because it was worth ten asses.[4] Livestock in the ancient herding cultures thus defined the value of gold and silver—food animals were the fundamental standard of wealth and power. This fact gives us insight into the political might of the ranching and dairy industries that continues to this day.

By commodifying and enslaving large, powerful animals, the ancient progenitors of Western culture established a basic mythos and worldview that still lives today at the heart of our culture. Riane Eisler's *The Chalice and the Blade* and Jim Mason's *An Unnatural Order* summarize and digest the work of historians and anthropologists, providing some interesting perspectives on the fundamental value shifts that occurred when humans began dominating large animals for food, and how these changes affect us in the present day.

It's important to note here that the study and interpretation of history is notoriously subjective. We can notice in our own individual lives that our experience and understanding of our past changes as we change. This is obviously also true of the vast and complex collective pasts generated by millions of people. When we move into trying to understand prehistory—cultural pasts before written records—it becomes even more subjective. As historian Cynthia Eller writes, "[P]rehistory is still a huge and largely blank canvas. Thus incredibly diverse scenarios can be painted upon it, depending on the predilections of individual thinkers."[5]

Riane Eisler draws on the work of many anthropologists and writers, particularly Marija Gimbutas, Jacquetta Hawkes, and Merlin Stone, to argue that there have been basically two types of societies, which she refers to as partnership and dominator. In partnership societies, men and women are essentially equal and work together cooperatively, and Eisler attempts to demonstrate that this was the norm for many tens of thousands of years of human life, prior to the expansion of patriarchal dominator cultures that were based on herding animals. This relatively recent occurrence, five to seven thousand years ago, was due to what Gimbutas calls the Kurgan invasions by warlike herders from central Asia into eastern Europe and the Mediterranean basin.

Bringing a culture in which men viewed women as chattel, they apparently came in three waves over roughly two thousand years, violently attacking, destroying, and fundamentally changing the older, more peaceful partnership societies.[6] According to Eisler, Gimbutas, and others, these older cultures tended to eat foraged and gardened foods, worship fertility goddesses, make communities in fertile valleys, use metals to make bowls rather than weapons, and did not engage in war. The invading dominator cultures herded animals and ate mainly animal flesh and milk, worshipped fierce male sky gods like Enlil, Zeus, and Yahweh, settled on hilltops and fortified them, used metals to make weapons, and were constantly competing and warring. Violent conflict, competition, oppression of women, and class strife, according to Eisler, need not characterize human nature but are relatively recent products of social pressure and conditioning brought by the invading herding cultures whose dominator values we have inherited.

Where did these invading patriarchal cultures come from and what made them that way? In a later book, *Sacred Pleasure*, Eisler cites the research of geographer James DeMeo, who ascribes the expansionist migrations of the Kurgan invaders and other herders to harsh climatic changes that "set off a complex sequence of events—famine, social chaos, land abandonment, and mass migration—that eventually led to a fundamental shift" in human cultural evolution.[7] Herding livestock, Eisler points out, "tends to lead to aridity," and to "produce a vicious cycle of environmental depletion and increasing economic competition for ever more scarce grazing grounds—and thus a tendency for violent contests over territorial boundaries."[8] She adds that the practice of herding animals produces the psychological hardening characteristic of dominator cultures:

> . . . pastoralism relies on what is basically the enslavement of living beings, beings that will be exploited for the products they produce . . . and that will eventually be killed. . . . This would also help to explain the psychological armoring (or deadening of "soft" emotions) that DeMeo believes characterized the origins of patrist or dominator societies. . . . Moreover, once one is habituated to living off enslaved ani-

mals (for meat, cheese, milk, hides, and so forth) as practically the sole source of survival, one can more easily become habituated to view the enslavement of other human beings as acceptable.[9]

Whether there actually were earlier cultures that were more peaceful, partnership-oriented, and egalitarian, as Eisler and many others assert, or whether violent conflict, males, and competition have always dominated human socioeconomic cultural structures is still a hotly contested issue among academics. What seems undeniable, though, is the effect on human consciousness of commodifying and enslaving large animals for food. Jim Mason takes Eisler's work farther in this regard, developing some more historical and psychological connections between domination of animals and domination of other people. He points out that the agricultural revolution introduced profound changes into the ancient forager cultures, transforming their relationship with nature from one of immersion to one of separating from and attempting to control her. Out of this separation, two types of agriculture emerged—plant and animal—and the distinction between them is significant. Growing plants and gardening is more feminine work; plants are tended and nurtured, and as we work with the cycles of nature, we are part of a process that enhances and amplifies life. It is life-affirming and humble (from *humus*, earth) work that supports our place in the web of life. On the other hand, large animal agriculture or husbandry was always men's work and required violent force from the beginning, to contain powerful animals, control them, guard them, castrate them and, in the end, kill them.

Mason also emphasizes the important influence that animals seem to have in human psychological development and health, as well as the violent psychosocial characteristics researchers find in observing cultures around the world that herd large animals. Citing anthropologists Paul Shepard and Anthony Leeds, he notes that Shepard

. . . ticks off the mainstays of herder cultures the world over: 'Aggressive hostility to outsiders, the armed family, feuding and raiding in a male-centered hierarchical organization, the substitution of war for hunting, elaborate arts of sacrifice, monomaniacal pride and suspicion.'[10]

Mason points out the similarities in these respects among desert tribes of the Middle East, Chukchi reindeer herders of eastern Siberia who "love to boast of 'feats of strength, acts of prowess, violent and heroic behavior, excessive endurance and expenditure of energy,' " and our American cowboy/rodeo culture.[11]

Building on the work of Eisler, Mason, and others, we can see that the culture we live in today is a modern continuation of the herding culture that arose in the Middle East and eastern Mediterranean basin, and that the central defining belief of this culture is still the same: animals are commodities to be owned, used, and eaten. By extension, nature, land, resources, and people are also seen as commodities to be owned, used, and exploited. While this seems logical to us today as modern inhabitants of a herding and animal-consuming capitalist culture, this is a view with enormous consequences: the commodification of animals marked the last real revolution in our culture, completely redefining human relations with animals, nature, the divine, and each other.

In the old herding cultures animals were gradually transformed from mysterious and fascinating cohabitants of a shared world to mere property objects to be used, sold, traded, confined, and killed. No longer wild and free, they were treated with increasing disrespect and violence, and eventually became contemptible and inferior in the eyes of the emerging culture's herders.[12] Wild animals began to be seen merely as potential threats to the livestock capital; likewise, other human beings too began to be seen as threats to livestock, or as potential targets for raiding if they owned animals. Battling others to acquire their cattle and sheep was the primary capital acquisition strategy; the ancient Aryan Sanskrit word for war, *gavyaa*, means literally "the desire for more cattle."[13] It appears that war, herding animals, oppression of the feminine, capitalism, and the desire for more capital/livestock have been linked since their ancient birth in the commodification of large animals.

The larger and more powerful the animals were that were herded, the more fierce, cruel, and violent the cultures had to be to successfully dominate them and protect them from marauding wild animals and peo-ple.[14] The largest animals were cattle and horses, and the cattle-herding cultures that established themselves in the Middle East and eastern Mediterranean engaged in unimaginably vicious warfare with each other and against weaker people for millennia, gradually and forcibly spreading their culture and herding values throughout Europe and most of Asia. From Europe, this same cattle culture eventually spread to the Americas. It continues to spread to this day through transnational corporations like ConAgra, Cargill, Smithfield, and McDonald's as well as through projects sponsored by the World Bank and the U.N., religious missionaries, and charities that propagate animal slavery like the Heifer Project.

At the living core of this ancient culture that became what we call today Western civilization was the absolute supremacy of humans over animals, reinforced through daily meals. Wealth and prestige for men began to be measured in terms of how many livestock animals were owned and how large an area of land was controlled for grazing. The role model for young boys became that of the successful proto-capitalist, the macho herder and warrior: tough, cool, emotionally dis-tant, and capable of unflinching violence. Women, livestock, and cap-tured or conquered people were property objects contributing to the total amount of capital; wars, though horrific to combatants and the general population, were potent methods used by the wealthy aristocracy to increase its accumulation of cattle/capital, land, power, and prestige.

It's helpful to realize that the mentality of domination characteriz-ing the culture into which we were born thrives on seeing and empha-sizing differences and ignoring similarities, because this is what enslav-ing and killing animals requires us all to practice. As herders and dom-inators of animals, we must continually practice seeing ourselves as sep-arate and different from them, as superior and special. Our natural human compassion can be repressed by learning to exclude others and to see them as essentially unlike us. This exclusivism is necessary to racism, elitism, and war, because in order to harm and dominate other people we must break the bonds that our hearts naturally feel with them. The mentality of domination is necessarily a mentality of exclusion.

It's obvious if we look closely that many of the root assumptions and activities of the ancient herding cultures still define our culture today. The single most defining activity of these ancient cultures was, as it is today, feasting regularly on foods provided by the bodies of dominated and excluded animals. Wars still enrich a wealthy elite class while millions bear the burden of them, and the world's rich feed on animals fattened on grain and fish while the poor go hungry. Our capitalistic economic system and its supporting political, legal, and educational institutions still legitimize our commodification and exploitation of animals, nature, and people; our domination of the underprivileged and foreign; and an unequal and unjust distribution of goods based on predation (often euphemized as "competition" and "free trade"), oppression, and war. As we have evolved socially, we have made some undeniable gains in reducing certain excesses, and in providing some protection to the weak and vulnerable. On the whole, however, we have to wonder why our progress has been so slow and difficult. The answer to this is on our plates and extends from there to feedlots, slaughterhouses, research laboratories, rodeos, circuses, racetracks, and zoos, to hunting, fishing, and trapping activities, and to prisons, ghettos, wars, and the military-industrial complex and our ongoing rape and destruction of the living world.

The Pythagorean Principle

"As long as men massacre animals, they will kill each other. Indeed, he
who sows the seeds of murder and pain cannot reap joy and love."
—PYTHAGORAS

Over two thousand years ago in ancient Greece, the need for a positive revolution based on compassion for animals was clearly understood and articulated by Pythagoras. Recognized today as a genius whose discoveries are still of critical importance, Pythagoras remains an enigma, with some of his insights eagerly received and used and others ignored. His theorems laid essential foundations in mathematics and geometry and made possible subsequent progress in architecture, design, construction, cartography, navigation, and astronomy. Pythagoras and his students also discovered and applied the principles of harmonics that underlie vibrational tone intervals, so Pythagoras is credited with establishing the seven-tone scale on which Western music is founded, with its mathematically precise vibrational relationships.

In all these areas our culture has zealously taken and benefited from Pythagoras's genius, but the underlying principle that he taught and lived by—compassion for all life—has been much harder for us to accept. His unequivocal teaching that our happiness depends on treating animals with kindness inspired Plato, Plutarch, Plotinus, the Gnostics, and the early fathers of the Christian church, and until 1850, when the word "vegetarian" was coined, anyone who refrained from eating animals was called a "Pythagorean." The principle he proclaimed, that we can never reap joy and love while sowing seeds of pain and death in our treatment of animals, haunts us today.

Two thousand years after Pythagoras came the great Leonardo da Vinci, another genius whose art and discoveries helped usher in the Renaissance. Again our culture ignored his prescient words about the dire consequences of our meals: "I have from an early age abjured the use of meat, and the time will come when men will look upon the murder of animals as they now look upon the murder of men."[15] With Albert Einstein, who wrote, "Nothing will benefit human health and increase chances for survival of life on Earth as much as the evolution to a vegetarian diet," and Mahatma Gandhi, George Bernard Shaw, Emily Dickinson, Albert Schweitzer, and others, it has been the same—we gladly take their gifts except where they break the herding culture taboo and challenge the sacred cow of eating animal foods.

The Vegan Revolution

The core values of the old herding culture still define our culture, as does its main ritual, eating commodified animals. Our deep urge to evolve to a more spiritually mature level of understanding and living, and to create a social order that promotes more justice, peace, freedom, health, sanity, prosperity, sustainability, and happiness, absolutely requires us to stop viewing animals as food objects to be consumed and to shift to a plant-based way of eating. This would bless us enormously, liberating us from routinely practicing, denying, and projecting violence, and would help us cultivate equality and loving-kindness in our relationships as well as develop our capacity for inner serenity. By sowing and nurturing seeds of inclusiveness and sensitivity, we can reap an understanding of our interconnectedness and an ability to live in peace. This means doing a lot of inner weeding, because the herding culture into which we have been born has sown in us the seeds of competitiveness, hubris, anxiety, and disconnectedness. By viewing animals and people as Thous rather than as Its, and by cultivating awareness and compassion, we can nurture within us the seeds of cooperation and caring. We are blessed by blessing others; by using or excluding others or seeking to control or dominate them, we become enmeshed in suffering and further enslaved to the illusion of separateness, which is the herding culture's fundamental orientation.

When we cultivate mindful awareness of the consequences of our food choices and conscientiously adopt a plant-based way of eating, refusing to participate in the domination of animals and the dulling of awareness this requires, we make a profound statement that both flows from and reinforces our ability to make connections. We become a force of sensitivity, healing, and compassion. We become a revolution of one, contributing to the foundation of a new world with every meal we eat. As we share our ideas with others, we promote what may be the most uplifting and healing revolution our culture has ever experienced.

In fact, when we speak of the various revolutions that have supposedly transformed our culture, such as the Industrial Revolution, the Scientific Revolution, and the Information-Communications Revolution, we are missing the bigger picture. None of these are actually revolutions at all, for they've all taken place entirely within the context of a culture of commodification, exploitation, and domination. These "revolutions" have not changed these underlying cultural values; if anything, they have further reinforced them! A true revolution must be far more fundamental than these.

The revolution that is demanded by our yearning for peace, freedom, and happiness must provide a new foundation for our culture, moving it away from its herding values of oppression and disconnectedness toward the post-herding values of respect, kindness, equality, sensitivity, and connectedness. Above all, this revolution must change our relationship to our meals—our most practiced rituals—and to our food, our most powerful inner and outer symbol.

There is no action that more profoundly, radically, and positively embraces these revolutionary changes than adopting a plant-based diet for ethical reasons. There is no action more subversive to the established herding order than cultivating awareness in order to transcend the view that animals are mere commodities.

We *are* waking up from the bad dream of commodifying and preying on animals. The revolution of compassion that is growing in our consciousness and culture requires that we stop eating animals not just for self-oriented health or economic reasons, but also from our hearts, out of caring for the animals, humans, and vast web of interconnected lives that are harmed and destroyed by animal-based meals. The word that sums up this underlying ethic and motivation is "vegan," coined in 1944 in England by Donald Watson. Watson was dissatisfied with the word "vegetarian" because it does not account for motivation and refers only to the exclusion of animal flesh from the diet. He took the first three and last two letters of that word, but wanted it pronounced completely differently, "vee-gn," to emphasize its revolutionary import. Its definition in the Articles of Association of the Vegan Society in England reads,

> Veganism denotes a philosophy and way of living which seeks to exclude—as far as is possible and practicable—all forms of exploitation of, and cruelty to, animals for food, clothing, or any other purpose; and by extension, promotes the development and use of animal-free alternatives for the benefit of humans, animals, and the environment.[16]

The word "vegan," newer and more challenging than "vegetarian" because it includes every sentient being in its circle of concern and addresses all forms of unnecessary cruelty from an essentially ethical perspective, with a motivation of compassion rather than health or purity, points to an ancient idea that has been articulated for many centuries, especially in the world's spiritual traditions. It indicates a mentality of expansive inclusiveness and is able to embrace science and virtually all religions because it is a manifestation of the yearning for universal peace, justice, wisdom, and freedom.

The contemporary vegan movement is founded on loving-kindness and mindfulness of our effects on others. It is revolutionary because it transcends and renounces the violent core of the herding culture in which we live. It is founded on living the truth of interconnectedness and thereby consciously minimizing the suffering we impose on animals, humans, and biosystems; it frees us *all* from the slavery of becoming mere commodities. It signifies the birth of a new consciousness, the resurrection of intelligence and compassion, and the basic rejection of cruelty and domination. It is our only real hope for the future of our species because it addresses the cause rather than being concerned merely with effects. From this new consciousness we can accomplish virtually anything; it represents the fundamental positive personal and cultural transformation that we yearn for, and it requires that we change something basic: our eating habits.

It's funny how we want transformation without having to change! Yet the fundamental transformation called for today requires the most fundamental change—a change in our relationship to food and to animals, which will cause a change in our behavior. To some, simply becoming vegan looks like a superficial step—can something so simple really change us? Yes! Given the power of childhood programming and of our culture's inertia and insensitivity to violence against animals, authentically becoming a committed vegan can only be the result of a genuine spiritual breakthrough. This breakthrough is the fruit of ripening and effort; however, it is not the end but the beginning of further spiritual and moral development. Veganism is still exceedingly rare even among people who consider themselves spiritual aspirants because the forces of early social conditioning are so difficult to transform. We are called to this, nevertheless; otherwise our culture will accomplish nothing but further devastation and eventual suicide.

CHAPTER THREE

THE NATURE OF INTELLIGENCE

"It should not be believed that all beings exist for the sake of the existence of man. On the contrary, all the other beings too have been
intended for their own sakes and not for the sake of anything else."
—Maimonides

"If one looks with a cold eye at the mess man has made of history, it is
difficult to avoid the conclusion that he has been afflicted by some built-
in mental disorder which drives him toward self-destruction."
—Arthur Koestler

On the Taboo against Knowing Who You Eat

The suppression of awareness required by our universal practice of
commodifying, enslaving, and killing animals for food generates the
"built-in mental disorder" that drives us toward the destruction not
only of ourselves but of the other living creatures and systems of this
earth. Because this practice of exploiting and brutalizing animals for
food has come to be regarded as normal, natural, and unavoidable, it
has become invisible. Though it is fundamental, it continues to be virtually ignored in the ongoing public discourse about why we have the
problems we have and how we can solve them. This lack of mindfulness

is tragic in the classical sense.* It obviously derives from the fact that the writers, speakers, researchers, theologians, doctors, politicians, businessmen, economists, and those who are in positions of leadership and influence, as well as those who are not, all regularly eat foods derived from cruelly treated animals and would prefer to collectively ignore the disturbing consequences of this behavior.

Our culture encourages us all to be omnivores. "Eating everything" has become an apt description of our culture as it consumes and ravages global ecosystems. It is ironically true on an individual level as well. Because of the industrialization of food production, we eat artificially colored, flavored, refined, processed, irradiated, engineered, and chemical-laden products that confirm we will eat virtually anything and everything. We are relentlessly pressured by corporate advertising to swallow anything, and thanks to our well-practiced ability to insulate our awareness from the horror we regularly consume during our meals, it's easy for us to similarly block our awareness of the toxic chemical preservatives and residues in our food. We may even pride ourselves on not being choosy about what we eat. Besides leading to reliable profits for the medical and pharmaceutical industries, this mentality leads to our co-creation of a culture that is "omnivoracious." Its voracious appetite hungers to consume virtually everything, transforming the beauty and diversity of nature into the gadgets, toys, and foods we crave and that never satisfy our inner hunger but lead inevitably to distraction, addiction, frustration, and environmental devastation. Animals, ever vulnerable, bear the burden of our voracious hunger. Their suffering returns, in the end, to us as well.

Eating animals is thus an unrecognized foundation of consumerism, the pseudo-religion of our modern world. Consumerism can only flourish when we feel disconnected and yearn to placate this by consuming, which is a warped attempt at reconnecting with the larger order. Because our greatest desensitization involves eating—our most sacred, essential, and defining act of consuming—we inevitably become desensitized consumers with increasingly voracious appetites. Through com-

*In the ancient Greek tragedies, the protagonist invariably suffers downfall and destruction because of his character defects, the chief ones being hubris and obtuseness.

modifying animals, we have ironically and unavoidably constructed a system that ultimately commodifies us as well. Our net worth is measured in dollars, as cows are sold by the pound.

Because virtually all of us are omnivores, our cruelty is invisible and unmentionable, like an enormous family secret. John Bradshaw, Virginia Satir, and others who have been attempting to illuminate the psychological repercussions of dysfunctional families over the last twenty-five years have emphasized that the more dysfunctional a family is, the more secrets it has.[1] The secrets are the ongoing addictive and abusive behaviors that are never discussed. Child abuse, sexual abuse, drug addiction, and alcoholism have been cultural secrets that, in order to be healed, must be brought into the light, fully acknowledged, and then worked through in open discussion. In dysfunctional families, the secrets and shadows stay buried and painfully unresolved, manifesting as shame, suicidal behavior, aggression, violence, emotional distancing, and psychological numbing. The biggest secret our dysfunctional cultural family has is our horrific brutality against animals for meals, and this shadow drives us into violent and suicidal behavior. The secret is never mentioned or even recognized in our ongoing discussions of dysfunctionality because, being omnivores and thus complicit perpetrators of abuse, we don't want to talk about it. Our efforts to understand family dysfunctionality can thus raise consciousness only to a certain extent. These efforts are vital, though, because they're part of the necessary preliminary work for facing the larger, deeper, more fundamental, and more ruinous shadow secret: our relentless and hidden abuse of animals for food.

The remorse and grief we suppress about the horror we routinely and efficiently inflict on animals in order to eat them is natural and healthy. People who kill or torture others without remorse appall us, and we lock them up as sociopaths and psychopaths. Yet we torture and kill animals who feel pain and fear just as we do, and though we try to ignore and discount their suffering at our hands, we know, deep down, that it's unnecessary, horrifying, and immoral.

There is a German saying, *Übung macht den Meister*: practice makes the master. If we practice golf and tennis, we become proficient at golf and tennis, and golf and tennis become part of us and part of our way of being. If we practice music, art, drama, or martial arts, we become proficient in these, and they influence us and become part of our way of being. If we practice generosity, kindness, and thoughtfulness, we become skilled at being more generous, kind, and thoughtful of others, and these qualities become part of our way of being. If we practice killing, lying and stealing, we become adept at killing, lying and stealing, and these activities become part of us and part of our way of being. By relentlessly and assiduously practicing the ability to disconnect the reality of the flesh, cheese, or egg on our plate from the reality of the misery a feeling being endured to provide it, we have become masters at reducing feeling beings to mere objects, to tools, to means, to property. We have become skilled at being numb and switching off, at not feeling sympathy for the suffering that we demand by our desire to eat animal foods. We have become masters of denial, absolutely refusing to register in consciousness the consequences of our actions. This denial becomes a sort of paralysis that prevents effective and innovative action. Practiced since infancy, our daily rituals of eating have made us highly skilled in the art of objectifying others. This is an enormous tragedy and we have hardly allowed ourselves to become aware of it.

In our churches, ministers often speak about the tragedy of loving things and using people, when we must instead love people and use things. After the services, people eat meals in which animals have become things to be used, not loved. This action, ritually repeated, propels us into using people just as we use animals—as things. We all know in our bones that other animals feel and suffer as we do. If we use them as things, we will inevitably use other humans as things. This is an impersonal universal principle, and ignoring it doesn't make it go away. It operates with mathematical regularity as Pythagoras taught: what we sow in our treatment of animals, we eventually reap in our lives. Because it is a taboo to say this or make this fundamental connection in our herding culture, we can go to church assured that we will not be confronted by the discomforting entreaty to love all living beings and to use none of them as things.

This taboo against speaking about our treatment of animals for food is so strong that I can often feel it as a living force. For several years, I've been speaking on Sunday mornings at progressive churches and centers, primarily Unity churches, and giving seminars on developing intuition. I find in addressing groups of even apparently progressive people that when I begin to raise the topic of the inherent cruelty to animals involved in viewing them as things, and the ethical and spiritual ramifications of our cultural practice of eating them, it seems I must push through an invisible psychic wall that absolutely resists hearing these ideas articulated. It seems to be the unconscious collective denial of the group.

This is ironic, since the Unity movement's two founders, Charles and Myrtle Fillmore, were ethical vegetarians who decried the unnecessary cruelty to animals involved in viewing them as commodities, and who spoke against using leather-bound Bibles, wearing fur, vivisecting animals, or in any way harming "our little sisters and brothers of the animal world." They strongly encouraged people to refrain from eating animal foods. Charles wrote copiously on the subject, saying for example in 1915, "Therefore, in the light of the Truth that God is love, and that Jesus came to make his love manifest in the world, we cannot believe it is his will for men to eat meat, or to do anything else that would cause suffering to the innocent and helpless."[2] In 1920, he wrote, "We need never look for universal peace on this earth until men stop killing animals for food."[3] Together, Charles and Myrtle started the Unity Vegetarian Inn outside Kansas City, writing, "The idea and object of Unity Inn is to demonstrate that man can live, and live well, on a meatless diet."[4] Today, a mere seventy years later, we find animal foods now permeating the menu, and the vegan ethic that Unity's founders wove into the fabric of their teaching has been repressed and virtually forgotten.

What has happened with Unity is not an isolated case. We know that the Buddha taught compassion for animals and a vegan ethic of plant-based eating, and yet many people today call themselves Buddhists and eat animal foods. A strong argument can be made that Jesus and his original followers propagated a similar teaching of compassion toward animals, and—according to researcher Keith Akers in *The*

Lost Religion of Jesus, for example—this original teaching was subverted by Paul and later followers who had a desire for animal flesh.[5] It seems that we have an appetite for eating animals, but no appetite for hearing about the plight of the animals we eat, or of the plight of the humans who suffer in countless ways because of our appetite for animals.

Intelligence: The Ability to Make Connections

To more fully understand the impact of our food choices upon our consciousness and upon our culture, it's helpful to understand the nature of intelligence in the broadest and deepest way we can. Systems theory provides a well-accepted and useful framework for understanding intelligence. Although it uses scientific jargon, the principles that inform it are consonant with the world's ancient wisdom traditions. According to systems theory, all self-organizing systems are seen as having intelligence, and these systems interrelate with each other in complex ways that promote life. Simpler systems, like cells, make up larger and more complex systems, like organs and circulatory systems, which constitute even larger and more complex systems like oaks, ducks, tuna, sheep, and humans, which make up groves, flocks, schools, herds, and villages, which make up forests, riparian communities, marine ecosystems, prairies, and societies. These make up larger systems, like planets, which are parts of even larger systems. Each system is a whole contributing to larger wholes, and composed of smaller wholes.

Simply stated, intelligence is the ability of any system to make connections that are meaningful and helpful for that system in its relations with other systems. Ecologist Gregory Bateson, for example, defined mind as a pattern of organization that is essential to all living systems. Mind is not limited to certain life forms, but also pervades ecosystems and the universe as the interrelating and organizing "pattern which connects."[6] Systems theory acknowledges the obvious intelligence that ranges beyond individual human and animal intelligence to the intelligence of communities, species, ecosystems, the earth, and beyond, and in the reverse direction, to the intelligence of organs, cells, and their smaller constituents. It is not difficult to see that reality as we know and experience it is made up of wholes that are parts of larger wholes, and that these larger wholes are parts of even larger wholes. Every part is connected with every other part by including it or being included along with it in a larger whole. Intelligence lies in the ability of every whole part to receive feedback from and make connections with all the other systems that are related to it, and to thereby unfold its inherent potential to serve the larger wholes.

In an orchestra, as in a community, intelligence allows individuals to make their unique contribution while receiving feedback from the larger wholes and serving them in a meaningful, fully connected way. Joy blossoms through this experience of intelligent interconnectedness—and joy may actually be the ultimate purpose of the boundless, ever-blooming and transforming dance of becoming that arises through the universal interplay of countless nested systems, each and every one including and included within countless others. We can see that no being is ultimately separate; all are interconnected and all arise within larger systems of intelligence that are, to the parts, transcendent and life-bestowing.

The largest whole that includes every atom, every cell, every creature, community, planet, star, galaxy, and universe is, to the part, say an individual human, inconceivable, and is intuited as divine, infinite, eternal, omniscient, and beyond all dualisms. There is literally nothing outside this largest whole, nothing that "it" is not. Our language completely fails to describe "it," since by its very nature language makes objects and things, and the ultimate wholeness within which all appearances reside as nested wholes is not a thing in any sense—it is separate from nothing. The intelligence of this universal wholeness embraces all apparent parts down to the tiniest, and lives within all the parts as their intelligence. Our dualistic thinking cannot grasp this directly, for it is beyond existence or experience as we know them. This universal intelligence can only be sensed non-dualistically, through intuitive receptivity in inner silence that is not clouded by concepts and conditioned thinking.

Intelligence, Telos, and Chickens

All of the nested wholes—systems, planets, communities, people, animals, plants, cells, and so forth—are possible because they partake of the universal intelligence operating through and within them. This intelligence is their ability to make connections that are meaningful to their existence and that serve their purpose or *telos*. The telos of every whole part is to serve the larger wholes within which it has its being, and the universal intelligence we see in nature is the infinitely complex expansion of this web of interconnectedness and feedback. The intelligence of a particular being is thus specific to its own nature as a whole that is served by those parts that make it up, and as a part that serves the larger wholes within which it is embedded. We can see that intelligence is specific to all self-organizing systems, and that all have a unique teleology, or purpose, that their intelligence is suited to fulfilling.

For example, the intelligence that manifests as a chicken is particularly suited to fulfilling the chicken's purpose, and upon reflection, this intelligence is breathtakingly complex. It attends to and regulates the chicken's relationship with the wholes that serve her purpose, that is, the cells and systems within her body, allowing for digestion, elimination, proper blood pressure and circulation, seeing, hearing, and responding to her environment, reproduction, immune system protection, management of hundreds of hormone and enzyme levels, and so forth. The intelligence that manifests as a chicken also attends to her relationship with other chickens and with her environment, as she searches for food, establishes herself within the pecking order of her community, flies up onto branches at night for safety, mates with a rooster, builds her nest, protects her brood, teaches her young how to find food, and so forth. This intelligence also allows her to serve the larger wholes in her own unique way, contributing to her family, her flock, and to the ongoing expression of her species by raising young, participating in the southeast Asian jungle ecosystem community where chickens lived and evolved for millions of years, and contributing to the celebratory unfolding of life on this earth and in the universe.

We can easily see that there is an enormous amount of intelligence invested in a chicken. Besides all these outer and accountable functions of intelligence, there is also the inner, subjective world of the chicken, which may be an equally important purpose for the investment of universal intelligence. We can perhaps never fully know the inner feeling states of being a chicken, but it is obvious to anyone who has been around chickens that they have a huge range of feelings. What does it feel like to sit for days on several eggs, attending carefully to them, turning them regularly to keep them warm? And unhesitatingly risking life and limb to fiercely protect the little chicks from predators after they're born? Perhaps we humans cannot feel what the chicken feels, or we have lost the ability to respect or empathize with her, but that does not mean that the universal intelligence, the infinite creative presence, does not know and appreciate and enjoy and love the chicken and her life. She exists as we humans exist, with a unique intelligence that guides and fulfills her on multiple levels and allows her to fulfill her place in the larger order. Like ours, her intelligence includes awareness, emotions, yearnings, and a central nervous system with pain receptors.

Destroying Intelligence and Purpose

When we forcefully remove a chicken, fish, pig, cow, or any animal from her natural life in order to confine and manipulate her for food, we systematically thwart and frustrate her innate intelligence. The universal intelligence within her can no longer operate freely and contribute to and enrich the many levels of larger wholes that she serves. This is a massive and tragic assault against the core of her being and destroys her purpose. When we confine animals for food, destroying their family and community connections, obliterating their connection with the earth and with their habitats, and thwarting their intelligent drives, we commit extreme violence against not only these creatures, but against the whole interconnected system of intelligence that supports them and that they serve. In committing such violence, we damage our own intelligence as well. We could not even carry out such plans and operations without having already forfeited much of our true intelligence and sense of purpose. How could it ever be our purpose to rob another living being of his or her purpose?

As inheritors of a herding tradition, we naturally try to rationalize this, saying that the animals we raise for food never would have existed without our herding and factory farm operations, and that they therefore do not exist for their purposes, but for our purposes. As the saying goes, if God didn't want us to eat animals, He wouldn't have made them out of meat. Of course, the same could be said about humans to justify cannibalism. Or one might say that if God didn't want people to rape each other, He wouldn't have made them with suitable body openings. Because of our own wounding, we cannot see the blindness and cruelty that always accompany our thinking that others exist for our purposes. Slave owners in the South couldn't see it, either. And yet, if we humans were the ones born into miserable confinement and routinely castrated, branded, raped, shocked, mutilated, and driven insane because we were viewed merely as tasty meat by a stronger and more "intelligent" species, we would certainly hope that this "superior" species would recognize that we have a greater purpose than being mere commodities to be imprisoned, killed, wrapped, sold, and eaten. We likewise must regain the intelligence we have lost through desensitizing ourselves to the undeniable truth that from the perspective of the millions of terrified animals whom we see only as food commodities, we are vicious terrorists.

To the degree that any whole part loses its intelligence, it loses its ability to make the connections that provide it with meaningful guidance in its creative serving of the larger wholes—its true purpose. As our intelligence increases, our capacity for joy and compassion increases. We become more aware of our connection with the human family, the whole web of life, and the infinite source of all life, and yearn to serve these larger wholes. As our intelligence decreases, we disconnect from our serving of the larger wholes, becoming less sensitive to feedback from them, more self-centered and self-preoccupied. This insensitivity becomes stupidity, inevitably bringing violence, disease, unhappiness, suffering, and death.

This truth is not arcane or difficult to understand. We see it in our own bodies, as cells and systems cooperate together with astonishing intelligence to allow us, as the larger whole, to simultaneously: eat and digest food, read a book, monitor our environment for sounds, smells, and sensations, breathe, pump blood, heal a sunburn, destroy stray cancer cells, regulate the levels of hundreds of hormones and enzymes, and perhaps even nurture a growing fetus! Common activities like reading a book, playing the piano, engaging in a classroom discussion, or playing tennis would be inconceivable without the concentrated serving intelligence of millions of smaller whole parts, working together, making countless vital connections, and constantly monitoring feedback levels in an almost unimaginably intricate way. If cooperation and intelligence in the body break down enough, illness and death quickly and inevitably result.

Cells that no longer serve the whole or respond appropriately to feedback have become, in essence, self-preoccupied, and give rise to cancerous tumors that are dangerous and counterproductive. Our body's intelligence knows that these cells would eventually destroy the larger whole upon which they live and depend, and works constantly to eliminate them and to rectify conditions that lead to their proliferation. Our body's intelligence makes connections and serves us, the larger whole. In the same way, human intelligence is the ability to make meaningful connections, and if we are not serving the larger wholes, the larger wholes will let us know. Individuals who damage society are removed from it and, we hope, rehabilitated; what happens when societies irresponsibly damage the earth? If our intelligence is impaired, we lose sight of our purpose and become increasingly numb to the healthy feedback from the larger wholes that is vital to us as intelligent systems and subsystems. If our culture's intelligence is impaired enough, we become the rogue cancer cells that we fear so much within ourselves.

Intelligence Is Species-Specific

Intelligence in living systems is thus determined by the quality and quantity of feedback these systems are capable of receiving, and this ability to receive feedback is closely related to the ability to sense meaningful connections. Because every animal species is unique, it is clear that each species has its own particular type of intelligence that is distinctly suited to its telos, or purpose, and to the types of feedback it receives and the connections it makes. To say that one type of intelligence is higher than another ignores this by imposing an arbitrary standard, and is usually part of an assumption that enshrines the human mode of intelligence at the top of an imagined hierarchy.

Yet we know that there are literally countless varieties of animal consciousness, and that they have many types of intelligence that humans seem not to have. People with companion animals, such as dogs and cats, are often amazed by the intuitive abilities of these animals. For example, as studies show, these animals can often know the precise moment their human companion, many miles away, decides to return home. There are countless other examples of nonhuman animals having intelligence that we can only marvel at, in being able to home and navigate infallibly, to migrate thousands of miles, and to communicate in ways that are utterly unexplained by our materialistic science.[7] It is sadly ironic that while we look longingly to space in search of other intelligent life forms, we are surrounded by thousands of species of intelligent life sharing our earth with us whose awareness, abilities, and subjective experiences we have barely begun to understand and appreciate.

The diversity of intelligence in nature is astonishing because species, subspecies, and individuals all have unique qualities of intelligence. However, scientists, like most people in our culture, have typically been loath to recognize or respect the diversities of intelligence in nature because they participate both consciously and unconsciously in a society that requires an almost complete domination of animals. Parallels can be drawn to the pre-Civil War South, when slavery was legal. Black people, being slaves and the objects of domination and exploitation, were "known" by the dominating culture to have inferior intelligence.

The great irony is that by ignoring, trivializing, and repressing the intelligence in other animals, we have actively reduced our own intelligence. This is the crux of our cultural sickness today and the reason our path is so perilous. By denying the intelligence in animals, ignoring their extensive abilities to feel and to live as subjects in their own ways in the natural world, we have made our culture and ourselves less intelligent. Despite our technological prowess, our individual and cultural intelligence is so severely hampered that we create massive systems of violence and abuse that damage the earth and cause enormous suffering to both humans and animals, and simply ignore the damage and suffering we impose. When *any* living system ignores feedback and refuses to make the connections for which its unique type of intelligence is suited, that living system is less alive, less aware, less free, less able to respond or adapt, and is, from its own survival perspective, in a dangerous situation. The larger wholes, which the system is harming through its loss of intelligence and sensitivity, will naturally, as part of their intelligence, restrict and remove it.

It is as if our nerves have been deadened and we are cutting off pieces of our own limbs, feeling no pain, unaware of the damage being done, and are thus unmotivated and unable to stop the self-destruction. For example, Dan Kindlon and Michael Thompson discuss in their book *Raising Cain* the rapidly climbing suicide rates among adolescent boys, with fourteen percent of fifteen-year-olds contemplating suicide on any given day.[8] Yet does anybody know, or grieve, or even care about this tragedy? Ninety thousand acres of rainforest are destroyed every day, causing nearly one hundred plant and animal species to go extinct daily,[9] yet we have mastered the fine art of disconnecting and deftly ignore this and other ongoing human-caused tragedies. How can we remorselessly devastate oceans by overfishing, destroy wildlife habitats with toxic agricultural runoff, and decimate vast, intricate rainforests through cattle grazing, causing the extinction of many thousands of species every year? How can we be so reckless in our profit-driven quests, genetically engineering living creatures and increasingly despoiling our living planet with military and toxic waste?

It is the socially driven act of eating animals that is primarily responsible for this loss of cultural and personal intelligence. Confining, mutilating, and killing animals for food is so fundamentally cruel and ugly that we must deaden large aspects of our private and public intelligence to do it, especially on the grand scale that animals are slaughtered and abused today.

Beyond cognitive intelligence, there is ethical intelligence, which is the urge to act to relieve the suffering of others. Harming animals so we can eat their flesh, milk, and eggs is so inherently disturbing and repulsive to us as spiritual beings that, in order to get us to do it, the herding culture must systematically numb us from birth, reducing our natural compassion. This suppression of the healthy compassion that is basic to our true nature is perhaps even more serious than the withering of cognitive intelligence. There is substantial evidence that children in our culture, especially boys, are brought up to be tough and to disconnect from their natural feelings of empathy and protectiveness—a process that is essential in a herding culture in which boys will be routinely required as men to dominate and kill animals for food. Hard, tough men, disconnected from their inner wellsprings of intelligence and compassion, are a frightening and devastating force on this earth, and in a herding culture like ours, they are often the role models that boys naturally emulate.

The disconnectedness responsible for our loss of intelligence and compassion afflicts highly paid scientists, doctors, politicians, and clergy just as deeply as it afflicts working-class farmers and laborers. In all cases, it narrows vision, causes a preoccupation with personal and national self-interest, and creates an enormous reservoir of guilt and violence that feeds the fires of war, disease, oppression, and indifference to the suffering of others. What goes around comes around. If we sow seeds of domination and exclusion, we lose intelligence and compassion, and life becomes a burdensome and confused struggle.

As We Sow, So Shall We Reap

The most universal spiritual teaching, found cross-culturally in virtually all the world's religious traditions, is based on the truth of our interconnectedness. It is presented both positively, in what we refer to as the Golden Rule (to do unto others as we would have them do unto us), and more neutrally as the law of cause and effect (that whatever we do unto others will rebound to us). Simply stated, we can never expect to be happy if we cause suffering to others, to be free if we confine others, to be healthy if we cause sickness in others, to be prosperous if we steal from others, or to have peace if we are violent to others and cause them to be afraid. As the Buddhists say, whatever seeds we plant and nurture through the actions of our body, speech, and mind will grow, and we will experience their fruits in our lives as abundance, joy, love, and inner peace, or anger, misery, pain, and lack. "Blessed are the merciful," as the New Testament says, "for they shall obtain mercy" (Matthew 5:7). As we free others, we become free; as we love others, we are loved; as we encourage others, we are encouraged; as we bless others, we are blessed; as we bring joy and healing to others, we find joy and healing in our lives.

This timeless wisdom is the foundation of intelligence and compassion, because it is firmly based on the truth of interconnectedness. In its light we can see how our mistreatment of animals has painful repercussions for us. The irony is breathtaking. For example, animals in the wild are never fat, but animals raised for food are severely confined, fed special diets, and given drugs and hormones in order to make them unnaturally fat (they're sold by the pound, after all). Obesity is a serious problem among human omnivores, with sixty percent of Americans overweight and twenty-six percent obese.[10] The medical costs of this are estimated in the billions, and the psychological costs, while unquantifiable, are enormous. We sow obesity in billions of chickens, turkeys, pigs, and cows, and we reap it in ourselves. Butterball turkeys are bred, fed, and confined to be so fat they can no longer engage in sexual intercourse, something that may for that matter be happening to an increasing number of people.

In the wild, the animals we eat for food live in families and have complex, vital, and enriching social relationships with others in their herds, flocks, schools, and communities. In animal agriculture, all family ties are destroyed, babies are quickly removed from their mothers, and each animal is seen as a separate unit of production. This is what we sow, and what we reap in human culture we can see everywhere: the breakdown of the family. What we do to the animals, we do to ourselves. More than ever, families are breaking up, parents are separating, children are abandoned or leave, and people feel the alienation of being lone "units of production" in a heartless and competitive economic system.

Female animals raised for food are pushed into unnaturally early pregnancies by administration of hormones, especially in egg, dairy, and pig operations, because it's cheaper than having to feed them until they naturally reach sexual maturity. They are only youngsters when they are forcibly impregnated on factory farms. This practice supplies an unnatural load of estrogen and other hormones in the cheese, milk, and other dairy products eaten by our children—pushing them, especially girls, into unnaturally early sexual development and pregnancy. This is a basic driving force behind the trauma of teen pregnancies and abortions, but we rarely hear it discussed.

Another fascinating example of doing unto ourselves what we do to animals is our sexual mutilation of human infants. The young male animals born into our food production system are virtually all castrated without anesthesia to be more easily controllable before being fattened and killed. While we obviously don't castrate all our baby boys, it is quite telling that the most common surgical procedure in the U.S. today is the circumcision of helpless male infants. As Ronald Goldman shows in *Circumcision: The Hidden Trauma,* it's still done as a matter of course, even though it's been proven to be damaging and serves no useful purpose.[11] Like the female circumcision perpetrated by some herding cultures, the male circumcision practiced by our culture reduces the sensitivity of the sexual organ. The foreskin of the penis is a membrane similar to our eyelids that keeps the head of the penis protected and moist and, when the penis is erect, allows for greater skin contact in the sexual act. By cutting away the foreskin in infants, the sensitive head is perpetually exposed, and gradually builds extra layers of cells that protect it and reduce its sensitivity. The skin of a circumcised penis when erect is also unnaturally tight. Most men in our culture have actually been physically mutilated without their consent in a way that reduces their capacity to experience sexual sensations. It's difficult to know what the effects of this have been on relationships, sexual dysfunctionality, and the sexual experience of women, but it's certainly all connected.

Circumcision may persist partly because fathers tend to do to their sons whatever was done to them, and partly because the medical establishment often recommends it. Every surgical procedure means more revenue for the doctors and hospitals, and what happens to all those pieces of foreskin cut off of human penises? They're not just thrown away! They fetch quite a high price when sold to the pharmaceutical companies that use them in their products. It's a poignant reflection of the old practice of slaughterhouses selling their pig pancreases to the same pharmaceutical industry to produce insulin. Vulnerable animal infants are restrained and attacked so their body parts can be sold, and vulnerable human infants are likewise restrained and attacked so their body parts can be sold. Circumcision is by far the most painful surgical procedure done in hospitals without anesthesia, as Paul M. Fleiss, M.D., points out:

In fact, babies feel pain more acutely than adults, and the younger the baby, the more acutely the pain is felt. If an adult needed to be circumcised, he would be given anesthesia and postoperative pain relief. Doctors almost never give babies either of these. The only reason doctors get away with circumcising babies without anesthesia is because the baby is defenseless and cannot protect himself. His screams of pain, terror, and agony are ignored.[12]

Infants are helpless and cannot retaliate, so their fear and pain—*our* fear and pain—like the fear and pain of piglets and other food animals, are simply ignored.

Castrating millions of young male animals has another consequence for human males as well, for by eating the flesh and secretions of these castrated animals, men often gradually lose their sexual ability. Saturated animal fat and cholesterol residues inexorably clog the veins and arteries of their sexual organ, and eventually not enough blood can get through to maintain an erection. On top of this humiliating and poetic consequence of macho brutality, eating animal foods has been positively linked with prostate cancer[13] and with lowered sperm counts.[14] Eating cruelty and death may fit a man into the culturally accepted model of tough masculinity, but this absurdity is revealed in his limp, impotent organ.

The same principle plays out again and again in a striking variety of ways. We pump huge quantities of drugs into billions of defenseless animals. We experience drug addiction, drug abuse, drug dependence, and all the horrors and traumas of side effects, numbing, and the perils of living in a society increasingly drugged with both medical prescriptions and illicit substances. We force farmed animals to live in extremely polluted and toxic environments, to breathe air made noxious by the concentrated ammonia excrement of thousands of enclosed and overcrowded animals, to live in their own waste and eat contaminated feed. We find ourselves living increasingly in our own waste as our air becomes more polluted and our water and food are increasingly contaminated.

We force animals to live in extremely stressful conditions. We find we are living in increasingly stressful conditions. We confine and imprison animals. We find ourselves feeling more confined as social and economic pressures increase, and we see our prison population exploding.[15] We push animals unremittingly to produce, and find we're constantly pushed to produce. We force ill health on animals raised for food by cramming them into toxic, stressful, and hopeless situations, and we find our disease rates increasing. We force millions of factory-farmed animals into insanity through the complete frustration and thwarting of their natural yearnings and drives, and we find human mental illness escalating.

We terrorize millions of vulnerable and defenseless animals daily with painful shockings, beatings, brandings, debeakings, dehornings, castrations, ear notchings, nose bashings, and by forcing them to watch the killing of other animals before they are killed. As we terrorize, so we increasingly fear the shadow of terrorism, and we pour billions of dollars into campaigns to "prevent terrorism." We steal from and deceive animals on a massive scale: we steal their babies, their bodies, their milk, their eggs, their honey, and their lives, and we deceive them with baited hooks, lures, nets, and slaughterhouse tunnels. We find that we live in a society increasingly rife with deception and theft, where predatory capitalism and sophisticated advertising work together to create a climate that legitimizes deceit in the name of profit, and fraudulent cunning in the name of return on investment.

We force food animals into cages, and we find more and more of us living in gated communities, behind bars and locks. We overcrowd them and we're increasingly overcrowded. We torture them by the millions and Amnesty International reports that human torture of other humans is at an all-time high.[16] In fact, one of the most widespread techniques of human torture, preferred because it causes severe pain while leaving little physical scarring, is electroshocking. According to Amnesty International, this technology was pioneered by U.S. corporations in the 1970s for use on animals, and there are now over 120 companies in the world (70 in the U.S.) making electroshock devices that are used on both animals and humans.[17]

Animals raised for food are often purposefully starved—sometimes it's female chickens being starved as part of a "forced molt," to shock their bodies to begin another cycle of egg laying, and sometimes it's to save money on feed, or just negligence. We find our culture rife with anorexia nervosa as people, mostly women, starve themselves, sometimes to death. And, even with an overabundance of grain being grown—but fed to livestock for consumption by the wealthy—many thousands of poor people, mostly children, die every day of starvation.

For young female animals born into our food production system, the sexual abuse of repeated raping is a defining experience. It is euphemized as "artificial insemination," but it is forcible rape, and young female pigs, cows, sheep, goats, turkeys, chickens, ducks and other animals are all repeatedly raped by men to produce offspring before being killed. For these defenseless females, men are serial rapists and killers. Young female turkeys, for example, are raped an average of twice a week for twelve to sixteen months until they're slaughtered for turkey soup and baby food.[18] Besides the systematic sexual abuse of insemination, many animals, particularly pigs, are the victims of sexual abuse by workers on factory farms, as has been documented by undercover workers. Rape is a central metaphor of our culture and an enormously serious problem, with a woman or girl being raped or sexually assaulted in the U.S. an average of every two minutes.[19] As in animal agriculture, where the female and the maternal are brutally dominated and exploited for profit, in our human society feminine and maternal values are suppressed and women are denied equal status with men. This ongoing, invisible domination of the feminine and of female animals in particular has enormous consequences and goes a long way toward explaining the lower status of women in our culture. Viewing animals merely as meat and objects to be consumed, we find that women, like animals, are also often viewed merely as meat to be used sexually. As Carol J. Adams points out, animals and women are linked in our culture through pornography, advertising, and the popular media, with "food" animals being seen as sexualized females who want to be eaten, and women linked with animals as sexual objects that want to be used.

As we inflict disease on animals through the bizarre conditions we force upon them in factory farms, we find new and deadly diseases haunting and stalking us, like SARS, AIDS, mad cow disease, and a variety of aggressive influenzas, as well as drug-resistant strains of tuberculosis, strep, E. coli, and other debilitating pathogen-related ailments. By severely crowding animals in ways that would never occur in the wild, breaking social structures, compelling them to eat the feces, blood, flesh, and organs of animals they would normally never feed upon, and forcing them into routine cannibalistic behavior by feeding them foods "enriched" with the body parts of members of their own species, we make factory farm operations the breeding grounds of deadly viruses, bacteria, parasites, and proteins that would never have any chance of developing in nature. These pathogens, like the prion responsible for mad cow disease, are passed into us when we ingest foods or drugs sourced from the bodies of these tortured creatures. As Michael Greger, M.D., has pointed out, aggressive new influenzas are easily tracked to overcrowded food animal confinement and slaughterhouse operations,[20] as is the prevalence of diseases caused by salmonella, E. coli, listeria, campylobacter, and other pathogens. The intensive confinement of animals for food causes high levels of stress, disease, and pathogen infestation in the animals we eat, which the industry combats by administering large quantities of drugs and antibiotics so the animals can survive until slaughter weight is attained. This only compounds the problem for human health, because the antibiotics and other drugs encourage the evolution of ever hardier and more drug-resistant strains of bacteria and viruses. It's well known that this practice leads to new and deadlier strains of pathogens, such as the tubercule bacillus that is so resistant to drugs that the suffering caused by the massive amounts of toxic pharmaceuticals used to combat the disease is considered worse than the disease itself. This is not difficult to understand, but new diseases and ever-larger intensive confinement factory farm operations both continue to proliferate with little public questioning because both are highly profitable, and the public cannot bear to look at its food habits. Sowing disease in defenseless animals, we can only reap the same for ourselves.

In countless ways, the chickens come home to roost. Forcing horror on animals, we find horror in the mass media and in popular entertainment increasing. As we kill young animals for food, we find child and teen suicide skyrocketing. As we purposefully enrage animals, as in rodeos, we find our own rage increasing. As we purposefully induce fear in them, as in laboratory experiments on fear, we find our own chronic fear increasing. As we force osteoporosis on them by pushing them to overproduce milk and eeggs, we find ourselves suffering an epidemimc of osteoporosis. As we intentionally overfeed them to create the swollen and diseased duck and goose livers we eat as foie gras, we find ourselves chronically over-eating foods with toxic residues and thereby damaging our livers and other internal organs. As we force animals to be fat, diseased, overcrowded, anxious, and stressed, we become the same. As we feed them unnaturally processed, chemical-laden foods, we find our grocery stores filled with similarly toxic products posing as food. As we confine them to little boxes, we find ourselves confined in office cubicles of our own making. As we ignore animal suffering, we ignore each other's suffering. As we deny animals their dignity and privacy, we deny our own dignity and find our privacy being increasingly eroded. As we enforce powerlessness on them, we feel increasingly powerless. As we reduce them to mere commodities, we become mere commodities ourselves. As we destroy their ability to fulfill their purpose, we lose track of our purpose. As we deny them rights, we lose our own rights. As we enslave them, we become slaves ourselves. As we break their spirits, our own spirits are broken. As we sow, we reap.

The cardiac units of metropolitan hospitals have become assembly lines for heart bypass surgeries. Scores of people go through every day, one after another, to have these expensive and radical operations performed. They are typically people who have eaten many animals. Meanwhile, animals are lined up in slaughterhouse disassembly lines and stabbed, one after the other. People eat them and line up in hospitals to be stabbed, one after the other. As we stab, so shall we be stabbed.

Scientists are hard at work now breeding food animals who will be as dull, insensitive, and controllable as possible, in order to better survive the unimaginable pain and stress they are forced to endure on factory farms. They want to create animals with minimal feelings and awareness, animals born with broken spirits, with no zest for life and with no purpose other than to serve the ends of their dominators. That would be good for business. As we cause others to be, so we become— and, in this case, perhaps, are already well on our way to becoming.

May we ponder deeply the wisdom of the Golden Rule before it's too late, and begin to actually live it with respect to the animals who are at our mercy. Otherwise, our future may be horribly grim: all that we force others to experience, we will eventually end up experiencing ourselves.

CHAPTER FOUR

INHERITING OUR FOOD CHOICES

"People wish to be settled. Only as far as they are unsettled is there any
hope for them."
—EMERSON

"It is nothing less than a form of violence to attempt to win children
over to the toxic poisons, the coarse flavour and the unsympathetic texture of animal flesh."
—JON WYNNE-TYSON

"This is dreadful! Not only the suffering and death of the animals, but
that man suppresses in himself, unnecessarily, the highest spiritual capacity—that of sympathy and pity towards living creatures like himself—
and by violating his own feelings becomes cruel."
—LEO TOLSTOY

Our Inheritance: Infant Indoctrination

Instead of reducing our intelligence and compassion by denying and
destroying the intelligence and purpose of animals, we could celebrate,
honor, and appreciate the immense diversity of intelligences, beauties,
abilities, and gifts that animals possess and contribute to our world. We
could liberate ourselves by liberating them and allowing them to fulfill

the purposes that their particular intelligences yearn for. We could respect their lives and treat them with kindness. Our awareness and compassion would flourish, bringing more love and wisdom into our relationships with each other. We could live in far greater harmony with the universal intelligence that is the source of our life. To do so, however, we would have to stop viewing animals as commodities, and this means we would have to stop viewing them as food.

If we look at animals in general, we realize that there is probably no more fundamental and essential teaching given by parent to offspring than how to feed. In finding, preparing, and eating food, adults of every species teach their young both directly and by example. We humans are no exception. In fact, because we are as infants more vulnerable than other animals, food education is even more important to us. The earliest and most basic connections we have with our parents are around food and eating.

From birth we partake of our mother's milk. For us and all mammals, this feeding epitomizes being loved, nurtured, protected and bonded with our mother and with all that our mother represents. She has birthed us out of her body and feeds us from her breast. She represents the infinite matrix of life, the vast loving intelligence that is our source and the source of all life, that feeds and loves all creatures as manifestations of itself within its boundless being. Feeding at our mother's breast is one of the most powerful symbolic natural acts that we humans can engage in. We are safe, loved, nourished, and directly connected with the vast loving, mysterious source of our life. We utterly trust our mother and her milk.

As we grow older, stronger, and more independent, our mother prepares special soft foods for us. In an event that is highly significant for us as children, we are weaned from our mother's milk and are taught how to eat our own food and to feed ourselves. It's likely that the disturbing loss of breast-feeding imprints the replacement food we are given especially strongly on our young and impressionable minds. We lose the warm, intimate feeding of nursing and begin to be fed our parents' food as softened baby food—including chicken, veal, cheese, and other animal products. As we get older, the amount of flesh, dairy, and

egg we are fed increases and becomes gradually more obvious and undeniable. Our bodies and minds are conditioned by the most powerful
forces in our world (our parents and family) and in the most powerful
ways (through our care and feeding) to believe that we are by nature
omnivorous, even carnivorous, and therefore predatory. It's no wonder it's
so difficult to question the foods we eat, and that this taboo runs so deep!

We could not survive without the food our parents gave us, a tangible and consumable expression of their love and caring for us. As we
incorporated their food, we partook of them and their values and their
culture. At every meal, three times a day, their food *became* us. *Their*
culture and food became *our* culture and *our* food.

Most of us resist being told we've been indoctrinated. After all, we
live in the land of the free, and we like to think we've arrived freely at
the belief that we need to eat animal products and that it's natural and
right to do so. In fact, we have inherited this belief. We've been indoctrinated in the most deeply rooted and potent way possible, as vulnerable infants; yet because our culture denies the existence of indoctrination, the reality of the process is invisible, making it difficult for most of
us to realize or admit the truth. We may become irate that someone
would even suggest that our mother's loving meals and our father's barbecues were a form of indoctrination. Our mother and father didn't
intend to indoctrinate us, just as their parents didn't intend to indoctrinate them. Nevertheless, our old herding culture, primarily through the
family and secondarily through religious, educational, economic, and
governmental institutions, enforces the indoctrination process in order
to replicate itself in each generation and continue on.

The reason that indoctrinated beliefs resist being contemplated or
questioned is that we did not arrive at them freely, on our own. If we
are challenged in a belief that we have struggled within ourselves to
attain, we feel energized and welcome an opportunity to deepen our
understanding, to exchange, to grow. If the belief has been indoctrinated, however, we feel nervous and irritated if it's challenged. It's not *our*
belief, and yet we believe it. So we try to change the subject, and if that
doesn't work, we create a distraction, or close down, or leave, or attack
the one who would challenge our indoctrinated belief. We do whatever

we can to block feedback or questioning. Because we have accepted the belief unconsciously, we cannot defend or support the belief but must remain unaware of any inner or outer feedback that would challenge it.

This forced unawareness becomes a sort of armor, dulling the mind and deadening the vital spiritual spark within us that seeks higher awareness through increased understanding and inner freedom. The price we pay for unquestioned indoctrinated and inherited beliefs is enormous. By uncritically accepting culturally transmitted beliefs and blindly being their agents, we remain children, ethically and spiritually. Because our mind is conditioned and we are unable to question the conditioning, we find it difficult to mature or contribute our unique gifts. Our song may die within us without ever being fully sung, to the loss of everyone, especially ourselves.

The Importance of Leaving Home

If we are to mature spiritually and morally, and if we are to nourish within us the seeds of intelligence, compassion, and freedom, we must practice questioning the underlying assumptions of the family and culture into which we were born. This has been understood for centuries as fundamental both to individual spiritual awakening and to social progress. In Buddhism, this is called "leaving home." Jesus refers to the same practice when he asks rhetorically, "Who is my mother? And who are my brethren?" (Matthew 12:47) and when he says, "There is no man who has left home . . . for my sake, and the gospel's, but he shall receive an hundredfold now . . . and in the world to come eternal life" (Mark 10:29–30).

Leaving home is Buddhist shorthand for the spiritual practice of questioning our society's values and adopting a higher set of values. This is essential to spiritual progress because it brings the maturity that can lead to higher consciousness, greater compassion, and, ultimately, freedom from the delusion of being a fundamentally separate self and the suffering and violence this delusion necessarily causes.

In consciously contemplating and questioning the worldview and practices of our parents, family, and culture, we make leaving home a vital foundation of and prerequisite for our spiritual growth and for undertaking what Joseph Campbell termed the Hero's Journey. The hero's journey is the cross-culturally recognized spiritual quest in which we leave the confines of home and culture, undertake an inner (and usually outer) journey and attain higher understanding, and then return to our culture with new powers to reform, vitalize, and uplift our community through the inner growth attained on our journey.

In questioning our culture's most fundamental and defining practice, that of imprisoning and brutalizing animals for food, we practice leaving home and embark on a spiritual journey that will put us fundamentally at odds with our culture's values, but that at the same time makes it possible for us to be heroes who can help uplift and transform our ailing culture. By recognizing and understanding the violence inherent in our culture's meal rituals and consciously adopting a plant-based diet, becoming a voice for those who have no voice, we can attain greater compassion and happiness and live more fully the truth of our interconnectedness with all life. In this we fulfill the universal teachings that promote intelligence, harmony, and spiritual awakening. Our life can become a field of freedom and peace as we deepen our understanding of the sacredness and interdependence of all living beings, and practice non-cooperation with those forces that see creatures as mere commodities.

By questioning our inherited cultural conditioning to commodify, abuse, and eat animals, we are taking the greatest step we can to leave home, become responsible adults, and mature spiritually, and by actively helping others do the same, we return home with a liberating message of compassion and truth that can inspire and bless others. By leaving home we can find our true home, contribute to social progress, and help the animals with whom we share this precious earth have a chance to be at home again as well.

The Power of Social Pressure

As we can see, our culture's pervasive belief in eating, dominating, and commodifying animals is a living inheritance, passed from one generation to the next through our most powerful shared ritual, eating meals. Most of us, if asked why we eat meat, will have three basic reasons: we need the protein, everybody else does it, and it tastes good. The first reason is a good example of an inherited belief. We've been told from childhood that we need animal protein, and we believe it in spite of the overwhelming evidence to the contrary. Along with this deep indoctrination that we must eat animals, which we can question through our practice of leaving home, the two other primary reasons why people today eat animals boil down to social pressure and taste.

We humans are highly sensitive to social pressure. We are surrounded by a culture of omnivorism as fish live surrounded by water. We like to fit in and be part of the group with which we identify, so we are unlikely to seriously examine the culturally pervasive practice of eating animal foods. Meals carry powerful social significance, and we fear that others might be hurt or offended or not like us if we go against the food status quo. We are aware that by not eating animal foods, we will be seen as threatening and implicitly criticizing the overwhelming majority of people around us who do eat them. Because we naturally want to please our friends, family, colleagues, and co-workers and be accepted by them, we know instinctively not to question such a primary practice as eating animal foods during the shared meals that are so basic to our relationships. Talking about how delicious the food is, sharing recipes, having cookouts together, going on fishing expeditions, traveling together, sharing favorite restaurants, relaxing and enjoying the church barbecue: it's remarkable how our social lives revolve around shared food, and there is nothing more potentially disturbing to all this than rejecting the confining and killing of defenseless animals, which constitutes the foundation of our meals. There is nothing more subversive to a herding culture than refusing to view animals as commodities—or, more concretely, than refusing to eat animal foods. We know this in our bones, and the social pressure to fit in and eat what everyone eats is unremitting.

On top of this social pressure is marketing pressure that comes directly from the animal food industries. The meat, dairy, and egg industries are notorious for aggressively marketing their products, targeting children and health care professionals in particular. It's well known, for example, that the dairy industry has been providing free "educational materials" to schools for decades that shamelessly promote dairy products. The animal food industries also cultivate cozy relationships with the professional nutritionist, dietician, and medical associations by sponsoring programs and studies and in other ways helping them financially. These associations of course repay favors by recommending—or at least not questioning—the practice of eating animal foods.

We are surrounded by media images and messages promoting the eating of flesh, milk products, and eggs. Meat-based fast food restaurants are ubiquitous in our cultural landscape, and they spend billions of dollars annually in advertising and promoting their products. McDonald's, for example, reportedly spends as much as $500 million on just one ad campaign, while the National Cancer Institute spends only about $1 million a year to promote eating five daily servings of fruits and vegetables.[1] The dairy industry spends hundreds of millions in its highly effective advertising campaigns, and even gets financial and legal assistance from the federal government to promote its products! Food is the largest U.S. industry, and it is dominated by meat, dairy, and egg producers. As potential consumers, we are all being constantly bombarded with subtle and not-so-subtle messages to buy their products. The meat, dairy, and egg industries' greatest sales promoters are, of course, our parents, families, neighbors, and teachers as we are growing up, and our colleagues, families, and friends as we get older.

We internalize this and create a self-image—of someone who eats normally and enjoys certain foods—that determines our behavior. The advertising industry learned long ago that, while we resist attempts to influence us directly, we are easily influenced when we can be made to identify with a particular image. Once we identify with an image, the industry needs only to manipulate the image to manipulate our behavior. Viewing images that portray "successful Americans" eating certain foods, for example, we naturally want to buy the same foods because we imagine ourselves to be successful Americans as well. In this way, programming and advertising in the mass media work hand in hand to create a powerful and reliable demand for certain products.

It should be noted that another fundamental source of pressure to eat animal foods is the medical establishment, which shows almost universal antipathy toward plant-based diets. Medicine is the second-largest U.S. industry after food, and the pharmaceutical industry, like the fast food industry, spends vast sums of money on advertising and promoting its products. With its gargantuan investment in hospitals, research, equipment, doctors, medical schools, and the other aspects of its massive substructure, the medical industry (and the banking industry lurking behind it) demands a continuous and reliable flood of sick people. It's suddenly understandable why so many means are used to discourage people from questioning their omnivorous way of eating, given the overwhelming evidence that we would be much healthier and less reliable consumers of pharmaceutical products and medical services if we abandoned animal foods.

Thus, social pressure from friends, family, and associates together with market pressure from the food and medical industries exert a powerful force on all of us to eat animal foods and curb our awareness of the repercussions of our actions. These influential powers in our lives do not want us to leave home and think for ourselves about what we are eating and the consequences of our food choices. It is the height of irony that, amid all this pressure, we may respond angrily to people who question our eating of animal foods with, "Don't tell me what to eat!" We've already been told, and are being told in no uncertain terms, what to eat.

We can see that historically, social pressure has been a potent factor in retarding social progress and in promoting racism, intolerance, violence, and war. While social mores can certainly influence us in positive ways, it's obvious that they influence us in many negative ways as well. Social pressures among adolescent boys are powerful factors in, for example, encouraging drug and alcohol abuse, viewing girls as sexual objects, and stigmatizing homosexuality, which drives some boys to despair and suicide. It's well known that in Nazi Germany, social pressure played a key role in Adolf Hitler's ability to consolidate power, kill millions of Jews, gypsies, communists, and homosexuals, and go to war against millions of others. The medieval European witch-hunt that spanned several centuries, terrorizing women and savagely killing tens of thousands of people, is a particularly bleak example of the terrible power social pressure can wield.

Social pressure was certainly a powerful influence in the antebellum

South, reinforcing the racist white attitudes that slavery required with stereotypes and social rituals that reaffirmed white supremacy. Today, social pressure is similarly fundamental in promulgating the speciesist attitudes that animals are ours to eat, wear, and use. Stereotypes of animals used for food are exceedingly negative, blinding us completely to the intelligence and beauty of pigs, cows, chickens, turkeys, fish, and other animals. Social rituals of domination, like rodeos, circuses, and zoo exhibits, all reinforce the daily rituals of domination and exclusion known as meals. The intensity of this social pressure to collectively abuse animals is enormous: even the most avid Ku Klux Klan members don't burn crosses three times a day!

We often find that if we don't participate in the eating and dominating of animals, we are frowned on and excluded in a variety of ways. The pressure would probably be more overt in the cowboy culture of Wyoming than in the urban culture of Chicago, but the pressures are nonetheless pervasive and, for many of us, simply too daunting to resist, especially coming from family members or colleagues whom we are trying to please.

Contemplating Taste

Besides infant indoctrination and social and market pressure, there is the third factor that drives people to eat animal foods: taste. Is the smell of cooking flesh—the familiar smell of a pot roast, for example—really good, or does it trigger old childhood memories that are good? The smell may evoke our mother's kitchen and the warm feeling of the love we received through her home cooking. If our spouse wants to eat a plant-based diet and prepares a vegetable stir-fry with tempeh and baked potatoes, we may not think it smells so good because we never smelled it in our mother's kitchen. We'll resist the meal and exert social pressure on our vegetarian spouse to go back to "real food."

It's perhaps true, as the old saying has it, that taste cannot be disputed, but it can nevertheless be contemplated. In contemplating the taste of animal foods, several things become immediately apparent. One is that we detest eating flesh in its natural state. How ironic! Unlike plant foods, which are often delicious to us when uncooked, raw flesh is basically disgusting to us. It is virtually always cooked and carefully prepared in order to become food for us humans, unlike the raw flesh, blood, scales, skin, bones, and organs that are gobbled up by natural omnivores and carnivores. If we had to eat natural raw flesh or no flesh, I suspect we would all become vegetarians immediately.

Another thing we notice is that we don't like the flesh if it's soaked in blood, even if it's cooked. The main reason animals suffer so horribly in slaughterhouses is that they must be alive when their throats are slit so that their still-beating hearts can pump the blood out of their bodies and partially dry up their flesh. If they were killed by some other means and then their corpses were cut up, the flesh would be so drenched with blood that no one would want to eat it.

One fact we may not ordinarily consider is that the blood-drained and well-cooked flesh we smack our lips over is permeated with the waste products of the cells that make up the flesh. These waste products, or urea, are inseparable from the flesh, and were flowing into the blood when the animal was killed, to be filtered out of the blood by the kidneys and excreted as urine. In fact, what gives meat its distinctive and apparently appetizing flavor is the cooked urea in the flesh. Salty and "meaty," urea gives flesh the taste we've come to associate with fine dining and good-time barbecues.

A fourth thing we notice about the taste of animal products is that in many ways, the more we disguise them and hide them, the more we like them. We cook flesh and eggs and add salt, pepper, seasonings, herbs, and all manner of taste enhancers and modifiers. Most cheeses involve cooking animals' milk, and without all the added salt, most cheeses would be unappetizing to most people. We add all kinds of flavorings and fruits and sugars to make cream and milk more appealing in ice cream, chocolate milk, and flavored yogurts. We bury a salted, smoked, and tenderized ground flesh patty amid sliced tomatoes, onions, lettuce, mustard, ketchup, mayonnaise, and relish. We have to ask, is it *really* the taste of the flesh and animal products that we enjoy so much? Or is it rather all the plant-based sauces, seasonings, condiments, and dressings that camouflage and elevate the taste of the animal products we've been pressured into eating? Besides the condiments, the hamburger is well buried in propaganda; McDonald's tells our children it comes from a "burger patch."

When cooked and properly camouflaged, animal flesh, eggs, and milk products all have one taste factor going for them: they are high in saturated fat. We humans seem to easily develop cravings for fatty, creamy, greasy foods, and animal foods tend to fulfill these taste cravings, though plant foods can certainly be prepared in fatty, creamy ways if we should so desire, and without any of the toxic cholesterol of animal foods. Because the cooked fat and urea combination cannot be exactly replicated by plant foods, there are certainly tastes and textures in animal foods that aren't precisely duplicated by plant foods, but many of the more recent meat analogs come amazingly close. However, most people who were raised as omnivores and have switched to a plant-based diet for at least a year or two find nothing at all attractive about the taste or texture of animal foods. From my experience they do not crave it at all, but find it increasingly revolting.

According to Neal Barnard, M.D., "One of the most surprising discoveries in the science of appetite is that tastes require maintenance."[2] Since our taste cells turn over about every three weeks, he points out that "two or three weeks is all it takes" for our taste cells to forget the taste of animal foods, and that this will eliminate most of our craving for them, because the new taste cells will be accustomed only to the tastes of plant-based foods. The craving we have for animal foods is conditioned and maintained by repetition, and our typical diet—high in animal fat, animal protein, and cholesterol—is fundamentally toxic to our physiology.

But the elimination of cravings may not be so simple. As Neal Barnard discusses in *Breaking the Food Seduction*, a growing body of research is demonstrating that meat and especially cheese are physically addicting. When digested, cheese releases opiates called casomorphins as well as an amphetamine-like chemical called phenylethylamine, also found in sausage. Ham, salami, tuna, and other meats also appear to be addicting, because opiate-blocking drugs reduce people's desire for them.[3] Besides whatever physical addiction there may be, a lot of the craving for animal foods seems to be mental and emotional;

the smell of the pot roast cooking conjures up mom and security and self-image.

Eating food is a lot like sex in that the inner images and attitudes we have are more important to our enjoyment than the physical or objective reality of which or of whom we partake. Our taste is determined, ultimately, by our mind. I've found personally that my taste appreciation for foods has grown enormously since I began eating a plant-based diet thirty years ago, and as the years go by, the flavors are richer, more infinitely varied, and ever more delicious. Most vegans I've talked with find this to be true for them as well. There are probably two main reasons for this. One is that plant-based foods tend to be subtler in their tastes than animal-based foods. As we discussed, animal foods are salty from urea and added salt, and they are usually dressed with strong-tasting tenderizers, sauces, condiments, and flavor enhancers.[4] Our sense of taste may become somewhat numbed by the strong flavors, so in the beginning a plant-based diet often seems bland.[5] In a few weeks, though, as our taste buds turn over and become more sensitive because they aren't being chronically overwhelmed by the strong artificial flavors added to animal foods, we become more sensitive to the delicate flavors of vegetables, grains, legumes, and fruits, and all the endless ways of preparing and combining them. New taste vistas unfold endlessly.

The other reason plant-based foods taste better is that we feel better eating them and contemplating their origins. Eating slowly, we enjoy contemplating the organic orchards and gardens that supply the delicious vegetables, fruits, and grains we're eating. We grow to appreciate the nearly miraculous beauty of cabbages and cauliflower, the fragrance of roasted sesame seeds, sliced oranges, chopped cilantro, and baked kabocha squash, and the wondrous textures of avocado, persimmon, steamed quinoa, and sautéed tempeh. We are grateful for the connection we feel with the earth, the clouds, the nurturing gardeners, and the seasons, and the tastes are delicious gifts we naturally enjoy opening to, as we would open to our beloved in making love and appreciating the beloved fully. In contrast, eating animal foods is often done quickly, without feeling deeply into the source of the food—for who would want to contemplate the utter hells that produce our factory-farmed fish, chicken, eggs, cheese, steaks, bacon, hot dogs, or burgers? Feeling guilty, we just take the life force, without really opening to it, as if we were having sex with a prostitute, refusing to acknowledge that she is a unique and precious being, and distancing ourselves from her suffering. Just the pleasure, please—anything more would spoil our fun. Actually, the taste that we prize in animal foods is more like the sex we would have as rapists, for the prostitute may at least consent and profit from our cravings, but the animal is always forced against her will to be tortured and killed for our taste and questionable pleasure.

When we contemplate our tastes, we can see how conditioned they actually are. More importantly, though, we can see how utterly unsupportable they are as reasons to commit violence against defenseless, feeling beings. Self-centered craving for pleasure and fulfillment at the expense of others is the antithesis of the Golden Rule and of every standard of morality.

We know it is unacceptable to knowingly harm sentient creatures simply to satisfy our personal taste. If we see a man whose umbrella we find attractive, we know it's wrong to attack or kill the man and steal the umbrella just because our taste desires to have it. Or if we see a woman whose body we find attractive, we know it's wrong to hit her and rape her just because we may desire to do so. These actions are wrong because they cause suffering to others and violate their sacred integrity for purely selfish reasons. We also know that we must face social and legal consequences if we commit such acts. However, if we desire to eat the flesh or milk or eggs of an animal because we like how it tastes—and this means killing, beating, raping, confining, stealing from, and in other ways hurting the animal and violating her sacred integrity—we are fully encouraged to do so! The social consequences of harming animals for food are all positive. Since our culture denies animals used for food any inherent value in their own right, limiting their worth simply to their value as commodities to those who own them, animals have no protection. Ordering a steak earns us approving nods, and our friends rave over the barbecued ribs at the office picnic. The actual confinement, raping, mutilating, and killing are kept carefully hidden as shameful secrets that would make us profoundly uncomfortable if we had to witness them or, worse, perform them ourselves.

Two hundred years ago in the South, a slave could certainly be beaten, stolen from, confined, raped, mutilated, and killed by the master or his overseer with no feelings of compunction; such behavior was encouraged by the culture and the upbringing of the dominating class. This upbringing dulled natural human feelings of compassion, connectedness, and justice, inhibited people's intelligence, and allowed them to act brutally without a sense of remorse. Deep down, though, they certainly knew better, just as we know better today when we order a cheese omelet with bacon because we like the taste. Though our natural intelligence knows this is a profoundly immoral act, our knowing is suppressed and our hearts are hardened against the misery that a chicken, a cow, and a pig endured to satisfy our passing and conditioned taste pleasure. We prefer not to know and are comfortable in knowing that no one—not the waitress, nor our friends, nor the media—will in any way remind us of the enormous animal misery necessitated by our demand. The animals suffer out of sight and their cries are unheeded by us. They have no voice as long as we refuse to listen to our hearts.

Defending the Fortress

We can see that the three reasons that we eat animal foods—infant indoctrination, social and market pressure, and taste—reinforce each other and create a force field around our food choices that, like a sturdy fortress, resists any incursions. The walls are up, and they're well fortified. Yet the fortress may not be as strong as it looks. For one thing, it confines us and inhibits our natural urge to fulfill a higher potential and to evolve spiritually. For another, it is not founded upon the truth of our basic nature, which is kindness, nor on our sense of interconnectedness with other living beings, and it militates against our ability to awaken wisdom and live in freedom together. At the core of our being we yearn to reach higher in our understanding and to live in peace and harmony on this earth. The walls of the fortress are built of cruelty, denial, ignorance, force, conditioning, and selfishness. Most importantly, they are not of our choosing. They have been, and are being, forced upon us.

Our well-being—and our survival—depend on our seeing this clearly and throwing off our chains of domination and unawareness. By harming and exploiting billions of animals, we confine ourselves spiritually, morally, emotionally, and cognitively, and blind ourselves to the poignant, heart-touching beauty of nature, animals, and each other.

To be free, we must practice freeing others. To feel loved, we must practice loving others. To have true self-respect, we must respect others. The animals and other voiceless beings, the starving humans and future generations, are pleading with us to see: it's on our plate.

CHAPTER FIVE

THE INTELLIGENCE OF HUMAN PHYSIOLOGY

"My refusing to eat flesh occasioned an inconveniency, and I was frequently chided for my singularity, but, with this lighter repast, I made the greater progress, from greater clearness of head and quicker comprehension."
—BENJAMIN FRANKLIN

"Human beings are not natural carnivores. When we kill animals to eat them, they end up killing us because their flesh, which contains cholesterol and saturated fat, was never intended for human beings, who are natural herbivores."
—WILLIAM C. ROBERTS, M.D.,
Editor-in-Chief, *The American Journal of Cardiology*

"The pain and suffering inflicted on children by the American diet is so brutal that if it were administered with a stick, parents would be put in jail."
—JOHN MCDOUGALL, M.D.[1]

The Gift

A basic reason that billions of animals suffer confinement and slaughter is our cultural belief that we need to eat animal-derived foods to be healthy, yet one of the most common motivations many of us have to reduce or eliminate animal food consumption is improving our health! Illuminating this paradox requires us to investigate our human physiology and the animal foods we eat, and to reconnect with the perennial understanding that cultivating kindness and awareness improves physical and mental health, while harmfulness and unconsciousness lead ultimately to physical and mental disease. We can realize that we are meant to live in harmony with the other animals of this earth because we've been given bodies that actually function better *without* killing and stealing from them. What a liberating gift! No animal need ever fear us, because there is no nutrient that we need that we cannot get from non-animal sources. The evidence of this is abundant, and we'll look at some of it in this chapter in order to question the delusion that we *need* to eat animal foods to be strong, healthy, and real. Both medical studies and the obvious examples of healthy vegan people we see around us tell us that eating animal products is unnecessary, and in many ways is actually detrimental to our health.

Some of us may protest, "Wait a minute! How can eating animal products be unhealthy? It seems so natural!" Let's take a closer look at the human body. A good way to begin is by observing with fresh eyes how our bodies compare to some of the other animals with whom we share this planet. How soft, hairless, and delicate we humans are! And how physically weak! A human, for example, has only one sixth the strength of a typical chimpanzee.[2] We dominate animals not through physical strength, but by using implements and treachery.

We can notice our organ of eating, our human mouth. We see how small it is, how small our teeth are, and how we lack long, sharp canines to tear tough flesh as well as the strong, heavy jawbone and jaw muscles of carnivores and omnivores. We notice also how soft human teeth are, compared to the much harder teeth of carnivorous animals that are able to crush bones to gain access to bone marrow.[3] Our teeth and jaw are obviously not designed for ripping flesh and gnawing bones; like frugivores and herbivores we have incisors in the front with molars along the sides for biting off and grinding plant foods.

It is interesting to imagine trying to kill and eat another mammal without using any implements, just our delicate mouth and fine, clawless hands. Could we do it? Could our parents, children, or friends do it? Could *any* human being do it? Could anyone, or would anyone chase down, say, a deer, cow, pig, sheep, goat, or rabbit in the wild and then, somehow catching her (highly unlikely) fall on her neck with our small, flat human mouth, tear through the fur and skin into the living flesh with our small human teeth, and fill our mouth with the fresh, hot blood of the unfortunate creature? This scenario shows the complete absurdity of what we humans are doing when we eat animal flesh. We have no claws or teeth to rip and rend raw flesh, to bite through fur, feathers, scales, or bones, nor do we have an appetite for fresh blood in our mouths.

We may notice that our jaw is especially hinged to provide side-to-side movement. This is a jaw construction shared by herbivorous mammals for grinding various types of plant material; omnivorous and carnivorous mammals have jaws that are rigidly hinged and just snap up and down. We notice further that the purpose of the dominant enzyme in our saliva, ptyalin, is to break down the complex carbohydrates in plant foods into glucose for energy. These carbohydrates are the fuel our bodies were designed to use; animal flesh contains *none*!

Unlike carnivores, we don't have strong stomach acids to quickly dissolve flesh, or short, smooth-walled intestines to pass decaying flesh from our bodies quickly. Instead, we have the weaker stomach acids and the much longer and more highly convoluted intestines of herbivores and frugivores for slowly extracting nutrients from plant foods as they pass through and are broken down.[4] Our long and convoluted small intestine is decidedly herbivorous, with thousands of little pockets and countless tiny fingers, or villi, that give it an enormous overall surface area—larger than a tennis court!—for our food nourishment to be passed into our blood.[5] Our digestive system requires high-fiber foods to keep these intestinal walls clean and functioning properly. Animal foods are not only devoid of fiber but also tend to be more clogging than plant foods as they decompose, leading to constipation, hemorrhoids, colitis, diverticulitis, colon cancer, and other ailments. We have the circulatory systems of herbivores as well, which have difficulty tolerating saturated fat and cholesterol. If a cat, for example, eats a large quantity of fat and cholesterol in the form of animal flesh or eggs, she gets no build-up and blockage in her arteries, but if a rabbit, gorilla, human, or other frugi-vore or herbivore does this, the arteries become severely coated. If the practice continues, the arteries become clogged and unhealthy, leading to arteriosclerosis, high blood pressure, heart disease, and, in the case of humans, guaranteed demand for drugs and surgeries.

By ignoring the obvious fact that we humans are not designed to eat the large quantities of animal foods typical of our culture, the pharmaceutical-medical establishment actually contributes to the supply of sick people and guarantees what John McDougall, M.D., refers to as its "job security."[6] This is not to imply any sort of conspiracy or that the average doctor is not motivated by altruistic impulses. Yet the medical establishment, like any other industry functioning within our culture's economic framework, simply follows the path of least resistance and most reliable financial return. To those in the upper echelons of the medical industry pyramid, who help determine political strategies and media/education policies, maintaining the status quo must seem like a basically good idea, so they de-emphasize prevention in favor of drug and surgical treatments and encourage the continued acceptance of an omnivorous diet for humans.

Classifying the human physiology has always been problematic in our culture and continues to be controversial today. While it's obvious we're not basically carnivorous, it's also obvious that we're not grazing ruminant or ungulate herbivores like sheep, deer, horses, and cows, who can browse on grass and leaves because of having multiple digestive pouches. We may best be classified as frugivorous herbivores, designed primarily for fruits, seeds, vegetables, nuts, and succulent roots and leaves. Most physiologists, though, still claim humans to be omnivorous by nature. Yet even horses can be taught to eat venison, and cows, sheep, and goats are taught to eat and relish the flesh of fish, chickens and pigs in modern confinement feeding operations—how much of our daily food choices are the result of being taught what to eat?

Three points, at least, seem undeniable: that we have choice, that animals suffer because of our choice to eat them, and that the current high levels of animal food consumption are unprecedented and have deleterious effects on our health. It's well established by fossil remains that early hominids lived primarily on a plant-based diet, and that contemporary foraging cultures do so as well. Indeed, renowned anthropologist Ashley Montagu has stated that these cultures should be called gathering-hunting rather than hunting-gathering.[7]

Like all animals, we are essentially spiritual beings, manifestations of a universal, loving intelligence that has given us bodies designed to thrive on the abundant foods that we can peacefully nourish and gather in orchards, fields, and gardens. Our bodies reflect our consciousness, which yearns to unfold higher dimensions of creativity, compassion, joy, and awareness, and longs to serve the larger wholes—our culture, our earth, and the benevolent source of all life—by blessing and helping others and by sharing, caring, and celebrating. We have, appropriately, a physiology of peace.

The wholesale killing and abuse of other animals for food runs counter to our essential sense of compassion, so we disguise the disturbing truth of our meals through self-deceptive rationalizations and elaborate methods of cooking, grinding, mixing, coating, seasoning, and covering. At a deep level we know we've been given the precious gift of bodies that require no living being to suffer, fear, or die for their feeding—but we throw this gift back in the face of the benevolent universe with the violence required by our food choices.

The Constituents of Animal Foods

Eating the large quantities of animal foods typical of our culture's meals leads to many problems. As mentioned above, animal flesh is completely devoid of the fiber that we require in our digestive systems and of the carbohydrates that our cells are designed to burn for energy. The saturated fat and cholesterol endemic in flesh, dairy products, and eggs are basically toxic to human beings, contributing to vascular disease. An especially damaging feature of animal fat is that it contains trans fats, which are well recognized as unstable substances that increase the risk of cancer and heart disease. In fact, the National Academy of Science has concluded that "the only safe intake of trans fat is zero."[8]

The highly touted animal protein that we are all cowed into believing we must ingest in order to be healthy may have toxic properties also, especially in the large amounts consumed in our culture today. Animal foods contain more concentrated protein than plant foods, which can be unhealthy because it is more difficult for our bodies to derive energy from protein than from the naturally occurring carbohydrates in fruits, vegetables, whole grains, legumes, and other plant foods. It's also well established that our bodies can synthesize most amino acids from other amino acids, so that in practice there is little need for people who eat a plant-based diet to "combine" proteins or foods in any particular way in order to get the "right amino acid profile." That old myth of "complete protein" was based on erroneous conclusions drawn by scientists due to experiments done on rats in the 1920s.[9] Even conservative organizations like the FDA and the American Dietetic Association recognize officially in their dietary recommendations that plant-based diets afford humans ample high-quality protein. The ADA has found, "Scientific data suggest positive relationships between a vegetarian diet and reduced risk for several chronic degenerative diseases and conditions, including obesity, coronary artery disease, hypertension, diabetes mellitus, and some types of cancer." It has concluded that "appropriately planned vegetarian diets are healthful, nutritionally adequate, and provide health benefits in the prevention and treatment of certain diseases."[10]

According to T. Colin Campbell, Ph.D., professor of nutritional biochemistry at Cornell University and lead researcher of one of the largest human nutrition studies yet undertaken, animal protein is completely inferior to plant protein for human needs:

> Our study suggests that the closer one approaches a total plant food diet, the greater the health benefit. . . . It turns out that animal protein, when consumed, exhibits a variety of undesirable health effects. Whether it is the immune system, various enzyme systems, the uptake of carcinogens into the cells, or hormonal activities, animal protein generally only causes mischief.[11]

Since we humans actually need relatively little protein to function well, the excess protein inherent in animal foods drains our body's energy, which must find a way to dispose of it somehow. Nutritionists understand that our actual protein needs are relatively small: between four and eight percent of our calories should be in the form of protein.[12] Virtually all grains, legumes, and vegetables are between eight and twenty percent protein, with some foods, like tempeh, even higher.[13] Andrew Weil, M.D., writes,

> In our society, protein deficiency is practically nonexistent. Instead, most people consume too much protein, which can also affect health adversely. . . . Remarkably small amounts are enough to satisfy the minimal requirements of the average adult—perhaps two ounces, or sixty grams, of a protein food a day. Many people in our society eat much more than that at every meal. . . . Cutting down on protein will free up energy, spare your digestive system and especially your liver and kidneys from extra work, and protect your immune system from irritation.[14]

Elsewhere, Dr. Weil writes, "In my opinion, one of the healthiest dietary changes people can make is to substitute soy foods for some (or all) of the animal foods they now eat."[15]

According to microbiologist Robert Young, excess protein causes the pH of the body's tissues to become too acidic. He emphasizes that this acidic condition is unhealthy and signals to bacteria in and around the body that the body is weak, decaying, and dying.[16] When any animal dies, as the life ebbs out of it, its flesh becomes increasingly acidic, signaling microorganisms in the region that it is time for them to do their job and break the flesh down so that it can return to the earth and be recycled. According to his research, instead of harboring primarily beneficial bacteria that aid in the various life-support processes of the body, the bodies of human omnivores may tend to harbor primarily destructive bacteria that are simply trying to do their natural job of breaking the body down because it gives signals, by the high acid content of the tissues and the presence of putrefying animal flesh, that it is dying.

The response of the medical establishment, rather than advising us to stop eating animal protein, is to supply antibiotics and other drugs that try to help the beleaguered immune system by killing off pathogens within the body. The unfortunate effect of this practice is that antibiotics are indiscriminate and may also kill off beneficial bacteria as well. The so-called harmful bacteria, which are just performing their vital function in nature, often develop more resistance and thus require ever-increasing dosages of antibiotic drugs to dispatch. This bacterial resistance to drugs is also directly attributable to the routine administration of antibiotics to factory-farmed livestock and fish, and the meat, dairy products, and eggs derived from them may contain high concentrations of antibiotic-resistant pathogens.

One result of the stress placed on our bodies by animal products is an increased risk of cancer. It is well known now that every minute a few cells out of the trillions in our bodies become cancerous. A healthy immune system can and does routinely locate and destroy these cells, thus preventing any cancers from developing in a healthy body. When the immune system's forces are overworked, however, by the trans fats and pathogen load in animal foods, they may be spread too thin to detect cancers in the body and prevent them from developing. The World Cancer Research Fund concluded after it analyzed more than 4,500 cancer research studies that "Vegetarian diets decrease the risk of cancer," and its primary dietary recommendation was, "Choose predominantly plant-based diets rich in a variety of vegetables, fruits and legumes."[17] Cancer is clearly and positively linked with eating animal foods.

The body, in its wisdom, constantly regulates the blood's pH, which must stay within a narrow range. With modern Western diets, the body must work hard to keep the blood from becoming overly acidic from the excess animal protein being eaten. To do this, it uses alkaline bone tissue substances such as bicarbonates and calcium. This can lead to the loss of bone density and helps explain the high rates of osteoporosis in cultures where people eat large quantities of acidifying animal foods. Osteoporosis rates among the Eskimo people, who eat an almost completely flesh-based diet, are among the highest in the world.[18] Next are northern Europeans and North Americans, who eat high quantities of flesh, eggs, and dairy products.[19] While there are other factors that may affect bone health, such as vitamin and mineral intake, levels of load-bearing exercise, and mental and emotional factors, there is evidence that brittle bones and osteoporosis are correlated with eating the large amounts of animal protein typical of our meals.

Scientific studies have linked many other diseases with high intake of animal foods, such as heart disease; diabetes; breast, prostate, and colon cancer; gallstones; strokes; and liver and kidney disease. Many books and articles document these findings,[20] but there is little financial incentive to publicize the information, and enormous financial incentive to ignore it and fund pseudo-studies and advertising campaigns to confuse the public about the effects of eating animal foods. According to a recent Cornell University study, eighty-four percent of people are either frequently confused about healthy eating or have completely given up trying to make sense of it all.[21] This says a lot about the effectiveness of the propaganda tide generated by the food industry, as well as our tendency to block connections when it comes to the suffering on our plates.

The cholesterol and saturated fat in our blood may create other problems. Besides clogging our body's veins and arteries and contributing to heart disease and strokes, they may block the capillaries that carry blood to individual cells, resulting in cells that are weak, lacking oxygen and nutrients, and unable to completely cleanse the toxins and carbon dioxide that are the by-products of their aerobic processes. Swimming in this unhealthy environment, they may begin, over time, to degenerate and die off.

One example of this is the increasingly common occurrence of macular degeneration, which causes severe vision impairment and blindness, mostly in older people. Years of eating animal protein, fat, and cholesterol causes the tiny eye capillaries to become clogged with waste debris, and the millions of cells in the macular area of the eye's retina, the cells specialized for seeing, start dying off or are blocked by the body's efforts to build new capillaries. Vision deteriorates and macular degeneration follows.[22] The same type of scenario may explain many other health degenerations as well, such as cataracts and other types of vision loss, impaired hearing and, particularly, impaired mental functioning caused by clogged capillaries that service vital brain cells.

This clogging of brain capillaries by animal fat and cholesterol may also contribute to the diminished level of actual intelligence in cultures that eat diets high in animal foods. Clogged brain capillaries may reduce the brain's efficiency and hinder its ability to make connections effectively. This could reduce the intelligence necessary for creativity and spirituality, and may help explain why we act so self-destructively without being able to realize it. Vegetarian children have been shown to have significantly higher IQs than average[23] and it's well known, for example, that Thomas Edison, during the years he worked so hard to discover the secrets of electricity, abstained from eating flesh because he found he could think more clearly and make vital connections more easily on a plant-based diet. Other geniuses like Pythagoras, Leonardo da Vinci, and Mahatma Gandhi abstained from eating animals. Plutarch wrote,

> When we clog and cloy our body with flesh, we also render our mind and intellect coarse. When the body's clogged with unnatural food, the mind becomes confused and dull and loses its cheerfulness. Such minds engage in trivial pursuits, because they lack the clearness and vigor for higher thinking.[24]

Clogged pathways may also directly or indirectly cause low energy, chronic fatigue and a host of other ailments. In adult males, for example, the arteries in the vascular tissue of the genitals can become clogged by the saturated fat and cholesterol of an animal-based diet, diminishing the natural ability of many men to have an erection. Since disease is far more profitable to the influential pharmaceutical corporations than health is, as the drug industry's wealth grows, our culture's ability to recognize the real source of the problem is suppressed.

Kidney disease, kidney stones, and gallstones are another direct result of eating animal foods, since the kidneys have the difficult task of purifying our fatty, acidic blood. Large stones may build up in our kidneys from the excess calcium and uric acid caused by the animal protein in our meals. These stones interfere with the functioning of our kidneys and the body may, in its wisdom, try to pass them out through the urethra, an exceedingly painful process. The excess fat and cholesterol in animal foods can lead to gallstones and gallbladder disease. The liver, as the organ most directly responsible for dealing with the invasion of toxic substances, is overtaxed when we eat dead animals, especially those imprisoned under the abysmal conditions of modern factory farms. These animals' miserable bodies are so laced with toxins, artificial growth hormones, drug and chemical residues, steroids, tumors, and chronic illness that ingesting them poses a Herculean and unending work for the liver.

The skin, as the largest organ of elimination, is also severely burdened by the toxins in animal foods, and many of the skin maladies and allergic reactions we experience may be attributable to the body's attempt to cleanse itself by passing toxins out through the skin. Our skin may be adversely affected by the excess fat and cholesterol in dairy products, which can clog the pores and may contribute to acne, allergic reactions, and excess body odor. Many people comment about how switching to a plant-based diet not only helped them lose weight, but also gave them clearer, fresher-looking skin tone, reducing the need for cosmetics.

The Fat of the Matter

The cholesterol and large concentrations of saturated fat in animal foods increase our risk for heart disease and strokes. Their high fat content increases our risk for obesity and the whole panorama of health problems to which being overweight contributes, such as diabetes and cancer. With sixty percent of Americans now overweight, and a concomitant $100 billion (and growing) price tag in health services,[25] obesity now kills 330,000 Americans a year and will soon pass tobacco as the leading preventable cause of sickness and death.[26]

Though we are all unique genetically, it is not natural for any of us to have a high percentage of body fat or to be chronically overweight. We are fat because we eat more calories than we burn, and fat is particularly high in calories. Generally, fat concentrates in animal foods much more than in plant foods, and the animals raised for our plates are especially fat. They are specifically bred, confined, drugged, and manipulated to be as fat as possible. The Butterball turkey we devour for our Thanksgiving ritual feast is so fat she could barely walk and couldn't mate when alive, a caricature of the wild, sensitive bird that inhabits our forests. The pigs, cows, and chickens on modern factory farms and feedlots are forced to be similarly obese. Are we creating these creatures in our image, or are they creating us in theirs?

To understand obesity and body weight, we simply need to understand what agribusiness animal fatteners figured out long ago: eating excess calories and fat makes confined herbivore animals fat. The same is true for us. The key is to realize and remember that all foods have just three basic components: carbohydrates, proteins, and lipids (fat). Carbohydrates are the necessary fuel we burn for energy. Animal foods are high in fat and protein and have no carbohydrates, except for honey and the lactose in milk. Unrefined complex carbohydrates from whole grains, fruits, vegetables, and legumes, and the proteins from either plant or animal sources, are not typically fattening in themselves, because the body must first convert them to fat in order to store them as fat. This has been scientifically demonstrated, as Neal Barnard, M.D., points out: "Scientists have biopsied people's fat stores and found that virtually all of their fat has come from fat in the foods they have eaten, and almost none of it is produced by carbohydrate."[27]

Why do so many of us mistakenly believe carbohydrates are fattening? There are two main reasons. One is that our culture has created and mass-produced a completely unnatural type of carbohydrate, the refined white sugar and white flour that are used by the food industry to make junk foods that are also high in fat. These refined foods have a high glycemic index and break down too quickly in the body, contributing to sugar level imbalances in the blood. Nutritionists correctly agree they are best avoided. The second reason is that these unnatural refined carbohydrates have become the scapegoat of our herding culture, for the last thing we want to admit is that the source of our obesity and other problems is the animal foods that define us. So we erroneously blame "carbohydrates," which are actually the healthy and natural fuel on which our physiology of peace is designed to run. Low-fat, high–complex carbohydrate diets based on vegetables, legumes, whole grains, nuts, and fruits have been shown universally to be the healthiest for humans, as the Oxford-Cornell study under T. Colin Campbell concluded. A 2002 USDA study, for example, found that adults eating high-carbohydrate diets (with a high proportion of grain products, fruits, and vegetables) were more likely to be in the normal weight range category than those eating low-carbohydrate diets.[28]

Ending obesity will remain difficult, mysterious, complex, and a losing battle as long as we continue to eat diets rich in high-fat animal flesh, eggs, and dairy products. Of course it is *possible* to eat a high-fat plant-based diet if we consume large quantities of avocados, nut butters, refined oils, potato chips, or other high-fat foods, but it is very easy and quite natural to eat a low-fat, plant-based diet, and virtually impossible to eat a low-fat diet based on animal foods. We are a culture of naturally plant-eating people who consume far too much dietary fat, suffer because of it, and then go on "diets" to lose weight and suffer needlessly. We read millions of diet books, many of which reassuringly recommend eating the flesh and fluids of animals, and in the process become more enslaved to the meat-medical complex. In fact, the most popular diet programs—such as the Atkins Diet, the Blood Type Diet, the Zone Diet, the South Beach Diet, and the ironically named Carbohydrate Addict's Diet—predictably recommend high-protein, low-carbohydrate diets rich in animal-derived foods. They find such ready acceptance simply because our culture's living foundation is the killing and eating of animals and we naturally crave the voice of scientific and medical authorities to reassure us that this practice is required by our physiology.

Excess fat puts a considerable strain on our body, and, like a self-imposed prison we carry with us, it can reduce our ability to express, create, and move freely. The fat slows down blood flow, makes the blood gluey, and clogs veins and arteries, causing cells to deteriorate. Unnecessary weight makes the heart pump harder than it should have to, and increases blood pressure. It saps energy and puts a strain on the spine and nervous system. Diabetes is linked with excess fat. The immune system also has to work harder to patrol the host of unnecessary baggage cells that often become dumping grounds for the toxins that come in through eating, drinking, and breathing. They thus tend to be more likely to become cancerous, and indeed obesity has been linked to increased risk for cancer. Obesity often causes us low self-esteem and other psychological problems as well.

The fat we carry around under our skin is mainly the fat of miserable and terrified animals—it's not surprising we're anxious to be rid of it! If we based our diet on the whole grains, fruits, vegetables and legumes for which we are designed, we would find the obesity problem in our culture evaporating, along with many other problems. Albert Einstein was correct in saying that no problem can be solved at the level on which it was created. As omnivores, we must go to another level to solve our problem with excess fat, a level where we no longer kill and confine animals by proxy and consume their fat-laden remains.

Toxins

When we get our protein from animal sources, we bring into our bodies much higher levels of toxic contaminants than we do by eating plant foods directly, because livestock feed grains are heavily sprayed with pesticides and these poisons tend to concentrate in animal flesh, milk, and eggs, as Andrew Weil points out:

> One problem is that diets rich in animal protein put you high on the food chain, not a good place to be. . . . One consequence of eating high on the food chain is that you take in much larger doses of toxins, because environmental toxins concentrate as you move up from level to level. The fat of domestic animals often contains high concentrations of toxins that exist in much lower concentrations in grains, for example. An independent problem is that the methods we use for raising animal sources of protein further load them up with unhealthy substances.[29]

The unfortunate animals raised for food are forced to eat large quantities of fish meal and rendered animal flesh and organs, which is totally unnatural for them, in order to fatten them quickly. Manure is also used to "enrich" their feed, and these additives concentrate toxins to an even higher extent than the plant foods the animals are fed. The toxins in the animal foods we eat include carcinogenic heavy metals, deadly PCBs, chemical residues, antibiotics, and the human-created nightmare we now call the prion. Prions are thought to cause mad cow disease and the other transmissible spongiform encephalopathies that have raged through both human cannibal populations (such as the cannibalistic Fore people of Papua New Guinea where a type of human spongiform encephalopathy, called by them "kuru," was first documented in the 1950s) and animal cannibal populations (such as the farmed sheep and mink populations that developed scrapie and transmissible mink encephalopathy after being fed rendered animal flesh). Similar diseases such as Creutzfeld-Jacob disease (the human equivalent of mad cow) and, according to some researchers, certain forms of Alzheimer's disease, now threaten human omnivore populations as well because of perverse industry standards that have dictated feeding cows to other cows, and that still feed pigs to other pigs, chickens to other chickens, and pigs and chickens to cows.[30]

It is also well known that animal foods are heavily contaminated with viruses and bacteria such as salmonella, listeria, E. coli, campylobacter, and streptococcus, which can be harmful if not fatal to people, especially given our already overworked immune systems.[31] The urea in animal flesh also contains toxins. It has furthermore recently been shown that cooked animal flesh contains heterocyclic amines, which are carcinogenic chemicals that form during the cooking process. Thus, by not cooking flesh enough, we may expose ourselves to salmonella, E. coli, and other pathogens, and by cooking it, we end up eating cancer-causing chemicals formed by heating the animal fat.

The industrialization of food production has created large-scale Confined Animal Feeding Operations (CAFOs), also called factory farms, that imprison animals in crowded, toxic environments that reduce labor costs and allow for lower prices of animal foods by relying on cheap fossil fuels and subsidies. To lower costs, the confined mammals, birds, and fish are bred for rapid weight gain and given steroid hormones to further shorten the time between birth and slaughter. Chickens, for example, are now killed when just forty-five days old, compared with eighty-four days in the 1950s.[32] These hormones and growth promotants are illegal in Europe because research has shown they increase the risk for cancer and reproductive dysfunction in humans—yet they are approved and used on more than ninety percent of beef cattle in the U.S.[33] The stress, stench, insects, feces and urine buildup, insecticides, and overcrowding create ideal conditions for disease, and the antibiotics and other drugs routinely administered also end up in the animals' flesh, milk, and eggs. There is virtually no oversight on the drugs used on animals in factory farms. Researcher Gail Eisnitz writes,

> [U]ntrained workers, not veterinarians, administer drugs to sick animals, often by injection. According to one worker who administers medication, what drugs and dosages they use are a matter of "trial and error."
>
> "I'd use the same needle on a hundred pigs, till you couldn't poke it in the skin anymore. Or till it broke. Then I'd have to get a pair of pliers and pull the needle out." The residue of these drugs can wind up in the bacon next to the consumer's morning eggs.[34]

For all these reasons, the animal foods in our supermarkets carry high levels of toxic contaminants and pathogens. Because of the wretched conditions in battery egg operations, for example, over 650,000 Americans are sickened every year by salmonella bacteria in eggs; salmonella contamination is found in seventy-two percent of slaughtered chickens.[35] Campylobacter, which is the number one cause of gastroenteritis and is linked with Guillain-Barré syndrome, infects ninety-eight percent of store-bought chickens.[36] Listeria is a particularly dangerous pathogen frequently found in cheeses, eggs, shellfish, and meats, causing ninety-two percent of the people infected with it to be hospitalized. It is linked with brain damage and cerebral palsy in infants born to infected pregnant women.[37] And E. coli 0157 sickens hundreds of hamburger eaters and kills several daily, according to the conservative figures of the Centers for Disease Control and Prevention.[38] Like mad cow disease, this is due to the cruel and irresponsible practices that pervade factory farms, causing animals to arrive at slaughter plants diseased and covered in excrement.

The conditions in slaughter plants today guarantee even more toxic contamination in the meat we eat. Over the last twenty years, line speeds have been rapidly accelerating and USDA inspection and oversight has been diminishing; now with the passage of HAACP (Hazard Analysis of Critical Control Points) in 1996, the meat industry basically regulates and inspects itself. Eisnitz tells what workers in signed affidavits say about the slaughterhouse production of the meat we eat:

> "Every day I saw black chicken, green chicken, chicken that stank, and chicken with feces on it. Chicken like this is supposed to be thrown away, but instead it would be sent down the line to be processed."
>
> An employee at another plant said, "I personally have seen rotten meat—you can tell by the odor. This rotten meat is mixed with fresh meat and sold for baby food. We are asked to mix it with the fresh food, and this is the way it is sold. You can see the worms inside the meat."
>
> Another worker, "in the department where chicken bones were ground up and processed into chicken franks and bologna," reported that "almost continuously, the bones had an awful, foul odor. Sometimes they came from other plants and had been sitting for days. Often there were maggots on them. These bones were never cleaned off and so the maggots were ground up with everything else and remained in the final product."[39]

Because of the new "streamlined" inspection process, virtually anything is allowed. Affidavits from USDA inspectors who now have diminished authority in slaughter plants repeatedly tell the same shocking story about the dangerous health implications of animal foods:

> "I've seen birds with cancerous tumors come through regularly, sometimes all day long. While on quality control, I'd pull off those I saw, but I couldn't possibly catch them all. Right after I'd put them in the condemn barrel, foremen would have the floor workers hang the birds back on the line."[40]

Every day, carcasses fall on the floor and are not trimmed before the company puts them back on the line. Floors are filthy, covered with blood, grease, feces, pus from abscesses, and mud. A lot gets embedded into the meat from the high-pressure carcass sprays. . . . [41]

Instead of cutting away fecal contamination and tumors, workers now use high-pressure hot water spray, which has the effect of driving contamination particles more deeply into the flesh. In hog and poultry slaughter operations, scald tanks are used:

In the scald tank, fecal contamination on skin and feathers gets inhaled by live birds, and hot water opens birds' pores, allowing pathogens to seep in. The pounding action of the defeathering machines creates an aerosol of feces-contaminated water which is then beaten into the birds. Contamination also occurs when the birds have their intestines removed by automatic eviscerating machines. The high-speed machines commonly rip open intestines, spilling feces into the birds' body cavities. [42]

Chill tanks are also used:

Another example of high-speed contamination occurs when the chickens are immersed in the chill tank. "Water in these tanks has been aptly named 'fecal soup' for all the filth and bacteria floating around," GAP [Government Accountability Project] 's Tom Devine told me. "By immersing clean, healthy birds in the same tank with dirty ones, you're practically assuring cross-contamination." [43]

Eisnitz writes about going through GAP files from 1996 and discovering the kinds of things inspectors had stopped, but are no longer able to stop:

Rancid meat had been smoked to cover foul odor, or marinated and breaded to disguise slime and smell. Warm meat or sour product was added to acceptable meat then processed. . . . Chickens and hams were soaked in chlorine baths to remove slime and odor, and red dye was added to beef to make it appear fresh.

The files described meat packed in boxes with fist-sized clumps of fecal matter. Pieces of lungs, rectums, and dead insects had been found as well. . . . Maggots were breeding in transport tubs and boxes, on the floor, in processing equipment and packaging. Plant personnel shoveled food directly off the floor into edible sausage bins.[44]

This is just the tip of the iceberg. When we eat animal foods for protein or some other imagined benefit, we are inevitably bringing into our psychophysical being products that are profoundly contaminated. In an attempt to reduce the risk, in February of 2000 the USDA legalized applying nuclear radiation to meat products to kill the dangerous pathogens inherent in them; the long term effects of eating irradiated foods are unknown, but short-term studies show the possibility of creating carcinogens and mutant bacteria. Interestingly, the medical establishment has not been found protesting any of this.

The Meat-Medical Complex

We've been trained by our eating habits to look without seeing. As but one example of this, a self-induced sickness, adult-onset diabetes, is now reaching epidemic proportions. Although evidence clearly links diabetes with the consumption of animal foods, millions of dollars are spent searching for a pharmaceutical "cure" for diabetes. Ordinary citizens even good-heartedly donate time to go on walkathons to raise money for "vital diabetes research." Diabetes is rare among those who eat a plant-based diet but it is a significant risk among people who eat flesh, eggs, and dairy products. It is not difficult to understand why. The excess fat in an animal-based diet may, if not burned, force the body eventually to become resistant to the actions of its insulin, the hormone that pushes fat into fat cells. So the fat, metabolized into sugar, is removed from the body through the urine. As John McDougall, M.D., points out, "This loss of sugar (calories) is the body's adaptive response to excess calorie intake and storage (body fat)."[45] If we stop the intake of animal foods, the body can dramatically reduce or eliminate its diabetic condition, and this has been shown repeatedly.

Even more to be wondered at is the fact that, with armies of apparently intelligent people working on the diabetes crisis, doing all sorts of tests, applying for grants, writing research papers, and sharing their findings, few seem to make these obvious connections. Researchers hurry ever onward, spending money and torturing laboratory animals in the search for "mechanisms" and pharmaceutical bullets that can be patented to profit their employers. And yet, as McDougall writes in a rare instance of someone candidly stating the obvious from within the medical profession,

> It is no coincidence that the same diet that helps prevent or cure diabetes also causes effortless weight loss, lowers cholesterol and triglycerides, cleans out the arteries, and returns the body to excellent function. But no matter how much research appears saying the same thing over and over again, the tide is unlikely to change because of the economic incentives for the medical establishment of continued illness and profitable treatments.[46]

The toxic fat, cholesterol, and protein in our diets are the foundation of a huge medical complex that continues to reap profits from our sickness. Weight reduction is a large and expanding industry, with both alternative and conventional programs offered, most of which seem to distract people from the simple truths and complicate the subject to their own advantage. Lucrative pharmaceutical and surgical invasions, such as drugs, liposuction, stomach stapling and gastric bypass, are often preferred by the medical complex to the simpler measure of advising people to eat a more plant-based diet.

Besides causing obesity, the fat and cholesterol in animal foods clog our arteries, and we again find ourselves reluctant customers of the medical industry's ingenious, expensive, and marginally effective solutions. These include a whole range of drugs (complete with "side" effects) that artificially thin our cholesterol-laden blood. And there are the surgical procedures as well. These include reaming out arteries, angioplasty, and heart bypass surgery.

With fast-food chain franchises and menus rich in animal products setting the example in hospitals, the medical industry is assured that repairs are temporary and that as patients continue eating flesh, eggs, and dairy products, they will be repeat customers. A *permanent reversal* of heart disease and arteriosclerosis, as Dean Ornish, M.D., achieved by having heart patients adopt plant-based diets, exercise, and learn to reduce stress, is considered far too radical.[47] The enormous irony is that changing to a plant-based diet is considered more radical even than having one's body repeatedly stabbed, sawed, mutilated, drugged, and potentially killed. Perhaps it *is* actually more radical, for in a herding culture, nothing is more subversive to the established order of exploitation and privilege than consciously refusing to participate in buying and eating the animal foods that define the culture.

The Placebo Effect

The good news is that our bodies thrive on a conscious plant-based diet, and that this diet is infinitely more compassionate to animals and people and more environmentally sustainable than eating animal foods. Any and all of us can adopt a healthy, low-cruelty way of eating today and need never look back! Why don't we all rejoice at this discovery and immediately change, transforming our culture, our minds, our lives, our well-being, and our planet? Why do we avert our eyes, grumble, mumble excuses, and resist so strongly? Why are we so paralyzed? I met James Gibson, M.D., in his hometown of El Paso, and asked him if there is any human being on this earth whose physiology somehow requires eating any animal foods. His immediate response was that there is no one like this; every human has the same basic physiology and it is designed for plant foods. Why then, I asked, do people think they need to eat animal foods? "Everyone's been brainwashed" was his reply.

The power of shared, culturally molded belief is enormous. It forms a force field around us, determining our thoughts, attitudes, and actions. In the herding culture into which we were all born, the core attitude is exclusion and domination, and the core action that reinforces this attitude is eating animals. As our culture teaches our separateness from nature, animals, and the divine, it has also taught us that our mind and body are basically separate. Though this dualistic view is being challenged, it still dominates our worldview, making it difficult to understand that what we believe and how we think and feel have direct reverberations in our body, and that the state of our body intimately affects our mind as well. The power of the placebo effect is based on this unity of mind and body, and it's amazing how strong it is. There have been many studies done in which the patients given only sugar pills by their doctors showed equal or even greater change in their physical/mental condition than did those who received the actual drugs![48] Expectations are powerful forces. Some people being told they were put on a chemotherapy program for cancer even lost their hair, though they were only given placebos, not drugs. And according to Wayne B. Jonas, M.D., a leader in placebo research and director of the Samueli Institute for Information Biology, placebo surgery—telling patients that a surgery will be performed, but then not performing it when in the operating room—"is as effective or more effective than real surgery."[49] Though our culture's mechanistic biomedical framework is confused and threatened by the immense power of the placebo effect and sees it negatively, it's helpful to realize that it's not negative at all, but wonderfully positive. Understanding this unity of mind and body allows us potentially to unleash enormous healing and vitalizing forces through our thoughts, ideas, feelings, and insights.

Most of us switching to plant-based diets feel the positive effects like a heavy weight lifting off our physical, mental, emotional, and spiritual bodies, but some of us feel worse, especially at the beginning. The immense and unrecognized power of the placebo effect helps to explain why this is so, especially if we're making the switch alone and don't have the example of healthy, vibrant vegans around us every day. The old programming can easily be activated, reinforced by the ubiquitous advertising and promotion messages of the meat, dairy, egg, and medical industries. It was pounded into us practically from birth, by those closest to us and in the positions of highest authority, that we'd be weak or sick if we didn't get our "protein"—our cheese, eggs, and meat—and their voices naturally still live within us. Subconsciously, when we switch to a plant-based diet, we may expect we'll feel weak or get sick, and so our bodies may manifest this. Therefore, when we let go of eating animal foods, it's important to let go consciously of the ingrained cultural beliefs that we need animal foods to be healthy. We swim in an emotionally charged thought-sea created by generations of omnivores, and this mass consciousness may make it more difficult for some of us to believe at deep levels that we can and will be more vibrantly healthy without eating animal foods.

On top of this, researchers have noticed that placebos are more effective if they are unpleasant. Bitter-tasting and expensive placebos, for example, like bitter and costly drugs, "work" better—because we have to go through some trauma and sacrifice to ingest them, we subconsciously expect their effects to be more powerful. Eating the flesh and secretions of animals is so fundamentally repulsive to us as humans that these animal foods make especially powerful placebos. We find vultures repulsive because they eat carrion, but we eat exactly the same thing! Sometimes it's euphemized as aged beef. And yet, because we've been taught to attribute strength and energy to eating animal foods, that expectation helps our quite miraculous and flexible psychophysiology to partially overcome the essentially disturbing and toxic nature of these foods so we can survive and function. As children, we had no other choice.

There are two other reasons we may experience difficulty switching to a plant-based diet. One is that when we stop ingesting the saturated fat, cholesterol, and other toxins in animal foods, our body may take this as a welcome opportunity to clean house. Fruits and vegetables are natural blood cleansers and detoxifiers, and as our body switches from a mode of survival and of storing toxins away in our fat cells to a mode of cleansing, renewing, and reducing the fat cells, stored toxins begin to flow into our bloodstream to be eliminated. Instead of feeling better, we may feel worse for a week or two as drug and toxin residues are cleaned out. This is actually a cause for rejoicing because those poisons are no longer lingering in our tissues.

Keep in mind that if we go to a medical practitioner for advice during this cleansing time, we will probably find that he or she is antagonistic to a plant-based diet and may derail the beneficent cleansing, warning us of the dangers of "fad diets" and counseling us that we "need" animal foods to be healthy. We may unfortunately return to the mainstream of animal brutality, convinced that we "tried" being a vegetarian but our doctor said we weren't getting enough protein, or iron, or vitamin B-12, or yang energy in our food, or that our blood type requires us to eat some animal protein, or some other excuse that disempowers us from stopping the cycle of violence we are enmeshed in with our acculturated eating habits.

It's helpful to remember that with so much medical information to be conveyed in medical schools, teaching nutrition is a low priority. Most doctors know little about nutrition because less than a quarter of medical schools have a single course in nutrition, and what little they do learn is heavily influenced by the meat, dairy, and egg industries as well as by our culture's underlying orientation. This influence touches those who study nutrition as their profession as well. Marion Nestle demonstrates in *Food Politics* that the animal food industries have considerable financial resources and exert enormous influence on our government at all levels, and on science and on the health profession as well. There is no similar force advocating for plant foods. It's well known that the animal food establishment funds university research, publishes promotional pieces posing as educational materials, and engages in questionable arrangements with professional medical research organizations. To give but two examples of this, the American Cancer Society and other cancer research foundations work with the meat industry sponsoring annual steak banquets called "Cattlemen's Balls" to raise money for cancer research! And the American Heart Association has given the Subway fast food chain the rights to its "fighting heart disease and strokes" logo after receiving ten million dollars in "donations" from Subway, despite the chain's menu being made up primarily of the processed meat and cheese foods that are known to increase the risk for heart disease.[50]

An old saying has it that if we spend our money in the first half of our life on a rich, meat-based diet, we'll spend our money in the second half of our life on doctors. So when we stop eating animal foods, we may feel worse for a few weeks as we cleanse, but the benefits of the change are clear, as Andrew Weil observes: "Studies consistently show vegetarians to be healthier and longer-lived than meat eaters."[51]

The third reason some of us have difficulty switching to a plant-based diet is that we don't know how to prepare vegan meals that are tasty, nutritious, and convenient. It's quite easy to do, but there is learning and unlearning to go through. Fortunately, there is an ever-increasing supply of vegan and vegetarian cookbooks, cooking classes, groups, programs, and convenience foods. For one thing, we may give up flesh and continue to eat dairy products and eggs. These products contain at least as much cruelty, toxins, cholesterol and animal protein as flesh does, so little improvement will likely be noticed. (This is why it may be best for some not to switch gradually to a completely plant-based way of eating, but to do it all at once. Becoming a "pesco-vegetarian," for example, and continuing to eat dairy, eggs, and fish, we may find we've given up enough to be irritated but not enough to notice any appreciable improvement in our body-mind.) We are also unlikely to notice significant improvement if we switch to a complete-ly plant-based diet but favor vegan junk food—loaded with hydro-genated fats, white flour, white sugar, artificial sweeteners, preserva-tives, and chemicals.

It's simple and easy to get all the nutrients we need on a plant-based diet. Eating a variety of vegetables, grains, nuts, legumes, and fruits will ensure that we get the vitamins, minerals, and protein we need for opti-mum health. The two primary substances that a vegan diet may be lack-ing are vitamin B-12 and omega-3 fatty acids. Vitamin B-12 is a natu-rally occurring substance that is plentiful in our soil and water and that we now may have difficulty obtaining in sufficient supply only because modern methods of water purification and of industrial food washing remove it from our plant foods and drinking water. A regular supple-ment is therefore recommended, and is easily obtained in fortified soy milk and other vegan products. And because of our modern food refin-ing practices that over-supply us with omega-6 fatty acids, it's a good idea for vegans to eat walnuts and flax seeds or flax oil for essential omega-3 fatty acids. Two tablespoons of ground flax seeds daily is considered sufficient. A good resource covering the nutritional aspects of a vegan diet is *Becoming Vegan* by Brenda Davis and Vesanto Melina, two registered dieticians.[52]

It's ironic that the burden of justifying possible nutritional deficiencies rests on vegans ("where do you get your protein/vitamin B-12/etc.?"), because research shows that vegans typically have twice the fruit and vegetable intake of people eating the standard American diet. In recent studies, vegans had higher intakes of sixteen out of the nineteen nutrients studied, including three times more vitamin C, vitamin E, and fiber, twice the folate, magnesium, copper, and manganese, and more calcium and plenty of protein.[53] Vegans also had half the saturated fat intake, one-sixth the rate of being overweight, and, while vegans were shown to be at risk for deficiencies in three nutrients (calcium, iodine, and vitamin B-12), people eating the standard American diet were at risk for deficiencies in seven nutrients (calcium, iodine, vitamin C, vitamin E, fiber, folate, and magnesium).[54]

Buying organically grown produce, grains, beans, and nuts is important not just because they're higher in vitamins and minerals, but also because the toxic runoff from conventional agriculture poisons streams and people, and kills birds, fish, insects, and wildlife. The amount of toxins used to produce a head of lettuce or bowl of rice is still, however, far less than that used to produce a hot dog, cheese omelet, or piece of catfish because animal foods require enormous quantities of pesticide-laden feed grain to produce.[55]

As far as taste goes, those of us who follow a plant-based diet invariably report that we discover new vistas of delicious foods that we hardly knew existed. Plant-based cuisines from the Mediterranean, Africa, India, East Asia, Mexico, and South America all offer delicious and nutritious possibilities. As our taste buds come back to life, we discover more subtle nuances of flavor, and as our hearts and minds relax and rejoice in supporting more cruelty-free foods, the foods become increasingly delicious. Due to the mind-body connection, they also become more nutritious as we begin to enjoy partaking of the attractive and regenerating fruits and herbs of our earth. Mindful eating is the essential foundation of happiness and peace.

Our Body, Our Friend

When our intelligence is reduced, we use drugs to force our body as we would force an innocent animal. For example, when our body in its wisdom attempts to cleanse itself of the congestion and toxins introduced to it through our diet, and generates a cold or fever to aid in this cleansing process, we often ingest pharmaceuticals in order to try to suppress the uncomfortable symptoms, thus derailing the natural healing process. Intelligence would realize that our body is our most precious friend. It works ceaselessly to maintain health and harmony and is our vehicle for expression and experience in this world. What could be more valuable and worthy of care and protection? It never works against us, but always does its best with whatever it has to work with. It is a shame that so many of these immeasurably valuable gifts from the loving source of all life, beautiful expressions of spiritual creativity, are distracted and harmed unnecessarily, saddled with heavy burdens that were never intended or foreseen by nature, and tragically destroyed by ignorance, fear, and a lack of caring. Radiant physical health is such a treasure; yet how rare it is today, particularly among those of us who abuse animals for food.

It's actually quite obvious why heart disease and cancer "run in the family." Everyone in the family has their legs under the same dinner table![56] As children we not only eat like our family but also soak up our inner attitudes from them. Unless we metaphorically leave home and question our culture's food mentality and the enslaving propaganda of the meat-medical complex, we will find it difficult to discern our unique mission and grow spiritually. Spiritual health, like physical and mental health, urges us to take responsibility for our lives, and to dedicate ourselves to a cause that is higher than our self-preoccupations.

By relying on the meat, dairy, egg, pharmaceutical, and medical industries that have been unwilling to make the connections we've been discussing, our culture has created the conditions for escalating disharmony and bondage. Agribusiness is continually trying to produce more for less through breeding, intensive confinement, and use of hormones, antibiotics, drugs, and feed grains that are "enriched" with fish, manure, and rendered animal by-products. The irony is this: by unnaturally fattening and toxifying vegetarian animals on animal flesh, we unnaturally fatten and toxify our vegetarian bodies on their animal flesh, milk, and eggs, and abuse the animals and ourselves to sickness, slavery, and early death. It's all unnecessary, and it's in our power to stop it.

Many people, glimpsing the outlines of the above, give up "red meat" and feel that by so doing, they are basically vegetarians and thus eating a healthy diet. Nothing, of course, could be further from the truth. The flesh of pigs, chickens, turkeys, ducks, and other farmed animals is just as high in cholesterol, acidifying protein, misery, fear, adrenalin, and the toxic residues of chemicals and drugs as is the flesh of cows, and perhaps more so. If the flesh is certified "organic," it *may* have fewer toxic residues, but it still has all the rest. The flesh of more exotic animals, like pheasant, grouse, ostrich, emu, buffalo, deer, rabbit, horse, frog, alligator, and turtle, is similarly unhealthy and causes at least as much misery. All animals suffer enormously and unnecessarily so we can dine upon their brutalized bodies.

Others may go a step farther, giving up "meat" entirely but continuing to eat fish, shellfish, dairy products, and eggs—foods they believe are healthier than "meat." Before examining that belief more deeply in the following chapters, it may be helpful to recognize that concern about our own personal health, while necessary, is in some essential ways a shallow, self-preoccupied, and thus shaky reason for abstaining from animal foods. The most solid and enduring motivations for action are ultimately based on caring for others—in this case imprisoned animals, wildlife, starving people, slaughterhouse workers, and future generations, to name some of those damaged by our desire for animal foods. The health advantages of a plant-based diet are the perquisites of loving-kindness and awareness, and the diseases and discomfort caused by animal foods are some of the consequences that follow from breaking natural laws. If our only motivation for not eating animal foods is our own health, it's easy to "cheat" a little here and there and pretty soon go back to eating them again. When our motivation is based on compassion, it is deep and lasting, because we understand that our actions have direct consequences on others who are vulnerable. We never "cheat," because that means directly harming others, which we are unwilling to do. While there are thus many "former vegetarians," it's unlikely that "former vegans" were ever actually vegans; it seems doubtful that compassion authentically attained is ever lost.

The main reason for outlining some of the negative health consequences of eating animal products in this chapter was to help disabuse us of the incorrect notion that our bodies somehow "need" animal foods. This erroneous belief opens gateways into incalculable dimensions of misery. The suffering that food animals undergo, the suffering of those who eat them and profit by them, the suffering of starving people who could be fed with the grain that feeds these animals, and the suffering we thoughtlessly impose on the ecosystem, other creatures, and future generations are all interconnected. It is this interconnectedness of suffering, and its reverse, of love, caring, and awareness, that calls out for our understanding.

CHAPTER SIX

HUNTING AND HERDING SEA LIFE

"The living world is dying in our time. . . . When our forebears commenced their exploitation of this continent they believed the animate resources of the New World were infinite and inexhaustible. The vulnerability of that living fabric—the intricacy and fragility of its all-too-finite parts—was beyond their comprehension. It can be said in their defense that they were mostly ignorant of the inevitable consequences of their dreadful depredations. We who are alive today can claim no such exculpation for our biocidal actions and their dire consequences."
—Farley Mowat, *Sea of Slaughter*[1]

"Earth provides enough to satisfy every man's need, but not every man's greed."
—Mahatma Gandhi

Toxic Wastes, Toxic Flesh

When we look at fish, shellfish, dairy products, and eggs, the animal foods considered the least unhealthy by the general public, it may seem at first blush that these foods cause less suffering than eating the flesh of birds or other mammals. We'll look first at some of the consequences of eating the animals who inhabit the waters of our earth.

Like the flesh of all animals, the flesh of fish and shellfish is high in the three toxic elements described earlier: saturated animal fat, cholesterol, and animal protein. The percentage of saturated fat relative to unsaturated fat may be "better" in fish than in other animals, but fish is not, by any stretch of the imagination, a "low-fat" food. Besides being generally high in fat, cholesterol, and animal protein, and thus encouraging heart disease, cancer, obesity, diabetes, and the other negative effects of eating these substances, fish, because they live in water, are generally even more toxic than factory farmed birds and mammals. That is saying *a lot!* How could that be?

The basic reason is that the millions of tons of toxins that are produced by our culture all end up, eventually, in the water. The largest share of this pollution comes from animal agriculture in the form of herbicide, pesticide, fungicide, and chemical fertilizer runoff from fields, and sewage from factory farms, rich in drug residues and other toxins. Livestock produce 10,000 pounds of manure for every person in the U.S.,[2] and the excess phosphorous and nitrogen from this waste causes algal blooms, red tides, and the proliferation of deadly one-celled creatures like *Pfisteria piscicida* that kill billions of fish and cause grotesque sores on human swimmers.[3] Waters are further polluted by the whole range of carcinogenic dioxins, polychlorinated biphenyls (PCBs), toxic heavy metals from industrial wastes, and other residues from mining, tanning, paper, energy, petroleum, and industrial production, as well as noxious pharmaceutical residues and radioactive contamination from nuclear leakage. In addition to all this, the toxins that pollute the air are eventually washed into lakes and oceans, and solid waste sites and landfills are also leached by water, which carries their toxins into rivers and aquifers.

Water is our planet's universal solvent, and the whole range of environmental contaminants we produce ends up eventually in our rivers, lakes, streams, and aquifers, leading to the increasingly severe pollution of our oceans. There are large oceanic areas called dead zones where no fish can survive the water's extreme toxicity and its lack of oxygen, a condition known as hypoxia. This is the result of the massive amounts of nitrogen fertilizer and livestock manure running into rivers and oceans. This unnatural, "high-nutrient" water encourages the profusion of algae and a consequent depletion of oxygen, bringing suffocation to fish and sea life. One such dead zone of over 7,000 square miles is off the coast of Louisiana, where every day the Mississippi River dumps billions of gallons of water poisoned by agricultural runoff and industrial discharge into the Gulf of Mexico, wreaking havoc on its delicate and mysteriously interconnected marine ecosystems.[4] To eat animals who live in our earth's waters is to eat our own noxious pollution, concentrated many times.

We know that environmental toxins concentrate in the fatty tissue of all animals. This basic fact should give us pause. Both freshwater and saltwater fish amass and store toxic substances and carcinogenic chemicals in their flesh in concentrations that are actually hundreds of thousands of times greater than in the water itself. There are two basic reasons for this. First, fish breathe water, passing it over their gills to extract vital oxygen. Thus, through breathing, all fish consume an enormous amount of water, and the toxins tend to collect in their gills and end up in the fatty tissues of their flesh. Secondly, large fish are carnivores who live on smaller fish, who in turn live on even smaller fish, who eat still smaller fish. Unlike land animals and birds, who are mostly herbivorous, with a few "top carnivores" who may eat the much more plentiful mice, rabbits, deer, and so forth, fish live in a more carnivorous world. At each level the concentration of toxins multiplies exponentially. We like to eat mainly larger fish, like tuna, swordfish, shark, and salmon. Researchers know that the flesh of large fish contains extremely high concentrations of toxins, and that according to the Environmental Protection Agency, for example, carcinogenic PCB concentrations in fish are roughly nine million times the concentration in the water.[5] Shellfish also become highly toxic because they typically live closer to shore and are thus bathed in waters that have higher concentrations of noxious effluents. The more toxic agricultural and industrial runoff we produce, the more toxic the flesh of water-dwelling creatures becomes.

Because humans have become the planet's "top carnivore," our flesh has become perhaps the most toxic, reflected in our high cancer rates. It is an unfortunate beginning for a baby to drink the milk of an omnivorous mother and be deluged with the toxins that ride in her milk.

DDT, for example, is still in use throughout much of the world, and breastfeeding women who eat fish show significant levels of DDT and other pesticide contamination in their breast milk.[6] The babies of all mammals, particularly whales and dolphins, but also, of course, cows, goats, and sheep, may also be hurt by the high concentrations of toxins in their mothers' milk. The offspring of farmed animals typically get none of their mothers' milk anyway: it is stolen from them before they can get any. Before we go to the subject of cow's milk, though, we can look more closely at the implications of mistakenly interpreting fish, crabs, lobsters, oysters, shrimp, and other water creatures as food for humans.

Fish flesh is, as Michael Klaper, M.D., points out, "*very* concentrated protein." Because protein is basically only used to grow hair and nails, to heal wounds and rebuild tissue, and, in children, to grow, we typically take in more protein than we can use with a fish filet. Our bodies cannot store protein, so we must metabolize it, which causes stress on our liver, kidneys and immune system. Klaper also warns against consuming fish flesh and oil for other reasons:

> The fish oils that are promoted as providing protection to the arteries from atherosclerosis may also pose a serious hazard because they decrease the blood's ability to coagulate to stop bleeding. Fish oil has also been shown to inhibit the action of insulin. This is bad news for any diabetic trying to maintain normal blood sugar levels while taking fish oil capsules and possibly eating a diet high in fish flesh. . . . Another unpublicized but potentially important problem results from fish oil's apparent tendency to increase the length of a normal pregnancy. An overly long gestation time increases the birth weight of the baby, and thus the attendant risk of birth accidents, caesarian sections, and maternal deaths.

Despite current advertising campaigns, no one needs to eat the oil squeezed out of a fish's flesh or liver; in fact, the oil of a fish's liver is one of the strangest substances to consider eating. The liver of any animal is the chemical detoxifier for the body, and thus concentrates all the pollutants consumed by that animal. The oil squeezed from fish livers may contain high levels of hydrocarbon toxins such as PCBs and dioxins. People who use fish oil "to protect their arteries" may actually be poisoning themselves with hydrocarbons, and thus increasing their cancer risk from these dietary oils.

The better solution is to keep one's arteries clear, by not loading the blood with saturated animal fats in the first place. People who do not eat saturated animal fats generally have a much lower risk of clogging their arteries. Fish is *not* "brain food"—in fact, it now may well have become just the opposite—mercury poisons the brain and nerve cells. Because, in our current dietary understanding, a vegan diet can, in theory, meet all the human body's nutritional needs, and help protect against clogged arteries, heart attacks, strokes and cancers, you will do your health (and the fish!) a favor by letting them "off the hook."[7]

Becoming Vegan outlines in detail the plant-based sources of the omega-3 fatty acids that people often eat fish flesh or oil to obtain. The main sources are flax seeds, walnuts, soybeans, tofu, canola oil, hemp oil, dark greens, and seaweeds.[8]

Fish absorb and intensely concentrate toxins like PCBs, dioxins, radioactive substances, and heavy metals like mercury, lead, cadmium, and arsenic,[9] all of which are linked to cancer as well as nervous system disorders, kidney damage, and impaired mental functioning. They contain excessive amounts of cholesterol, animal protein, and hazardous, blood-altering oils. Besides contributing directly to human disease and suffering through the toxicity of its products, the seafood industry causes enormous damage to marine ecosystems throughout the world.

Herding Fish

Most people don't realize that the confinement and factory farming of fish and shellfish is a large and growing industry, euphemized as the "Blue Revolution." In fact, according to the United Nations' Food and Agriculture Organization, about thirty percent of worldwide saltwater and freshwater seafood production comes from commercial fish farm operations.[10] In the U.S., the percentages are somewhat higher, with approximately forty percent of shrimp, crab, and other shellfish, ninety percent of salmon, and sixty-five percent of freshwater fish consumed here coming from aquaculture operations.[11] Trout, catfish, tilapia, and other freshwater fish are forced to live in horrendously overcrowded concrete troughs. I talked with an investigator who visited a fish farm in Illinois, housed inside an enormous metal shed. When she went in, the air was so putrid she could barely breathe. The huge shallow pond inside was completely black and at first she couldn't see any fish. Then she realized the water was utterly full of fish, severely crowded together, and the blackness of the water was due to the concentration of their feces. I've seen abysmally overcrowded fish confined to feces-blackened water in outdoor fish farms in southern California and contemplated the miserable lives of these creatures, crammed inescapably in their own excrement, and then mercilessly slaughtered. People order this at local restaurants, ironically believing they're getting their healthy omega-3s or the fish that is recommended for their blood type.

Obviously, fish farmed in commercial aquaculture operations accumulate toxins from the water through gill breathing, and large amounts of antibiotics are routinely used, not only to unnaturally spur growth but also to control the disease that is an ever-present threat in such unhygienic conditions. The fish feed also contains high levels of contaminants, because besides grains it often contains feces, offal, and other by-products of the livestock industry, as well as fish and fish by-products not fit for human or pet consumption.

Saltwater fish farming also involves inhumane and unhealthy overcrowding of the fish, usually in offshore pens. These operations cause an enormous amount of water pollution, forcing thousands of fish to live in highly concentrated areas, with feces, antibiotics, pesticides, and toxic chemicals—such as the pigments that turn farmed salmon flesh from dull gray to appetizing pink—all flowing right into the surrounding ocean waters.[12] Scotland's caged salmon, for example, create an amount of untreated waste equivalent to that from eight million people, far more than Scotland's human population.[13] These fish farming operations have an ironically devastating effect on ocean fisheries because the fish being grown require large quantities of other fish in their feed.

For example, it takes three to five pounds of wild ocean fish to produce one pound of farmed saltwater fish or shrimp.[14] In addition to all this, fish farming fosters disease that can easily spread to wild salmon or other fish and wipe out whole stocks. This is what has happened with chronic wasting disease in wild elk and deer herds infected by cattle operations. As but one example, parasitic sea lice are rampant in the unnaturally concentrated populations of farmed salmon. The industry uses toxic pesticides and antibiotics in its vain struggle to control the lice, who spread in clouds in the surrounding water, stretching up to nineteen miles around the farms, infesting wild salmon populations in the area and decimating them.[15] Another practice that is wreaking havoc with wild populations is the introduction of non-native farmed fish species that escape into local ecosystems. Commercial shrimp farms are another particularly well-known and egregious ecological disaster, causing pollution that is killing precious coral reefs and coastal mangrove forests worldwide. The fish flesh obtained from commercial aquaculture factory farms is intensified misery, toxicity, and environmental devastation.

Floating Death Ships

The story behind the living beings pulled out of our earth's oceans is just as tragic, though in a different way. The world's marine ecosystems are being ruthlessly plundered. Long gone are the days when the first Europeans arrived on North American shores and wrote how the schools of fish were so vast and thick that they thought their ships would run aground on them before they reached the land.[16] These once-fecund waters have been, and continue to be, strip-mined for fish, using fishing trawlers with nets many thousands of feet in length, to meet the relentless demand of humans, fish farms, and enslaved food animals. (An amazing fifty percent of the world fish catch is fed to the needlessly imprisoned food animals, and not to people.[17]) All of the seventeen major global fisheries are depleted or in serious decline.

In most parts of the world, because of overfishing and near-shore water pollution, it is no longer possible to run profitable fishing operations close to shore. As boats go farther out, they stay out longer. When fish are hauled into the boats, they are dumped in tanks in the hull where they slowly die, defecating and crushing the fish beneath them. This often goes on for many days, the dead and dying fish piled atop each other with open wounds, workers pouring antibiotics into the fecal soup to keep infection in check. Seafood is the leading cause of food poisoning in the United States.[18] There is virtually no governmental inspection of seafood before it is sold to markets and the public, and recent studies by Consumer Reports showed that over twenty-five percent of the fish they examined for sale were "on the brink of spoilage," over half the grocery store samples of "red snapper" were actually other species, and half of swordfish samples exceeded the FDA's action level for nerve-damaging methylmercury. E. coli, histamine, and other dangerous substances were also detected.[19]

The carnage caused by modern factory fishing methods is horrific. Huge trawlers, using satellite and radar technology and even helicopters and airplanes, deploy nets that reach to the ocean floor and bring up virtually everything in their path. The fish are often pulled rapidly from such depths that they suffer decompression. Their internal organs may burst and their eyes pop out, as they die an excruciating death through suffocation, crushing, or evisceration. In the course of this marine strip-mining, an enormous number of sea creatures that are "unprofitable" are hauled in. This so-called "bycatch" of certain fish, turtles, dolphins, sea birds, and other animals is thrown back into the ocean mostly dead or severely wounded. Every year, this adds up to about twenty-five million tons of dead and dying sea animals, roughly a third of the total that's dragged in. A recent Duke University study, for example, found that over 300,000 sea turtles are killed annually just by commercial long-line fishing operations.[20] According to Environmental Defense:

> Bycatch can include juvenile commercial fish, sea turtles, whales, seabirds, dolphins and any other sea creature that's not commercially desirable. Shrimp trawling throws away an average of five pounds of bycatch for every pound of shrimp caught, including up to 150,000 endangered sea turtles every year. Methods of capture that can result in high bycatch are gill nets, purse seines and bottom trawling.[21]

Paul Watson, founder of the Sea Shepherd Conservation Society, describes the consequences of today's fishing methods:

The trawlers literally leave no stone unturned. Bottom draggers plow the benthonic depths taking ground-fish, mollusks, crustaceans, and damaging vegetation and structure. Mid-water draggers stalk those fish that dwell between the bottom and the surface. Surface trawlers maul the upper reaches of the seas. Those species of the deep that do survive the tri-level assaults must then run the gauntlet of longliner fleets, gill netters, purse seine netters, and crab and lobster pots.

The very foundation of the food chain is being shattered as large Japanese small-mesh plankton trawlers haul in krill by the hundreds of millions of tons. The krill, shrimp-like zooplankton, are then converted into a protein base to use as animal feed. The more krill exploited means less food available for fish and whales.

The global carnage inflicted on the world's fish species ranges from the horrendous waste and slaughter of the huge floating factory operations to the cumulative damage caused by millions of people fishing with rods, small nets and traps, and combing the shorelines for crabs and shellfish.[22]

Entire species of fish are being killed to the verge of extinction to satisfy the demand for fish meal for fattening livestock or factory-farmed fish, or for seafood for humans. According to Watson:

The rationalization for fishmeal production defies all logic. As animal food, about one hundred pounds, live weight, of fish is required to produce one pound of beef. Two hundred pounds of fishmeal used as fertilizer produces no more than three pounds of vegetable protein. Even more ironic is that over fifty pounds of fish meal is needed to raise one farm-raised salmon.[23]

Many other species of marine creatures suffer directly from our unnatural demand for fish flesh. Sea lions, seals, whales, dolphins, and seabirds suffer and often starve because their source of food has been destroyed by human fishing activity. The number of Stellar's sea lions in the Bering Sea, for example, is less than twenty percent of what it was in the 1950s. Besides stealing their food supply, fishers or their agents kill many of these creatures because they are seen as competition for the ever-decreasing number of fish in the over-fished ocean waters. The Canadian Department of Fisheries subsidizes the yearly spring slaughter of seal pups on the ice floes of eastern Canada—the brutal and bloody bludgeoning and shooting to death each year of over 300,000 helpless baby seals by local fishermen.[24] In recent years, the government has actually raised the limit on the number of seals that can be killed; the Newfoundland minister of fisheries has proclaimed his hope that the seals will be completely eliminated, because he believes they threaten Canada's fishing industry.[25] Biologists who have studied the situation report that the main threat to the fishing industry is its own rapacity, not the seals; there aren't enough young fish surviving the fishing nets to replenish the stocks. Iceland candidly justifies its killing of whales as a necessary step to protect its commercial fishing industry.

Cormorants and other water birds are hunted, trapped, and killed by both government agencies and private interests because of their perceived competition with fishers and the fishing industry. At least twenty thousand dolphins are killed each year by the tuna industry. Because dolphins tend to swim above schools of tuna, fishing operations use them to find tuna, and dolphins inevitably end up drowning in the nets. There is no oversight on many tuna fishing operations, and Galapagos National Park personnel, for example, caught a tuna seiner with its net deployed within park boundaries on May 3, 2002, with over fifty dead and dying dolphins and just eight tuna. Virtually no punishment was imposed.[26] Sharks are now being killed by the tens of thousands simply for their fins. They are hauled in, their fins chopped off, and their bodies thrown back into the water to die slow, agonizing deaths.[27] Sometimes their spines are also slit to remove the cartilage that is sold in health food stores as a cancer remedy; this has been shown to have little effect other than as a placebo, but still the sharks die for it. Some species, such as swordfish and grouper, are approaching extinction in the wild, as are most sea turtle species, drowned in the nets used by commercial shrimp trawlers.

In addition to all this commercial fishing, which has destroyed nine-ty percent of the ocean's large fish such as tuna and swordfish, there is the toll taken by recreational and "sport" fishermen on both freshwater and saltwater fish.[28] Recent research shows that anglers kill a far larger percentage of threatened species than previously thought, causing, for example, over twenty-five percent of the deaths of over-fished saltwater species. Whether they kill the fish to eat or throw them back, the fish suffer intensely. The whole intent of sport fishing is, as Barry MacKay points out, "to engage in a battle between the fisher and the fish—a bat-tle never asked for by, or in the interest of, the fish."[29] Studies have shown that fish who are hooked and thrown back are so traumatized that many die from the experience. The pain of being hooked in the mouth is excruciating—Thomas Hopkins, professor of marine science at the University of Alabama, has compared it to "dentistry without Novocain, drilling into exposed nerves."[30] This pain is compounded by being pulled and "played" on the line, which for the fish is an agoniz-ing struggle leading to utter exhaustion. Being handled by the fisher damages the protective mucus layer on the fish's scales; then, after inflicting more trauma removing the hook, the fisher tosses the wound-ed fish back to "fight" again another day. The estimates of "catch and release" fish mortality vary depending on a variety of factors, including the species and age of the fish, the depth at which they're caught, how severely they're hooked and how much they're handled, and how exhausted they are by their life-and-death struggle. In a study of Coho salmon, twenty to thirty percent died from the ordeal; in other studies, the percentages of catch-and-release fish that die shortly after being returned to the water are between five and ten percent, and with others it's fifty percent and even up to one hundred percent.[31]

Besides the suffering of the fish, there is also the extreme cruelty to creatures used as bait in fishing, as Joan Dunayer explains:

Animals used as live bait range from shrimps, lizards, worms, and frogs to mackerels, salmons, crickets, and crabs. "Baitfish" are hooked so that they won't die quickly: through their lips, their nose, their eye sockets. . . . If large, they may be impaled on two or three hooks. Sometimes, to reduce drag, fishers sew a fish's mouth shut before towing them as bait. Because a fish who struggles and bleeds is especially likely to attract predators, fishers often break a "bait-fish's" back, cut their fins, or notch them with multiple razor slits.[32]

The scope of suffering caused by the demand for the flesh of sea creatures is vast, almost incomprehensible. Whereas records are kept of the number of individual birds and mammals killed each year for food (in the U.S., that number is now over ten billion annually), for "seafood," only the tonnage is reported. Eighty million tons of water creatures per year: how many individuals is that? Every individual fish is a vertebrate with a central nervous system and pain proprioceptors, like we mammals have. Marine biologists have proven that fish definitely do feel and avoid pain and that they learn to evade painful stimuli, even to the degree of selecting the option of food deprivation over pain. Researchers have also proven what is really quite obvious, that fish can be fearful and learn to anticipate pain. Besides this, scientists have discovered that fish and also sea-dwelling invertebrates "generate opiate-like pain-dampening biochemicals (enkephalins and endorphins) in response to injuries that would unquestionably be painful to humans, as further proof of the ability of fish to feel pain."[33] Like us, they would not survive if they didn't feel pain. Their pain sensors are especially dense around their mouths, where they are often cruelly hooked and pulled.

In addition to feeling pain, scientists have discovered that fish are far more intelligent than had been presumed. For example, British experts say that fish, as the most ancient of the major vertebrate groups, have had "ample time" to evolve complex and diverse behavior patterns that rival those of many other vertebrates. They report that there have been huge changes in science's understanding of the psychological and mental abilities of fish in the last few years, adding, "Although it may seem extraordinary to those comfortably used to pre-judging animal intelligence on the basis of brain volume, in some cognitive domains, fishes can even be favorably compared to non-human primates."[34] Recent research has shown that fish are "steeped in social intelligence," recognizing individual "shoal mates" and social prestige, and scientists have observed them using tools, building complex nests, cooperating, and exhibiting stable cultural traditions and long-term memories.[35]

Sylvia Earle, former chief scientist of the U.S. National Oceanic and Atmospheric Administration, has written, "[Fish] are our fellow citizens with scales and fins. . . . I would never eat anyone I know personally. I wouldn't deliberately eat a grouper any more than I'd eat a cocker spaniel. They're so good-natured, so curious. You know, fish are sensitive, they have personalities, they hurt when they're wounded."[36] Fish are sensitive and intelligent creatures, and their flesh, filled with pain, fear, and toxins, is obviously unhealthy for us to eat; yet we persist. Pursuing, confining, slaughtering, and eating them as mere objects to be consumed, we inevitably deaden ourselves spiritually and emotionally as well. Paul Watson has noted,

> Seafood is simply a socially acceptable form of bush meat. We condemn Africans for hunting monkeys and mammalian and bird species from the jungle yet the developed world thinks nothing of hauling in magnificent wild creatures like swordfish, tuna, halibut, shark, and salmon for our meals. The fact is that the global slaughter of marine wildlife is simply the largest massacre of wildlife on the planet.[37]

Chefs know that fish who die with great resistance, struggling against the net or the hook and line, have a more bitter taste because of the lactic acid that remains in their muscles. In eating fish, we eat the lactic acid the fish produce in their death throes, and the fear-induced adrenalin and other hormones. It should be amply clear that in unwisely eating fish because of an imagined benefit, we bring into our body a host of toxins and cause suffering and negative effects that far outweigh their potential benefit. We can all get ample high-quality protein from plant sources without causing unnecessary misery and trauma to other living creatures.

Finally, in exterminating the fish from our waters, we are destroying the earth's system for cleaning the waters. It is well known that fish clean the waters of toxins and impurities: they can be seen as the earth's kidneys, absorbing contaminants into their flesh. This is a natural function and an important reason why it is so damaging to the health of the earth that we are drastically reducing their numbers—and to our individual health to actually eat them. It is common, for example, to see fish congregated around the sewer pipes that dump untreated sewage into the ocean in countries that still allow this. The fish eat the human feces as it emerges from these pipes. As fecal eaters and flesh eaters, fish are completely inappropriate for human food, "unclean" in every way imaginable. In violently entering their world, imprisoning, manipulating, and killing them, and harming seabirds and marine mammals with them, we are committing crimes against nature on a gigantic scale. It shows our disrespect for life and the benevolent source of all life, which has blessed us with bodies that require not one fish, dolphin, turtle, albatross, lobster, shrimp, or crab to suffer and die for their feeding.

CHAPTER SEVEN

THE DOMINATION OF THE FEMININE

"Can one regard a fellow creature as a property item, an investment,
a piece of meat, an 'it,' without degenerating into cruelty towards
that creature?"
—KAREN DAVIS[1]

"Milk was destined to feed the animal's offspring and not that man
should take it with force for himself. The kid has the right to enjoy its
mother's milk and its mother's love, but hard-hearted man, influenced by
his materialistic and shallow outlook, changes and perverts these true
functions. Thus the gentle kid is unable to partake of its mother's love
and rejoice in the splendor of life."
—RABBI ABRAHAM KOOK, Chief Rabbi of Israel, 1865–1935

"The wrong done another reacts most heavily against one's self."[2]
—MARY BAKER EDDY

The Dairy Nightmare

There are two other large categories of animal products that we eat even
though they are not food for humans: dairy products and eggs. Many people who take a close look at dairy and egg operations say that they are in
some ways more toxic and cruel than those dealing only with the flesh of

animals, because the cows and chickens are severely abused for longer periods and inevitably slaughtered when their productivity declines.

Dairy products, to begin with, constitute an exceedingly large and complex topic. The enslavement of the female dairy cow has contributed to the enslavement of humans in a range of ways, so the damage caused by this practice extends far beyond the negative physical effects of consuming milk. Though many of us stop eating dairy products just for health reasons, it's important to see the larger context of the ongoing tragedy, for this truth is as old as time: we cannot sow seeds of slavery and cruelty and reap the fruit of freedom and health.

Fundamentally, cow's milk is a substance designed by nature for baby cows, not for humans. We are the only species that drinks the milk intended for the young of other species, and we are the only species that insists on drinking milk beyond the time of weaning. It seems we cannot bear the thought of growing up and leaving home. Perhaps we long for infancy and the peaceful oblivion of our mother's breast, and if hers isn't available, then we'll use the breast of any lactating mother, even if she's a cow and we have to kill her babies to get to it. Just as the complete unnaturalness of humans killing and eating animals is obvious if we contemplate trying to do it without implements, so is the drinking of milk. The easy availability of veal cutlets and cheap hamburger masks their true cost and the cruelty of their dairy-farm origin, as do the tidy packages of cheese, milk, cream, and butter in the refrigerated dairy sections.

In the wild, it is doubtful we'd ever be able to get close enough to a lactating cow, in a forest or grassland somewhere in Asia where cows naturally live, to obtain any milk. Wild bulls are ferociously protective and would gore us or chase us off first. If we managed to get by the bulls, it is unlikely any cow would allow us to get under her and suck on her teats. We would have to compete with the cow's own baby, the rightful recipient of her milk, and push or kick the calf away, and somehow get the mother to hold still for us while we sucked or squeezed on her teats. The whole image is so absurd that not even the most committed milk-bibber would ever contemplate attempting it.

It is only through an ongoing tradition of vicious domination that humans can drink cows' milk, an unhealthy and perverse action at its core. The dairy products in our grocery stores are the result of many centuries of human manipulation and horrific brutality against cows—a brutality epitomized by today's mechanized dairy operations, both large and small.

Pushing Cows to Produce

Cows today are forced to produce a far greater quantity of milk than they ever would in the wild. This is accomplished through two types of manipulation—of food and of hormones.[3] In the wild, a cow, like all mammals, will produce milk after giving birth to a baby, and does so in a classic bell curve for about seven months, beginning at less than ten pounds of milk per day, climaxing at about twenty-five pounds per day, and then tapering back to ten pounds and then to zero as the calf begins to eat solid food. On today's dairies the newborn calf is immediately removed from the mother, causing enormous anguish to both, and the mother is artificially forced to produce from *90 to 110* pounds of milk per day for a full seven to eight months. Dairy cows are impregnated at a much younger age than would ever occur in the wild, and are kept pregnant virtually continuously, even while they are lactating from the previous pregnancy. The enormous strain of being pushed so hard to produce such abnormally large quantities of milk quickly destroys the health of these cows. Though they would naturally live twenty-five years in the wild, after about four years of this dairy abuse their "productivity" drops off. They are then forced to endure the brutality of the slaughterhouse and be reduced to inexpensive hamburger meat, leather, and animal feed.

The enormous and continuous abuse to which dairy cow mothers are subjected makes their milk extremely unhealthy for humans. Besides the naturally occurring human toxins in cows' milk, like IGF-1 growth factor, casein, estrogen, soporific hormones, lactase, pus, bacteria, parasites, and the apparently addictive casomorphins discussed in Chapter 4, there are the toxins that are a direct result of pushing the cows so hard: artificially introduced growth hormones, milk-increasing hormones, antibiotics, tranquilizers, and feeds high in pesticide residues. So-called organic milk may contain smaller quantities of the artificial toxins, but not of the natural ones, whose presence in cow's milk reminds us that this is a food that is designed for calves, not for humans.

How are the mother cows actually pushed to produce such gigantic volumes of milk? They are forced to eat cholesterol in their feed and are injected with a blend of hormones, including estrogen, progesterone, prolactin, and testosterone. Dairy consumers receive little protection from these hormones, since regulations on using them are minimal. As Mason and Singer demonstrate in *Animal Factories*, the Food and Drug Administration and the Department of Agriculture exist to serve and protect agribusiness interests rather than consumer, environmental, or animal interests.[4] As but one example, while Canada and all European governments banned the use of rBGH, Monsanto's controversial, genetically engineered, milk-increasing recombinant bovine growth hormone, the FDA dutifully approved it in 1985. It has been used on dairies in this country ever since, despite scientific evidence that it may increase cancer risks in both consumers and cows.[5]

Dairy farmers also discovered long ago that if cows were fed cholesterol-rich foods, they would give a lot more milk. Of course, an adult cow in the wild is a complete herbivore and would never eat animal flesh, milk, or eggs (the only sources of cholesterol, which is absent in all plant foods). But dairy cows, like many other farmed animals enduring the debasement of modern industrialized agriculture, are given feed "enriched" with animal flesh and offal, by-products from the slaughter of fish, birds, and other mammals, including perhaps other cows and even their own calves. It is all unspeakably perverse, yet it has been standard procedure on dairy operations for years. According to former dairyman Tom Rodgers, even the smaller dairy operations feed their cows "enriched" feed to boost output so they can compete economically.[6]

Because each dairy cow is forced to produce far more calves than can be used on the dairy, her calves are immediately slaughtered, auctioned to veal operations, or auctioned to build beef herds and killed at one to two years of age. In all these cases, parts of their bodies will end up at the rendering plant, mixed with the offal and unusable body parts of fish, pigs, poultry, road kill, laboratory animals, and euthanized dogs, cats, horses, and other animals, and then cooked, ground up, and added to corn, wheat, soybeans, and other grains to be fed back to the cows. Cows have thus been routinely forced to eat other cows, and quite possibly the flesh and organs of their own young, in their "enriched" feed. The only reason this may now be stopping is the outbreak of mad cow disease, a direct result of such mad agricultural practices. Although the FDA's ban on feeding the flesh of ruminants to ruminants has reduced the likelihood of cows eating other cows, they are still fed pigs, chickens, turkeys, fish, dogs, and other animals. Considering the reputedly lax enforcement and inspection of this FDA policy, some are likely still forced into cannibalism.

This bizarre and outrageous cruelty lurks behind every milk mustache. It is considered business as usual, and no one has questioned it because the animals involved have been reduced to mere objects by the dairy industry, with the sole overriding goal of producing the most milk at the lowest price. (And with the USDA guaranteeing to buy milk surpluses, the industry maximizes production.[7]) This whole industry is obviously both a result of—and a contributor to—a severely reduced cultural intelligence that has lost its ability to make basic connections.

The Toxins in Milk

As discussed earlier, ingested chemicals, pesticides, fungicides, fertilizers, and heavy metals accumulate in body tissues, especially in the fatty tissues and organs. Dairy cows thus concentrate not only the toxins that are sprayed on the grains and hay they eat, but also the more concentrated toxins that have accumulated in the rendered body parts of the animals they are forced to eat as well. All this accumulates in their milk, because milk is high in fat and toxins ride in fat. Dairy products, particularly butter, cheese, cream, and ice cream, are clearly unhealthy and dangerous to eat, especially for children and pregnant or nursing women.

Besides all this, there are potent naturally occurring toxins in milk. Nature never intended us to drink milk intended for the offspring of another species, particularly cows. Cow's milk is specifically suited to the nutritional needs of herd animals who double their weight in only forty-seven days, weigh three hundred pounds within fourteen weeks, and grow four healthy stomachs! Cow's milk contains three times as much protein as human milk and about fifty percent more fat. Dog's milk, for example, is nutritionally much more similar to human milk than cow's milk. Cow's milk is far too coarse, especially for young children who are growing delicate brain, nervous system, and other tissues. Human children are not calves! Infant brain and nerve tissue are best grown with the nutrients in human milk. The main protein in human milk, lactalbumin, has a molecular weight of 14K. It is perfectly suited to building sensitive human tissue. The basic protein in cow's milk, casein, has a molecular weight of 233K[8] and, because it is so durable and sticky, is used as a binder in paint, and as the glue that holds plywood together and sticks labels to bottles.[9] It is perfect for building a calf's tissues but causes incalculable harm to humans. Casein is an immense and unwieldy protein, difficult for a human child (or adult for that matter) to properly break down, creating a lot of acidic residue when metabolized, and in the case of young children, causing many serious problems.

We are concerned not only about the host of childhood symptoms that have been linked with dairy products, including colic, earaches, sore throats, colds, fevers, anemia, diabetes, tonsillitis, appendicitis, allergies of various kinds, inflamed mucus membranes, diarrhea, gas, and cramps.[10] We are also concerned about the damage done to the early development of tissues of young children who are forced to eat and drink dairy products. Can the sensitive human tissues that make up the young child's mind-body system possibly be properly formed with the gluey and cumbersome casein and excess fat that are meant for growing young bovines? It's like trying to create a delicate landscape painting with house-painting brushes as tools! This may certainly affect the early psychological development of our children—and with the bovine hormones, toxins, and misery in milk, one of the effects may very well be a basic desensitization of the child. How tragic to pollute and damage the miraculously sensitive human vehicle at an early age, reducing its ability to be a conduit for spiritual energy, wisdom, and compassion, and perhaps diminishing its ability to sense the subtle interconnectedness that it is created to perceive, explore, and celebrate. To continue to eat

dairy products into adolescence and adulthood compounds and reinforces the tragedy.

At a deeper level, forcing young children to eat dairy products
brings into their impressionable minds and bodies a most unfortunate
and terrible vibrational energy of the profound sadness, grief, panic,
suffering, and fear that mother cows always experience on dairies,
organic or not. The whole dairy business is founded upon stealing:
forcibly stealing calves from their mothers and mother's milk from
calves. We have become desensitized to just how cruel this actually is,
and how it underlies, perhaps in large measure, our culture's basic
repression, confinement, and exploitation of the female and the feminine principle.

The mothers of all mammals feel terrible emotional stress if their
newborn offspring are endangered and will do everything in their power
to protect them. Human mothers know how deep this feeling is, and
how devastating it would be to have their children taken from them.
Mother love will often give its own life for its child. We can see this deep
maternal caring in dogs, bears, elephants, monkeys, deer, lions, whales:
in all mammals it is a defining and obvious characteristic of mothers.
For scientists, agribusinessmen, or theologians to deny this, or discount
its importance, only shows how reduced their intelligence and sensitivity have become through their cultural woundedness and consequent
skill in disconnecting.

Of all the mammals, it is the cow whose maternal instinct has been
perhaps the most obvious and celebrated: her gentle and patient eyes,
her natural mothering way with her calf, licking and feeding and watching over her baby, and her loud lamenting when the calf is taken from
her. She cannot fight the hands that steal her offspring away, or speak
to us in human words, telling us how deeply it hurts her. But it is obvious to anyone with eyes to see and ears to hear. For us to ignore her suffering, and the suffering of her calf—hundreds, thousands, millions of
times over—is to ignore and deny our own decency. There is a deep and
terrible transgression in this, the unnatural coveting of the calf's mother's milk several thousand years ago, and the building of a whole culture
around the stealing of milk, the killing of the mother and her children,

and justifying the whole horrific thing by mythologizing it: the Lord promising us the land of milk and honey. This violent theft of milk from enslaved mothers planted seeds of war and exploitation that are tragically almost completely invisible. Today, our culture takes milk for granted! It is aggressively promoted around the world. How can we ever hope for peace when we practice such shameful violence on such a massive scale?

Four Pathways to Hell

The calves taken from their mothers are always destined for brutal mistreatment, and the mother cow certainly has an awareness of this. Animals are remarkably sensitive, as countless cultures have recognized and as scientific evidence is increasingly showing. Mother cows are aware that the hands that confine and rape her and push her so hard for her milk cannot mean well for her children. The dairy-born calf will go down one of four doomed pathways.

If she is a female, she may be raised to be, like her mother, a slave in the dairy. She will be removed from her mother as early as possible so as not to waste the mother's marketable milk. She will be dehorned, usually by the use of a red-hot electric iron applied to her horn buttons. This is described in a modern dairy management textbook:

> . . . lay the calf on its side and put your knee on the neck. . . . The dehorner has to be left on the button for approximately five to twenty seconds. The time will seem longer, because of the combined unpleasantness of burning hair and a struggling calf . . . dehorning may be complete . . . when you hear a squeaking sound as the dehorner is twisted. It is the sound of the dehorner tip rubbing against the bone of the skull.[11]

According to the dairy industry, about half the calves are born with "too many" teats on their udders, and these extra teats, which are "unsightly" and may interfere with the electric milking machines, are also removed from the calves with no anesthetic, as described again in the dairy management textbook: "Grasp the teat between your thumb and forefinger. Even in small calves, the nerve supply to their teats is well developed. Make sure the calf is well restrained before you proceed. Pull the teat outwards and take a generous bite with the scissors."[12] Dehorning, tail docking, and teat removal not only cause intense pain but also increase the risk of infection and thus the spread of disease. They help account for the widespread problem of Bovine Leukemia Virus, which infects cows in an estimated eighty-nine percent of U.S. dairies[13] and, according to researchers at the University of California, may pose a cancer threat to consumers.[14]

Whereas in the wild a heifer would not be ready to have her first calf for at least three to five years, that is far too long to feed her without getting milk money from her. Cow feed is expensive, so operators want to get her into production quickly, which means getting her pregnant as soon as possible, in just a year or less, when she is still a mere child in human terms. This is accomplished through hormone manipulation, administering excessive amounts of estrogen and other hormones, as well as prostaglandin, a hormone that is used to bring cows into heat when dairy operators want to have them inseminated. In the vast majority of cases, the dairy cow will be confined to a stall or milking paddock year-round, often exposed to extreme temperatures, with nothing to do but eat and stand in one place, reduced to the status of a milk-producing machine. She will be inseminated by a sperm gun shoved elbow-deep into her vagina and fired. The sperm comes from a special bull who also exists to be milked—for his sperm—and will be slaughtered when his productivity declines.

As soon as she gives birth, the cow's baby will be quickly stolen from her, and she will be milked two to three times per day by the milking machines. No longer something done *by* her, milking is something inflicted upon her. The machines often cause cuts and injuries and can lead to mastitis, infection of the udder, which is rampant in modern dairies. Sometimes the milking machines give electrical shocks as well, causing considerable discomfort and fear. The cow may also be "drenched," a procedure routinely performed on some cows after giving birth to reduce metabolic diseases in early lactation. Many gallons of nutrient-dense solution are forced into her through a seven-foot tube shoved down her throat. She may drown if the liquid is pumped too fast or if the tube is stuck into her windpipe. A similar procedure called lavage may be imposed on her newborn calf as well, to administer colostrum.

Right after the cow begins to be milked, she is again inseminated on the "rape rack" by the sperm gun. She is thus both pregnant and lactating simultaneously, and will be taken off the milking machine only during the last two months of pregnancy. As soon as she gives birth, the baby is again taken away, and she goes back on the milking machine and is raped and inseminated again.

All this causes enormous suffering for the mother cows, and their health breaks down quickly. The lactogenic hormones and cholesterol-laden feed and unnatural milking schedules cause the cows' udders to become painful and so heavy they sometimes drag on the ground and in their own feces, increasing the painful mastitis and leading to overuse of antibiotics. Their udders are permanently stretched far beyond what they would be in nature, their ankles swollen and sore from standing constantly on concrete. After three to five years, these mother cows, dairy slaves, are worn out and sent off in overcrowded trucks to face the final insulting brutality of the slaughterhouse. The majority of "downed" cattle arriving at slaughterhouses are dairy cows. These are animals too weak, diseased, or injured to walk off the truck. Their bones may break easily because of osteoporosis brought on by high-protein feed and forced high-volume milk production. Transport may last for several days with no food or water through bitter cold or extreme heat. Sometimes the cows are literally frozen to the inner sides of the trucks. If they have collapsed, these "downers" are shocked with excruciatingly painful prods. If they still can't move, they are literally dragged by chains, often tearing skin, ripping tendons and ligaments, and breaking bones in the process. They aren't humanely euthanized because they're seen merely as meat, and dead carcasses aren't supposed to be butchered (though that also happens, according to worker affidavits in Gail Eisnitz's *Slaughterhouse*). They're dragged to the killing floor, where their bodies will be ripped apart to produce hamburger meat, animal feed, pet food, leather, gelatin, glue, and other products.

The same scenarios apply to dairies that produce so-called organic milk products, except that the feed is organic, there is a limit to some of the hormones and other toxins, and there may be a little more space in the prison stall. The cows are still slaughtered after a few years, and the same pricing mechanism drives the industry: to get the most milk for the cheapest price. Individual cows are worth very little, since maximizing pregnancies boosts milk production and there are always more calves on hand than can be used.

This brings us to the second possible path for calves born on the dairy: they may be killed shortly after birth if the veal industry and beef industry demand is low. The rennet in their young stomachs is valuable for making cheeses. Their bodies are then ground up for animal feed, and their skin is used for more expensive leather. Sometimes pregnant cows are sent off to slaughter. In this case, the fetal calves that fall out of them when they are sliced open must be killed separately by the slaughterhouse workers. These unborn babies are skinned for the soft leather on their small, wet bodies, which fetches quite a high price.

The third possible path for dairy-born calves is to be auctioned to the veal industry. Both males and females are forced down this dark and miserable path when they are not needed on the dairy (this includes organic dairies). The abuse these poor creatures must endure for their short lives is well known and documented. They are forced into veal crates and chained at the neck as soon as they arrive at the veal operation, only days or weeks old. These crates are built small, to confine the calves so they cannot move, causing their muscles to be undeveloped and their "meat" more tender. They are kept in darkness and fed a diet purposefully deficient in iron so their flesh will be pale, which brings a higher price. They will frantically suck on or lick any iron, like nails that happen to be within reach. They endure this cruel confinement, often covered with their own excrement. Their naturally joyful and frolicsome temperaments are destroyed by the pain and hopelessness of their situations. Their liquid diet is laced with chemicals, drugs, and antibiotics, and after three to four months, they are trucked to the slaughterhouse to be killed for the veal and calfskin markets.

The fourth path for dairy-born calves, if they are male, is to be auctioned to the meat industry and raised for beef. In this case they will face the intense pain of unanesthetized castration when they are still young. These poor animals may also be branded—often several times, inflicting extremely painful third-degree burns—and dehorned, which is also highly painful. They spend one to one and a half years either confined or grazing, growing to a size that makes them profitable to slaughter, and then are sent to the feedlot to be fattened.

On feedlots, hundreds or thousands of castrated cattle are crowded together for a few months with little or no shelter, in fetid confinement, and fed whatever the feedlot operators can devise to make them gain as much weight as quickly and cheaply as possible (when they are sold, the operators are paid by the pound). The unfortunate creatures, mere objects in the meat complex, are given artificial steroid growth pro-motants such as Ralgro, Synovex, or Rumensin so they will grow to be much heavier much younger than they ever would in nature.[15] While cows are natural grass eaters who would never eat grain in the wild, feedlot operators, like dairy operators, have found that feeding them grain boosts growth and profits. Because grain (mainly corn, soybeans, wheat, and oats) is relatively expensive, it is supplemented with cheap-er additives to add even more weight to the cattle. Well-known cattle feed additives are sawdust, cement dust, chicken manure, and petrole-um by-products. All the toxins in the grain, as well as in the other sub-stances, concentrate in the fat and flesh of the steer. Other feed additives are equally unpleasant to contemplate: the ground-up bodies and parts of animals obtained from the rendering industry. These animal products are especially high in concentrated toxins, as well as fat, cholesterol, and animal protein, which helps produce the marbled fat that brings a high-er price. The young steers are not allowed to move around, since that would burn calories and toughen their flesh. Agribusiness has also dis-covered that if animals are fed antibiotics routinely in their feed, they grow faster, with the result that, according to the Union of Concerned Scientists, over seventy percent of all antibiotics produced in the U.S. are administered to animals imprisoned for food.[16] Antibiotics are also administered to help combat the infections and diseases that are ram-pant in the overcrowded feedlot environment where the steers are imprisoned. And while it is comical to think of cows wading into streams to catch fish, the bizarre truth is that entire fish populations have been decimated in both the Atlantic and Pacific oceans by large-scale net-trawling fishing operations simply to supply fish to the livestock feed industry. This fish contains the fat and cholesterol that work so well to unnaturally fatten these unfortunate steers in the feedlots.

As soon as they can, the feedlot operators send the fattened steers to the slaughterhouse so their flesh can be eaten by humans and other herbivores, all imprisoned by a macabre fatten-and-kill operation that encompasses and pollutes the entire planet. Oceans, fields, pastures, forests, highways, zoos, ranches, circuses, laboratories, animal control agencies, pet breeding companies, and schools are linked to rendering plants and slaughterhouses in this web of violence, and the animals dominated or killed in these places contribute to the fattening of these steers so they can be more profitably killed. Their flesh is home to a defiling misery that may curse us in a variety of ways if we support the industry by patronizing it at the ubiquitous meat outlets that define our culture.

All four of the possible paths that a calf born on a dairy may take are paths of abuse and early death. Since bovines in the wild easily live twenty to thirty years, the industry, in killing calves, steers, and dairy cows at the ages of several months to several years, is really killing infants and children. In this it is the same as the industries that confine and kill lambs, pigs, chickens, turkeys, and fish: all are pushed to grow abnormally quickly and are slaughtered young. Similarly, in the wars we inflict upon each other, children suffer and die the most, and more than ever they are even forced to do the killing. The animal food culture promotes domination and exploitation of the female and the feminine, which are full of life-giving and nurturing powers, and of infants and children, who are full of the powers of innocence and growth.

The Mustache Mask

That innocent-looking and effective marketing tool, the dairy industry's milk mustache, is thus actually a mask that hides the most sickening and inhumane industry practically imaginable. These docile vegetarian mothers and their unfortunate children are dominated from birth to death, unnaturally fattened on animal flesh so humans can fatten themselves on dairy products and cow flesh. One would almost hope that for their enormous sacrifice, the dairy cows would at least be supplying humans with something beneficial. And yet the deeper justice is inescapable: by killing them, we kill ourselves; by enslaving them, we enslave ourselves; by sickening them, we sicken ourselves.

Mother cows, like all lactating mammals, produce high levels of estrogen in their milk. It is not healthy for humans to take in this high estrogen load at any age. One obvious result is that young girls' bodies are unnaturally pushed to become sexually mature at an early age. The average age of menarche, of first menstruation, instead of being seventeen as it was in the mid-nineteenth century, is now 12.5 years.[17] This was made startlingly clear in Japan after World War II, where in the space of just one or two generations after dairy products were introduced there, the average age of menarche went from 15.2 to 12.5.[18] According to researcher Kerrie Saunders, "Both African villages and the Chinese have retained many of their dietary traditions of eating plant-based foods, and they both average an onset of female puberty at seventeen years of age."[19] The unnaturally early menarche in our culture causes untold anguish, with unnecessary teen pregnancies, abortion dilemmas and debates, and unnatural physical, psychological, and social stress that is simply a result of pushing our girls into sexual maturity too early, just as we do to the young cow slaves on the dairy.

Even as they eat milk products, instigating the rape, exploitation, and death of other female animals, women may be viewed simultaneously by men as meat, mere objects to be used. Ironically, just as cows are forced to have unnaturally large and swollen mammary glands to overproduce milk for the dairy industry, the resulting foods produce unnaturally large mammary glands in the women who consume them—a feature that is prized in our herding culture and further reinforces women's status as mere objects for the eyes of men. The interconnected dairy and meat industries perpetuate the patriarchal herding mentality that sees both animals and women as "meat," to be milked and eaten in one case and used sexually in the other.

There are other disasters linked with human consumption of cow's milk products. Charles Attwood, M.D., and T. Colin Campbell, Ph.D., have written,

> Human epidemiological studies have strongly related animal protein consumption to various cancers. Of all animal protein, there is strong experimental evidence that casein, the principal protein of milk, is especially capable of promoting cancer development. . . .
>
> What are the other problems with milk and dairy products? The majority of practicing pediatric allergists insist that more than half of their patients are allergic to one or more of milk's more than two dozen proteins. Their allergy symptoms include eczema, asthma, middle ear infections, sinus infections, rhinitis, gastroenteritis, and allergic colitis—conditions responsible for eighty to ninety percent of doctor's office visits. . . . [20]

Eighty to ninety percent of doctor's office visits—it's not surprising that dairy products are promoted so heavily by the pharmaceutical-media-banking complex and that plant-based diets are discouraged.

The huge pathogen load that is permissible in pasteurized milk—five million pathogens per cup, more than two hundred times the load found in grains, vegetables, fruits, legumes, and nuts if uncontaminated in handling[21]—is a constant stress on the immune system and may increase risks for a whole spectrum of diseases as well as cancers of all types, especially breast and prostate cancer.[22] Cow's milk contains large amounts of pus, which is inevitable due to the high levels of bacteria in the traumatized udders of dairy cows, and pasteurization does not stem the incoming pathogen tide. Some pasteurized milk samples bought and tested by Consumer Reports contained as many as 30 million to 700 million microbes per cup![23] These pathogens, besides increasing risks for gastroenteritis, strep, and a variety of other illnesses, are also known to promote tooth decay, and babies who go to sleep nursing a bottle with cow's milk are well known to risk partial or even complete dissolution of their teeth![24] According to researchers cited by Frank Oski, M.D., eating dairy products is linked with diarrhea, iron-deficiency anemia, gastrointestinal bleeding, kidney disease, eczema, bronchitis, allergies, asthma, hay fever, rheumatoid arthritis, hives, allergy to penicillin, leukemia, multiple sclerosis, and dental decay, as well as to the diabetes, obesity, and atherosclerosis caused by the high fat and cholesterol content.[25]

The protein in milk, particularly casein, while perfect for calves, is too large and difficult for us to digest. Calves have a particular enzyme, rennin, not present in humans, that coagulates and helps breaks down casein. According to renowned nutrition researcher T. Colin Campbell, "Cows' milk protein may be the single most significant chemical carcinogen to which humans are exposed."[26]

On top of this, cow's milk is rich in natural growth hormone, to induce the newborn calf to grow many hundreds of pounds in just the first year of life. This growth-inducing substance, named by scientists insulin-like growth factor one (IGF-1), is absolutely identical, molecularly, to the IGF-1 in humans that spurs our growth as children. The extra dose of growth factor we receive in cow's milk causes us to grow unnaturally, and not just in height. I remember, as a child raised in a typically heavy dairy-eating household, that my teeth were way too large for my mouth and my orthodontist, in sizing the bands needed to straighten them, exclaimed, "Wow! Looks like you've got cow's teeth!"

In adults, studies have shown that excess IGF-1 from eating dairy products may increase the risk of cancer.[27] Since we are not growing, as adults we normally have very little, if any, IGF-1 in our blood to promote the growth of new cells. The IGF-1 that enters our bloodstream when we eat dairy products has serious consequences. Recall that in the trillions of cells in our bodies, there are naturally some cancer cells erupting here and there all the time; with a healthy immune system, these cells are easily discovered and destroyed. Enter IGF-1 from cow's milk. This growth factor is like gasoline thrown on a fire, stimulating sudden, rapid cell division in a small, easy-to-handle cancerous cell growth. The immune system, already overworked by the pathogen load and toxins in the dairy products, may not be able to contain it. The IGF-1 in dairy products may actually be promoting cancer—yet famous people, including health professionals, appear in expensive advertising campaigns sporting milk mustaches, supporting the dairy industry!

Eggs: More Domination of the Feminine

As with dairy products, when we buy eggs we instigate theft and violence against horribly abused females and contribute to environmental contamination, social pathology, and disease. In egg agribusiness, the same principles apply that we have been discussing with the dairy industry, taken to even further extremes. Sentient females are categorized and reduced to mere monetary units of production, imprisoned in unimaginably crowded, stressful, and filthy conditions, their eggs stolen—and then, when they are no longer capable of producing at a high enough level, they are brutally killed.

Chicken eggs are toxic for humans in the manner of all animal products. First, they are made up of animal protein, saturated fat, and cholesterol, all three of which clog arteries, acidify blood and tissues, impair the immune system, and stress the body in a variety of ways, as has been discussed. Eggs, in fact, are *the* most concentrated packets of cholesterol available in supermarkets. Second, eggs concentrate noxious pesticide, chemical, hormonal, and bacterial residue. Third, eating eggs is eating the vibrations of misery, as will become evident below when we look at methods of egg production.

Like all the animals whose bodies are used to produce food for our dining tables, chickens are seen as mere commodities. Individual chickens in egg-laying operations are so cheap to replace that they are virtually worthless and are treated as such. They spend their lives in battery cages, small wire prisons fourteen to sixteen inches high and eighteen to twenty inches across, each containing four to eight hens packed in so tightly that they can never spread their wings. The wires of the cages chafe most of their feathers away, leaving them naked, wounded, and unprotected.[28] They may get their heads, wings, or legs stuck between the wires and thus starve to death, their rotting corpses endured by the other hens in their cage. Their feet are painfully cut by the wires, which can become embedded in their flesh as their feet grow around them. The battery cages are stacked four or five rows high, with the feces and urine from those above falling on the heads and bodies of the birds beneath them, finally landing in a stinking waste pit into which some chickens who manage somehow to escape their prisons fall and slowly die.

As with the dairy industry, the egg industry is founded upon the total domination of the feminine, and upon the manipulation of female bodies to maximize profits with no regard to the outrageous cruelty involved. And because chickens are smaller and held in even lower esteem than cows, they are brutalized even more blatantly in the quest for cheap eggs. Female chicks are routinely debeaked, an exceedingly traumatic operation in which about half of the beak is chopped off. The hot blade cuts through the most sensitive nerve tissue in their beaks, causing such acute pain that the birds' heart rate increases by over one hundred beats per minute. Many die on the spot. For those who survive, the chronic pain from this procedure may last their whole lives and interfere with eating. Male chicks are unneeded, so workers mass-annihilate them, either by live suffocation and crushing in large plastic trash bags or by dumping them living into machines with rotating blades like wood chippers that turn them into instant chicken feed or fertilizer. Hens who no longer produce enough eggs have also been disposed of by being thrown living into the spinning blades of wood chipping machines.

The egg industry acknowledges the huge number of diseases and syndromes that are inherent in the battery system: painful foot and leg deformities, as well as broken and tangled wings and legs, from the wire cages; calcium deficiency, as well as painful prolapsed and distended uteruses, from being forced to produce unnaturally large quantities of eggs; caged layer osteoporosis, which is the loss of bone tissue directly attributed to being immobilized; fatty liver syndrome and swollen head syndrome due to poor-quality food and air and being forced to live constantly in filth and stress; lung and eye problems from the ammonia-drenched air; lost eyes from henpecks by desperate cagemates; and salmonella, in which the hen's oviducts become infested with salmonella bacteria, passing the infection to consumers through the eggs. It is well established that antibiotics are given to battery hens in basically one hundred percent of egg operations to control the bacterial diseases that thrive in these squalid conditions. Antibiotics are also found to increase egg production, but, as with all creatures, including humans, antibiotics increase other problems, since they disrupt and kill the intestinal microflora that are necessary for digestion and elimination, thus weakening the immune system. Toxic pesticide residues from the feed, antibiotic residues, and hormonal, chemical, and pathogenic bacteria residues all concentrate in the fat and eggs of these hens, making them extremely unhealthy to consume.[29]

The tens of thousands of chickens crammed into one egg production shed have nowhere to move and no way to nest, establish social order, or in any way express their natural intelligence or purpose. The artificial lighting schedule that keeps them in almost continuous darkness, and the feed and drugs are all designed with only one goal: to cut costs and maximize the number of eggs that drop from the hens' uteruses and roll down the slanted wire cage bottoms to be whisked away on the conveyor belt. On modern chicken operations, this is over 250 eggs per year, more than two and a half times the number hens would lay under more natural conditions.[30] In nature, a hen is particular about her nest and often chooses the right place to lay her precious egg in partnership with a rooster. When she actually lays the egg in her carefully prepared nest, it is "obviously for the hen a moment full of pride and satisfaction."[31] Contrast this with the following description of egg laying for a caged chicken.

> The frightened battery hen starts to panic as she vainly searches for privacy and a suitable nesting place in the crowded but bare wire cage; then she appears to become oblivious to her surroundings, struggling against the cage as though trying to escape. . . .
>
> Take a moment to imagine yourself as a layer chicken; your home is a crowded cage with a wire floor that causes your feet to hurt and become deformed; there's no room to stretch your legs or flap your wings and they become weak from lack of exercise; but at the same time, you can never be still because there is always one of your miserable cell mates who needs to move about; one of the other chickens is always picking on you and you cannot get away—except by letting others sit on top of you; the air is filled with dust and flying feathers that stick to the sides of the cage splattered with chicken shit from the inmates in the cage upstairs; it is hard to breathe—there is

the choking stench of ammonia in the air from the piles of manure under the cages and you don't feel at all well; the flies are unbearable despite the insecticide sprayed in the air and laced in your food—to kill the fly larvae before they mature; the food—never green and fresh—seldom varies and tastes always of the chemical additives and drugs needed to keep you alive; eventually, despite your wretchedness and anguish, and the tormented din of thousands of birds shrieking their pain together, you lay an egg and watch it roll out of sight; but the joy of making a nest, of giving birth, of clucking to your chicks is absent—laying the egg is an empty, frustrating, and exhausting ritual.[32]

All family and social and natural life is destroyed. These hens know neither mothers nor children, neither mates nor earth nor sun. They are born in hatcheries, debeaked and then sentenced to the caged slavery of egg production.

When a population of thousands of hens in an egg operation is at the end of its laying cycle, the hens will either be gassed and killed, since their tortured bodies have so little flesh they aren't worth the trouble of shipping to slaughter, or they may be slaughtered for the low-grade meat used in chicken soup and pet food. Often, though, the hens are force-molted first, to shock their bodies into another cycle of egg laying. This is done by withholding food and water and administering a combination of drugs, including hormones. The forced starvation may last up to two weeks, typically killing many birds in the process. After they have been force-molted once or twice, soon to be slaughtered for chicken soup, the birds are roughly yanked from their cages, tossed into trucks, and taken away to make room for the next wave of hen slaves. We can perhaps be born into no worse hell in this universe than being a female chicken on an industrial egg farm in the United States.

In so-called free-range egg operations the hens are all typically debeaked, as in standard egg factories, and males are all brutally killed at birth. The chickens are still treated as objects, pushed to produce, and killed cruelly when they are no longer profitable. The term free-range has surprisingly little legal meaning, and there are thus no rules governing the amount of space a free-range hen must have, so though their confinement may be less extreme than the usual battery cages, they are nevertheless typically crammed together in enormous, stinking sheds where they never see the light of day.[33]

The Web of Connections

Female cows and chickens are ruthlessly dominated to provide products that are vital and healthy for their offspring, community, and species but cause disease, pollution, hunger, and suffering when consumed by humans. When we steal their milk and eggs and kill their children, we set up the conditions for the same to happen to us. The fates of cow mothers and human mothers, cow babies and human babies, ultimately run parallel. If we allow corporations to steal, use, and kill cow and chicken babies, it will happen to our babies also. In fact, it is already happening.

The negative effects of consuming dairy products and eggs on individual health are linked to negative consequences for our world ecosystems and our culture. Everything is connected; the consumption of dairy products and eggs is linked with: allergies, skin disorders, cancer, heart disease, strokes, diabetes, and a laundry list of other ailments; the arsenal of products and procedures marketed by the medical industry to combat these unnecessary ailments (all of which are major sources of pollution and disempowerment); the enormous profits accumulated by the agribusiness, chemical, pharmaceutical, and banking industries from our domination of female animals; the social inequality and injustice that this promotes, giving rise to elitism and further conflict; the environmental and human health effects of agricultural runoff, which is poisoning rivers, killing fish, contributing to human cancer, and causing red tides that inflict respiratory disease; the lives lost in wars caused by spiraling demand for petroleum and by desperation, as water rights go to rich agribusiness dairy and chicken operations funded by U.S. banks in Third World countries while poor people face chronic thirst and contaminated water. . . .

The web of connections surrounding our consumption of dairy products and eggs is vast and includes all beings. When we feed on other animals' milk and eggs, we are feeding on their fear and despair, on the violence that a patriarchal mentality systematically enforces on them. If we look deeply, we'll see that this mentality breeds violence in our lives as well. Should we, who long for mercy, freedom, and joy, and for a more enlightened society that supports peace and respect for our earth and the sacredness of all life, be the agents of such violence? When we make the connection between our culturally induced desire to eat dairy and egg products and the cruelty to vulnerable mothers that this will necessarily entail, our intelligence and compassion are nourished, and we naturally begin to make new choices. There are plenty of substitutes for animal-derived milk products and eggs, and they are becoming increasingly available as more of us make these connections.

Reviving Sophia

Dominating others requires us to disconnect from them, and from aspects of ourselves as well. In exploiting dairy cows and hens, we dominate them not just for their flesh, skin, bones, and the other body parts that we can use or sell; we specifically exploit their uteruses and mammary glands. This inhumane desecration of the most intimate and life-giving functions of the feminine principle, that of giving birth to new life and of tenderly nourishing that life, harms us perhaps as deeply as it does the cows, though our wounds may be less obvious. Many spiritual teachers have pointed out that when we harm others, we harm ourselves even more severely. The hard-heartedness of the killer and exploiter is in itself a terrible punishment because it is a loss of sensitivity to the beauty and sacredness of life. That loss may go unrecognized, but the life itself, armored, violent, and competitive, is lived as a struggle of separateness and underlying fear, and its relations with others are poisoned.

By enslaving and cruelly exploiting cow mothers and babies in dairy operations, we attack and injure the sacred feminine within ourselves as well as in nature. This is an attack on our essential being, on our sense of nurturing life and protecting the vulnerable. These are truly terrible seeds to be sowing, for the feminine principle within us all is the seat of loving-kindness, receptivity, caring, and the urge to nurture and protect.

In attacking our own inner feminine principle, we become as a culture harder and more separate, competitive, aggressive, and self-centered. Ironically, we become commodities ourselves, controlled and enslaved by a system of our own making, yet we don't realize it because we've been taught to disconnect. We learn to cover our ears to block out the plaintive cries of cow mothers on dairies. We block out the cries of human mothers whose babies are taken from them—thousands every day—by easily preventable starvation. We block out the cries of mothers whose babies are killed by bombs and bullets fired by boys serving the military death machine. Who will hear or heed our cries if we don't heed the cries of these mothers?

Liberating and honoring the feminine principle is perhaps the most pressing task in our culture's evolution toward peace, sustainability, and spiritual maturity. The feminine principle, cross-culturally, is concerned fundamentally with nurturing, receptivity, making connections, intuition, and bringing forth new life. In our herding culture, these qualities are not respected because the work of herding animals requires men to become hard and cruel, and to emphasize their separateness from and superiority to animals, nature, and the life-giving processes of the feminine. This has led to a patriarchal mentality concerned fundamentally with domination, control, separation, rational analysis, commodification, war, and killing. Its basic dictum in human affairs follows from its fundamental herding orientation toward animals, which is that might makes right. And yet the feminine principle is still alive, longed for, and beloved, because we know at the deepest levels that this is a vital aspect of our essential nature.

Veneration of the sacred feminine goes back many millennia, predating the rise of our herding culture, and we still remember this even though the ancient goddesses have been supplanted by the decidedly male deities now recognized by conventional Western religion and science, the Lord God/Jehovah and Reason. The Greek term for the third person of the Trinity, the Holy Spirit, *Hagia Sophia* or Holy Wisdom, was feminine, though this was lost when translated later into Latin as the masculine *Spiritus Sanctus*, which made all three aspects of the Christian trinity male to the detriment of women, animals, nature, and our culture's spiritual depth. The loss of Sophia—Holy Wisdom—was inevitable as the domination and male violence required by commodifying animals continued to spread and intensify. But Sophia, though repressed, could never die, and has lived on, disguised as Mary, as Beatrice, and as the *Paraclete*, another term for the Holy Spirit, Greek for "Comforter." One form this takes is the resilient archetype of the Fairy Godmother, symbolizing the benevolent feminine process mediating between the visible and invisible realms. *Philo-sophia*, literally the "love of wisdom," was originally a quest for Sophia as intuitive wisdom that would be spiritually liberating and significant. As the feminine principle and intuition were increasingly trivialized and despised, however, Western philosophy lost much of its potential depth and eventually became a shallow accomplice to science.

Sophia's symbol is the cup, grail, or chalice, which, unlike the traditional symbol of male divinity—the sword, spear, blade, or thunderbolt—is nonviolent and non-threatening. It holds, nurtures, fills, mixes, connects, and gives birth. The cauldron and bowl represent the feminine receptivity that is essential to intuitive wisdom and spiritual maturity. Sophia's cup eventually became the central image of one of our most fundamental stories, that of the Holy Grail, in which sword-bearing knights searched in vain to find the lost grail cup. At deep levels, we recognize that what has been lost is the feminine approach to wisdom and that an unbalanced masculine approach of unbridled reductionism brings war, disease, and perversity to the degree it has repressed the feminine principle and spurned a partnership with the wisdom that connects, nurtures, and gives form to life.

In myths, fairy tales, poetry, drama, art, and other deep cultural expressions, we can see the loss mourned everywhere, from Odysseus, Orestes, Antigone, and the Ramayana through Faust, Galahad, Lear, and Parsifal to modern epics like *Star Wars* and the *Lord of the Rings*. The true self or radiant indwelling Christ-nature is repressed or lost and is replaced by a false self, a persona or mask that is insecure, fragmented, proud, and convinced of its separateness and need to dominate and control. In fairy tales, one way this is expressed is through archetypal tales involving a wrongful ruler who usurps the throne and drives the country and people into war, poverty, and ruin. We sometimes see this mythic archetype thrust strikingly into reality on the world's political stage, with false and rigged elections and the disastrous consequences of administrations that further the oppressive and violent herder mentality by propagating war and the interests of a privileged elite at the expense of disadvantaged people, animals, ecosystems, and future generations.

At a deeper symbolic level, the mask and the usurper represent not only the deluded and conniving ego, but also our native herding culture, which has spread and conquered less aggressive cultures and still enforces its mentality of domination and its core practice of commodifying and eating animals. The usurper continues today, attacking nature, women, animals, and the vulnerable as it strives to consolidate control in a few elite hands. It derives power from the public's regular daily meals of hidden violence. Consuming and killing have become defining activities, fed by the disconnectedness and repressed guilt that accompany our suppression of the feminine principle. Beings who are the subjects of their lives are forced into the role of mere objects, and both people and animals end up becoming things. The way hunters, fishers, and herders look at animals, the way corporate developers look at nature, and the way men are typically taught to look at women, and how women typically learn to be looked at by men, are all part of this process.

Enormous suffering is inevitable in all this, polluting relationships and eroding the spiritual sensitivity that sees beyond materialistic, I-it dualisms to the sacred subjects that are always present in living beings. As individuals and as a culture, our ability to heal, transform, and evolve beyond this old defiling mentality is tied to our food choices more than to anything else. To meditate for world peace, to pray for a better world, and to work for social justice and environmental protection while continuing to purchase the flesh, milk, and eggs of horribly abused animals exposes a disconnect that is so fundamental that it renders our efforts absurd, hypocritical, and doomed to certain failure.

We are hearing a call from our inner wisdom to reawaken respect for the feminine principle. Can we ever be successful in answering this call while still imprisoning, raping, abusing, and killing millions of mothers just for our pleasure, continuing our subservience to social pressure and indoctrination? The inner feminine is our intuition, our sensitivity, and our ability to sense the profound interconnectedness of events and beings, and it is vital to peace, wisdom, joy, intelligence, creativity, and spiritual awakening. With every baby calf stolen from her mother and killed, with every gallon of milk stolen from enslaved and broken mothers, with every thrust of the raping sperm gun, with every egg stolen from a helpless, frantic hen, and with every baby chick killed or locked for life in a hellish nightmare cage, we kill the sacred feminine within ourselves. By ordering and eating products from the industrial herding complex that dominates the feminine with an iron fist, we squelch our opportunities for maturing to higher levels of understanding, sensitivity, and compassion. We remain merely ironic in our quests.

Our welfare is ultimately dependent on the welfare of others. By freeing and encouraging others we are liberated and encouraged. We can never sever our connection to all beings, but we can ignore and violate it, planting seeds of tragedy and suffering. Honoring our natural place in the web of life by eating the foods intended for us will plant seeds of abundance, love, and freedom, whatever our religion may be. Our prayers for peace will bear fruit when we are living the prayer for peace and, most importantly, when we offer peace to those who are at our mercy and who also long for peace and the freedom to live their lives and fulfill their purposes.

Achieving peace among human beings, from the household to the international battlefields, depends upon treating each other with respect and kindness. This will be possible when we first extend that respect and kindness to those who are at our mercy and who cannot retaliate against us. If we are sincere in our quest for human peace, freedom, and dignity, we have no choice but to offer this to our neighbors, the animals of this earth. Cultivating awareness, we can transcend the imposed view that animals are mere food objects. With this, we will see consumerism, pornography, and the disconnectedness that leads inexorably to slavery and self-destruction evaporate. As the mentality of domination and exclusivism fades, we will be able to heal divisions of gender, race, and class.

CHAPTER EIGHT

THE METAPHYSICS OF FOOD

⇝

"There's nothing more difficult than waking someone who is only
pretending to be asleep."
—BISHOP DESMOND TUTU

"All beings tremble before violence. All fear death. All love life. See
yourself in others. Then whom can you hurt? What harm can you do?"
—BUDDHA

"Everybody, soon or late, sits down to a banquet of consequences."
—ROBERT LOUIS STEVENSON

Eating Vibrations

Animal foods concentrate both physical and metaphysical toxins. The
physical toxins in animal foods such as the trans fats, pathogens, and
pesticide, drug, and hormone residues, besides injuring our bodily
health, can also disturb us mentally and emotionally. Mood swings, irritability, and loss of attentiveness are well-known side effects of drugs
and chemicals and the power of psychoactive substances is well documented. We are rediscovering what Pythagoras taught us: that eating
animal foods has negative effects on our consciousness; one recognized

biomechanism for this is the sex hormone testosterone. Consciousness theorist Ken Wilber writes,

> Studies on testosterone—in the laboratory, cross-culturally, embry-onically, and even what happens when women are given testosterone injections for medical reasons—all point to a simple conclusion. I don't mean to be crude, but it appears that testosterone basically has two, and only two, major drives: fuck it or kill it.
>
> And males are saddled with this biological nightmare almost from day one, a nightmare women can barely imagine (except when they are given testosterone injections for medical purposes, which drives them nuts. As one woman put it, "I can't stop thinking about sex. Please, can't you make this stop?")[1]

Studies have repeatedly shown that high levels of testosterone are associated with aggressive-destructive behavior, impatience, and irritability.[2] In addition, it's now understood that diets high in animal fat and low in plant fiber lead to a retention and concentration of sex hormones like testosterone in the body. The fiber of vegetables, grains, and other plant foods binds these circulating hormones and "keeps them in check"[3] through SHBG (sex hormone binding globulin), which increases with plant food intake. Neil Barnard writes,

> In the Massachusetts Male Aging Study, a large, ongoing study of middle-aged and older men in the Boston area, researchers have found that those men with more SHBG in their blood are less domineering and aggressive. It may well be that a better diet can make you an easier-to-get-along-with partner.[4]

Research has also shown that children with the nutritional deficiencies often found in diets low in vegetables, fruits, grains, and legumes are more disposed to violent and antisocial behavior as they grow older.[5]

Beyond this physical level of biomechanisms such as hormone levels, toxins, and nutrients, there are metaphysical forces at work that though ignored are nevertheless operating. Metaphysical toxins—i.e., the concentrated vibrations of terror, grief, frustration, and desperation permeating these foods—are invisible and completely unrecognized by conventional science, yet they may be even more disturbing to us than physical toxins because they work on the level of feelings and consciousness, which are more essential dimensions of ourselves than our physical vehicle.

By purchasing or ordering animal products we directly cause misery and sow seeds of despair and cruel violence. It would be naïve to think these seeds simply disappear into thin air. The terror, pain, and frustration we cause to feeling creatures, whose bodies and minds are tormented beyond imagining, are extremely powerful forces that affect us, their causative agents, in many ways. When we nourish the cells with which we think and feel with the flesh and secretions of these terrorized animals, we absorb the vibrations of fear, disease, and violence, no matter how we try to disguise this with euphemisms and distractions.

Physicists are beginning to glimpse the truth that mystics and sages have been pointing toward for centuries, that the world that appears to us through our senses is a vibrational phenomenon. Energy that vibrates within a certain range becomes perceptible to us as "matter," and vibrations outside that range, though not necessarily perceptible by our senses, still exist. Standing in a dark, quiet room, for example, we may not see or hear anything, but if we turn on a radio or television, we will suddenly become aware of the music, conversations, ads and TV programs that have been with us in the room, unperceived because we lacked the equipment to perceive them. In a similar way, we may look at an egg and see just a material thing, but if we had the necessary intuitive equipment, we could become much more aware of the egg as a vibrational entity. Though our mind may be blocked from seeing, feeling, or sensing the egg as a vibrational energy system, our body, which is also a vibratory system, will be affected by it at the essential vibratory level. Our body knows what vibration it is eating, as does our mind at the deeper levels beyond conscious awareness.

We have probably all experienced being in a physically beautiful place and noticed that if we are angry, jealous, or afraid, or if the people with us are, then the physical beauty cannot be appreciated. The converse is also true. Joy, nobility, compassion, high energy, and pure vibrations can transform any physical surrounding into a paradise, and fear or anger can make any paradise (for example, our earth) into a hell or a prison gulag. Our inability to fully recognize, appreciate, and protect the inexhaustible, spectacular beauty of our earth and of her creatures is due to our inner desensitization to vibrational energy frequencies—the numbness that keeps us from screaming or weeping when we bite into a hot dog or cheeseburger.

At the level of vibrational frequency, our bodies know and respond to the vibrations of environments and situations, of relationships, of emotions, and especially of what we eat. It has been well known for generations that the milk of a mother who is angry or disturbed will often make her baby sick. While most scientists continue to restrict their search to materialist explanations for phenomena, modern physics, for example, is demonstrating that matter is energy and that consciousness is fundamental, far more fundamental than energy-matter.

Both the uncertainty principle and the observer effect, foundational to quantum physics,[6] imply that the appearance of energy-matter is inseparable from and conditioned by consciousness; the universe is not fundamentally physical but is an arising in awareness, in consciousness. Max Planck, the Nobel Prize-winning father of quantum theory, wrote, for example, "All matter originates and exists only by virtue of a force. . . . We must assume behind this force the existence of a conscious and intelligent Mind. This Mind is the matrix of all matter."[7]

These apparent three—consciousness, energy, and matter—are finally slowly being recognized for what they are: a unity. Consciousness and energy-matter are mutually conditioning, interpenetrating, and interdependent in utterly profound and mysterious ways. Consciousness is primary and essential, and what appears as energy-matter is ultimately a manifestation of consciousness. It is consciousness, for example, that ultimately heals; the huge variety of healing methods may all be seen as placebos, as Andrew Weil has discussed at length in *Health and Healing*, because they work to the degree that the mind believes in them, from shamanism to herbs to acupuncture to surgery and drugs.[8] Some spiritual forms of healing recognize this basic truth, yet our culture's established institutions still reflect the overwhelmingly materialist and reductionist prejudice of our underlying mentality, desensitized by the constant practice from childhood of blocking awareness and sensibility during our daily meals.

As we become more alert to energy and to vibrations, we see directly the link between consciousness and matter. Our lives on the physical level are an outpicturing of our thoughts and feelings—our consciousness. Some intuitive humans and many nonhuman animals may be much more sensitive to subtle energy information than most of us are; their natural intelligence senses energy vibrations in situations and individuals, and they may directly know the consciousness that is giving rise to a particular situation, or that is manifesting as a group or individual. For example, observers are often amazed to see impalas and lions relaxing in close proximity to each other and wonder how the impalas routinely sense when lions are dangerous and when they're satiated. It's well known that intuitive people, as well as cats, dogs, pigs, and many other animals, are sensitive to the vibrations of feeling and intention that they perceive in people, and that they have access to information to which most of us are oblivious.[9]

If we take another look at the egg, bacon, or cheese we are purchasing and eating, we see clearly that it is a living vibratory embodiment of cruelty, violence, enslavement, terror, and despair. The tormented consciousness of the animals and the hardened consciousness of those humans who abuse sentient creatures and exploit them for money have blended to create a "food" that is toxic at the deepest levels. It generates turmoil and disease in the physical, mental, emotional, spiritual, and social dimensions of our being. If we could look at eggs, at dairy products, and at processed animal flesh with enlightened eyes that see beyond physical appearance, we would shrink, horrified, from the idea of causing such misery, much less actually serving it as food to our loved ones and to ourselves.

Many cultures recognize that food that is prepared with love and caring attention to detail is more healthful than food that is prepared with indifference or, even worse, with irritation or anger. For this reason, for example, in many Zen monasteries, only the most senior and advanced meditation monks are allowed to prepare food in the monastery kitchen.

In India, mothers have been encouraged for centuries to cook in a loving, calm, and meditative mood so that the food they prepare for their children will nourish them not only physically but also emotionally and spiritually. They believe that it is the universal energy, or *prana*, in food that gives us energy. The vibrational field of the person preparing the food is also a form of prana and can increase or decrease the food's healthy vibration. There are many other cultures and religions that recognize that food is an intimate vehicle of energy and consciousness, and that when it is prepared with love, mindfulness, and gratitude, these vibrations bless and support the fortunate recipients of the food.

It's also widely recognized that when food is eaten in an attitude of mindfulness and appreciation, it's more nourishing than if eaten in a distracted, hurried, or irritated frame of mind. The Zen Buddhist teacher Thich Nhat Hanh writes, for example, in *Peace Is Every Step*, "Contemplating our food for a few seconds before eating, and eating in mindfulness can bring us much happiness."[10] Monastic and yogic traditions have long recognized the benefit of eating mindfully and prayerfully as a meditation, being fully in the present moment of eating, and contemplating the origin of the food and giving thanks for it. This practice is believed to increase the energy and nutritional value of our food by opening us more fully to it.

Eating is an act of connecting. Even if we eat alone, we are not alone. The food we are eating connects us with the rhythms, forces, and abundance of nature and of our universe, and with the presence of those who nurtured and gathered the foods we are eating. Fields, forests, oceans, rivers, wildlife, farmers, and grocers are all with us and become part of us as we chew and digest the food. People we think of while we are chewing and digesting our food become a part of us also. Cross-culturally, meals are events of social bonding and communion. When we eat together as a family or a community, and especially if we do it in an attitude of appreciation of the food and the opportunity of being together, we strengthen the bonds of understanding and love between us.

If we consume animal foods, all of these elements of energy and consciousness are diminished by the violence and fear inherent in the vibration of the foods we are eating. Thich Nhat Hanh says it plainly:

When we eat an egg or a chicken, we know that the egg or chicken can also contain a lot of anger. We are eating anger, and therefore we express anger. . . . So be aware. Be careful what you eat. If you eat anger, you will become and express anger. If you eat despair, you will express despair. If you eat frustration, you will express frustration.[11]

Since there is such an obvious and overwhelmingly strong vibration of violence, fear, and despair in animal foods, when we prepare the food we are not likely to do so mindfully, but mechanically and quickly, in order to avoid awakening our natural sensitivity. We tend to eat these foods in a disconnected way as well. To maintain our pretense that we are oblivious to the obvious horror on our plates, we eat quickly and keep ourselves busy and distracted. Fast food and the industrialization of eating are understandable outcomes of eating animal foods over an extended period. The aggressive busyness of our culture and our outward-looking expansionist orientation are rooted historically and currently in our discomfort with how we treat the animals we eat and the hardness we cultivate toward their suffering.

Food, like all apparently physical matter, is energy and vibration and is a manifestation of consciousness, and though it is important to prepare, eat, and share food mindfully, we can see that it's important to look more deeply than this, to the actual source of our food. When we instigate violence and slavery with our food purchases, it is inevitable that the consciousness of violence and slavery will be planted in our psychophysical being, dulling our feelings and undermining our possible attempts to prepare and eat the food mindfully and thankfully. Matter, energy, and consciousness are inseparable, and the cruelty unavoidably embodied in animal foods is a potent and unrecognized toxin, damaging not just to our physical health, but to our emotional and spiritual health as well.

With the Eyes of an Angel

Animal foods are also toxic to us and our world for another reason. Just as we must harden and desensitize ourselves to produce and eat them, our culture must produce certain hardened people to manipulate and kill the unfortunate creatures. When we make it a goal to cultivate cruelty and remorselessness in some people, all of us are hurt. In conspiring to pretend that we do not recognize the pain we cause, we deaden the compassion, intelligence, and creativity of our children and of all our people.

We silence our compassion at the circuses, rodeos, racetracks, zoos, and other places where animals are imprisoned and used for our entertainment. In these places most of the violence and cruelty is kept hidden from public view. If we contemplate these places deeply and educate ourselves, however, the inherent violence becomes obvious and disturbing. The only way, for example, to get non-domesticated animals like elephants, monkeys, tigers, dolphins, seals, and orcas to do tricks or work is by inflicting pain and fear through beatings and electroshocks, and/or through food deprivation. Circus trainers are taught to dominate elephants by beating them with bullhooks, bears dance because as babies they were forced to remain on hot metal plates while their "trainers" played music, and dolphins do tricks only because they otherwise face the pain of hunger. Zoos imprison innocent animals, buying and selling them to increase their revenue and the number of "baby" animals, which are by far the most lucrative attractions, while older animals typically end up in "canned hunt" facilities where they are shot as trophies by sportsmen at point-blank range. We dull our sensitivity when we use animals for clothing, furniture, jewelry, and other products, shutting down our awareness of the horror and torment inflicted on living beings to provide them. And we stifle our empathy in scientific research and education, where we teach each other that the suffering of non-human animals is of little consequence. It starts perhaps with school chick-hatching projects, progresses through biology lab frog dissection, and culminates in the millions of animals tortured by researchers working for the military, industrial, scientific, and educational establishments.

Underlying this cultural deadening, of course, are our meals, our fundamental social activity. And to create these meals, we must undergo the further deadening of choosing and buying animal products. Every time we make the decision to purchase the eggs, fluids, or flesh of animals, we enforce the disconnection between consumer and what is consumed. When we take out our wallets and pay for an animal's flesh or secretions, at that moment we directly instigate violence, fear, slavery, death, and the spread of toxic pollution. At that moment the seeds are actually sown. We are the mafia boss paying the hired gun to kill, and even if we're not using the knife, our white shirt is spoiled.

If we could look over the world we live in with the eyes of an angel, an intuitively awakened being, and see energy vibrations rather than just physical forms, we would see that the wars and violence on our earth are generated from a vast complex of venues where deadening takes place: the countless kitchens and dining rooms, inns, hotels, restaurants, resorts, cafeterias, mess halls, fast food outlets, supermarkets, stores, butcher shops, malls, ice cream stands, snack bars, ships, campgrounds, racetracks, picnic areas, circuses, convention centers, fairs, schools, sports stadiums, churches, casinos, prisons, military bases, nursing homes, nursery schools, hospitals, zoos, and mental institutions where animal flesh, eggs, and dairy products are bought and sold, prepared and eaten. Compassion is deadened and truth ignored in virtually every home, shopping plaza, and institution in our culture. Until we see them for what they are, these inescapable forces will continue to foster denial and violence in every apparently unsuspecting patron. That we cannot see this, and assume our way of living is sane, humane, honorable, and kind, only shows how blind we have become.

Our intuitive angel, looking over our world, would see not only these millions upon millions of deadening venues throughout the cities, suburbs, and rural communities we have erected. She would also see enormous pulsating centers radiating fear, violence, horror, and frustration: the tens of thousands of factory farms, slaughterhouses, stockyards, feedlots, and aquaculture and fishing operations where animals are enslaved, tormented, and brutally killed by the billions every year. Most of these operations, though they are enormous, imprisoning and killing tens and even hundreds of thousands of individuals, are hidden from public view. Huge floating death ships work far out at sea. In the countryside, animal processing facilities are purposefully located far from main roads and population centers, fenced off from public entry.

Their names are vague and euphemistic, like the "Carolina Protein Products" sign I once saw on a large, ominous-looking building far from the highway. But to our intuitive angel, they are not hidden at all, but rise gigantic, towering over the landscape, the intensity and thunderous volume of the suffering within their walls billowing high as roiling vibrational fields of grief, terror, panic, and despair. Radiating thought forms of abuse, domination, and enslavement darken the sky, spreading into the surrounding communities, polluting the energy fields and consciousness fields that connect us all, humans and animals alike. This massive and unremitting negative energy, the despair and pain of the millions upon millions of sensitive individuals imprisoned and killed needlessly for our conditioned cravings, is perhaps the most serious pollution we humans create. Its repercussions ripple out through the vast and intricate webs of thought, energy, and consciousness that form our human relationships with each other, with animals and nature, and with our children, our dreams, and our aspirations.

Many people have understood the tragic implications of this pollution of the earth's vibrational field with the agony of our animal brothers and sisters. Tolstoy, for example, wrote that as long as we have slaughterhouses, we will have battlefields. According to Nobel Prize–winning novelist Isaac Bashevis Singer, "As long as people will shed the blood of innocent creatures there can be no peace, no liberty, no harmony between people. Slaughter and justice cannot dwell together." Charles Fillmore, the co-founder of the Unity School of Practical Christianity in Kansas City, wrote in 1903,

In San Francisco a number of years ago many people were made violently ill from eating meat bought at a certain shop. Physicians investigated and they found that the carcass of a certain steer was the source, and it was presumed that it was diseased. Further inquiry developed this to be an error—the animal was unusually healthy and vigorous—in fact so vigorous and forceful that he fought for his life for over an hour after the attempt to kill him began. He was in a frenzy of terror and anger; his eyes were bloodshot and he frothed at the mouth while the butchers were trying to slay him. The physicians decided that the anger and terror of this steer poisoned his meat in a manner similar to that of the angry mother her milk, which is well known to make the infant sick.

This instance was but an exaggeration of conditions that exist in milder form in all animal flesh offered for food in our markets. Before they are slain these poor brutes are maltreated in ways almost beyond enumeration. Visit shipping pens, stock-trains, stockyards and packinghouses, if you want evidence of the sufferings of the poor beasts of the field. And these very sufferings are through the law of sympathetic mental vibrations transferred to the flesh of those who eat the bodies of these animals. The undefined fears, the terrors of the nightmare, and the many disturbances in stomach and bowels that man endures may be in a measure traced to these unsuspected sources.[12]

Fillmore was writing a hundred years ago in a time that seems quaint, when we could actually track meat to a particular animal. Eric Schlosser, author of *Fast Food Nation*, says that in one of our hamburgers there may be the flesh of dozens of different animals, from all parts of the hemisphere. The suffering the animals must endure is certainly much worse today as well, with the extreme confinement, bizarre drug manipulations and excruciating mutilations practiced on industrialized factory farms. And while we may guardedly discuss the cholesterol and artificial hormone residues in animals foods, the sheer misery we eat and its toxic effect is never seriously considered. We are blinded by our culture's materialism, a natural outgrowth of our eating habits.

In 1910 Fillmore elaborated on his earlier ideas, writing:

Every animal will fight for its life. What then can be the mental condition of the animal that has been cruelly forced into contracted pens and cars, and finally deprived of its body amid the most terrifying surroundings? Can it be otherwise than that its entire consciousness is permeated by violent vibrations of terror that act and react upon all planes of animal life with which they come into contact? You think that you eat a material thing called meat, but the fact is there is no such thing in reality. The flesh may seem to your outer sense to be a dead, inert mass, but, could your soul eye be opened, you would behold mental currents pervading its every atom, acting and reacting upon each other in a wild, bewildered manner, like the animal of whose body it formed a part. You are taking into your temple elements that will unsettle it, elements that you will have difficulty in harmonizing.[13]

Even if we attempt to prepare and eat animal foods slowly and mindfully, both the reality and our thought of what we are preparing and eating are disturbing to our natural sense of compassion for other living creatures. By desecrating animals, we create energy fields that desecrate us and block our purpose on this earth: to unfold wisdom, love, and understanding. Instead, we have become agents of ugliness and death, serving the interests of enormous industrial conglomerates and corporations that exist primarily to maximize their own self-centered profits and power. And we have hardened ourselves and our children, who, like innocent sponges, soak up our attitudes and beliefs and pass them on to their children as our parents and grandparents have done.

Masks and Fear

Our psychological hardening is an armoring that protects us from feeling the grief and pain we would naturally feel. It desensitizes us and masks our true nature from ourselves. With this in mind, it is fascinating to examine the phenomenal success of the potent and costly milk mustache advertising campaign, which was generated and promoted by our government through the Fluid Milk Promotion Act of 1990.[14] The milk mustache can be seen as an archetypal mask, and the campaign appeals to our deep knowing that in order to abuse animals and eat their bodies and secretions we must wear a mask. The little white mustache triggers an unconscious recognition that dairy products mask terrible cruelty, yet the goodness associated with the color white provides the emotional relief we crave. Working on the unconscious levels of archetypal symbols the dairy industry thus promotes its products by exploiting our deep ambivalence about animal foods, signified by the mask, and transforms that ambivalence into a psychological release or catharsis by showing the milk mustache masks being worn by the gods of our culture: the most prominent figures in athletics, entertainment, science, and politics. The mask represents our culture's covering up of the hidden misery in the dairy industry and its brutal domination of the feminine, and because this is the last thing we want to support and partake of, we pretend to be oblivious to the suffering involved.

This unseen shadow of violence generates an irrepressible energy field within our culture. All animal researchers know that fear is one of the most powerful and basic emotions for all animals (including us), and extreme fear is an inescapable reality for the animals in our factory farms and slaughterhouses. Albert Schweitzer, in urging kindness to animals, wrote, "Pain is a more terrible lord . . . than even death himself.[15] By inflicting massive amounts of both acute pain and chronic pain on the animals we eat, we generate similarly massive amounts of acute fear and chronic fear. We eat terror and are thus fascinated with it, lured by the lurid, the grotesque, and the violent. Our fascination with blood, death, terror, and violence is a manifestation of the repressed shadow of our wholesale brutality and killing of animals, sublimated and projected into countless expressions in the mass media and in popular entertainment. Violence and horror in movies, novels, and music fascinate and attract us only because we are regularly eating violence and horror and are therefore complicit. The knives, swords, and guns that permeate the popular media reflect the killing and stunning guns fired around the clock in slaughterhouses and the long knives that bleed the animals there and carve their flesh for our consumption. Though we hide and repress the violence of our meals, it erupts on our movie screens and televisions, undeniable, fascinating, and irresistibly interesting to us.

By celebrating and cultivating terror and cruelty in the media, we sow those same seeds in consciousness and they bear fruit in further violence. Increased violence in the media, especially television, has been conclusively linked with increased violence in child TV viewers. The violence we practice against animals for food, sublimated and projected through the TV as violence against people, then becomes violence by children, with animals being the easiest and most vulnerable targets.

Fishing, hunting, and abusing pets and caught wild animals are some of the ways children express this acculturated violence, which further legitimizes the most pervasive practice of violence against animals—slaughtering and eating them. The link between children's violence against animals and their later violence against humans, now well established, is yet another reminder of the Pythagorean principle that our mistreatment of animals inevitably boomerangs as cruelty to each other and the untold suffering this causes.

Cultivating Compassion

The cycle of violence that starts on our dinner tables reverberates through our families, our communities, and through all our relations, rippling into the field of our shared awareness. If we had the clear vision of an angel, we would see that it reverberates around the planet in incalculable ways and into incalculable dimensions. What we are, and what all beings and manifestations ultimately are, is consciousness. Consciousness manifests vehicles, which are sacred embodiments for the expression, growth, and development of consciousness. All of us are parts of something far greater, and we all have a unique purpose and contribution to make. The idea that consciousness is merely an epiphenomenon of matter is an erroneous reversal. It is the myth of materialism that the shallow, terrorized and terrorizing mentality of domination has invented and propagates in order to maintain its blindness to the painful but liberating understanding of the interconnectedness of all life and the fundamentally spiritual nature of all beings. No being is merely a material thing or object, and no being can thus ever be a commodity or article of property. We are all infinitely mysterious manifestations of consciousness, and spiritual maturity is an awakening from the crippling limitations of materialism and separatism, accompanied by a sense of love and compassion for all creatures.

This idea has been articulated by mystics, saints, and sages from all traditions and cultures since time immemorial. Two contemporaries 2,500 years ago in India—Mahavira, founder of the Jain tradition, and Gautama Buddha—preached the fundamental spiritual necessity of cultivating an attitude of *ahimsa*, or non-harmfulness, in their followers' relations with both humans and animals. The Buddha says, for example, in the *Mahaparinirvana-sutra*, "Eating meat destroys the attitude of great compassion."[16] The twelfth-century Tibetan Buddhist poet-saint Milarepa sings, "Accustomed long to contemplating love and compassion, I have forgotten all difference between myself and others."[17] The seventh-century Christian mystic Saint Isaac the Syrian asks,

> What is a charitable heart? It is a heart which is burning with love for the whole creation, for men, for the birds, for the beasts . . . for all creatures. He who has such a heart cannot see or call to mind a creature without his eyes being filled with tears by reason of the immense compassion which seizes his heart; a heart which is softened and can no longer bear to see or learn from others of any suffering, even the smallest pain being inflicted upon a creature. That is why such a man never ceases to pray for the animals . . . moved by the infinite pity which reigns in the hearts of those who are becoming united with God.[18]

John Wesley, the eighteenth-century founder of Methodism, writes, "I believe in my heart that faith in Jesus Christ can and will lead us beyond an exclusive concern for the well-being of other human beings to the broader concern for the well-being of the birds in our backyards, the fish in our rivers, and every living creature on the face of the earth."[19]

The ninth-century Islamic Sufi saint Misri says, "Never think of anyone as inferior to you. Open the inner Eye and you will see the One Glory shining in all creatures."[20]

Albert Einstein articulates it in this way:

> A human being is a part of the whole, called by us the "Universe," a part limited in time and space. He experiences himself, his thoughts and feelings, as something separated from the rest—a kind of optical delusion of his consciousness. This delusion is a kind of prison for us, restricting us to our personal desires and to affection for a few persons nearest to us. Our task must be to free ourselves from this

prison by widening our circle of compassion to embrace all living creatures and the whole of nature in its beauty.[21]

By breaking the blinding grip of materialism, we can see the subtle connections that link us all to each other. We all know that thoughts and feelings have power. We've seen, in both our private and public lives, how effective a strong feeling and a clear thought can be in manifesting an outcome—for an energy field is thus created that will attract others with similar vibrational tendencies, further reinforcing that energized thought form. These thought fields will reproduce after their kind. It is apparent, for example, that Adolf Hitler understood the power of thought fields on mass consciousness, and that his colleagues consciously used symbols, slogans, and focused thought to create a vibrational field of pride and conquest that was irresistible to millions of people in what was, ironically, perhaps the most highly educated and apparently rational society of the time.

The oneness of human consciousness has been demonstrated in positive ways as well, and the effect of people joined in loving thoughts and prayers for peace has been widely documented. Some researchers refer to this effect as "the Maharishi effect," since people trained in Transcendental Meditation have conducted many experiments on the effects that a group of meditators radiating a focused field of peace and harmony have on the crime rate and other social indicators of particular targeted cities.[22] The results have been impressive and significant. Some researchers, like Larry Dossey, M.D., are documenting and exploring the consequent effects of prayer on bodily healing.[23] These uses of materialistic science to prove what we already know are ironic. Materialism has covered over and ignored the truth that we are all connected, that rather than separate material objects with brains that give rise to consciousness, we are infinite consciousness manifesting as beings in time and space. The evidence for this is overwhelming, both in the utterances of spiritually illumined people and in our own hearts, minds, and daily life experiences, if we open our eyes and see! The undeniable effect of prayer (consciousness) in promoting physical healing is but one example of this.

Thus, the pollution of our shared consciousness-field by the dark agonies endured by billions of animals killed for food is an unrecognized fact that impedes our social progress and contributes gigantically to human violence and the warfare that is constantly erupting around the world. Joining together to pray for and visualize world peace is certainly a noble idea, but if we continue to dine on the misery of our fellow neighbors we are creating a monumental and ongoing prayer for violence, terror, and slavery. It is the prayer of our actions, and it is the experienced reality of billions of sensitive creatures who are at our mercy and to whom we show no mercy.

Until we live our prayers for peace and freedom by granting peace and freedom to those who are vulnerable in our hands, we will find neither peace nor freedom. Joy, love, and abundance are always available to us, and will manifest in our lives to the degree that we understand that they are given to us as we give them to others. The price we must pay for love and freedom *is* the ice cream cone, the steak, and the eggnog we casually consume. We are conditioned mentally to disconnect our food from the animal who was mindlessly abused to provide it, but the vibrational fields created by our food choices impact us profoundly whether we pretend to ignore them or not. Practicing mindful eating illuminates these hidden connections, cleanses our mind, heart, and actions, and removes inner masks and armor so that it becomes quite plain to see.

CHAPTER NINE

REDUCTIONIST SCIENCE
AND RELIGION

"Estrus control will open the doors of factory hog production. Control of female cycles is the missing link to the assembly-line approach."
—Earl Ainsworth, *The Farm Journal*, 1976

"There is no religion without love, and people may talk as much as they like about their religion, but if it does not teach them to be good and kind to beasts as well as man it is all a sham."
—Anna Sewell, *Black Beauty*

"'Tis said that the view of nature held by any people determine all their institutions."
—Ralph Waldo Emerson, *English Traits*

Sons of the Herding Culture

Science and religion are fundamental institutions in our culture that embody many of our highest ideals and contribute to our lives and well-being in a wide variety of ways. Science derives from *scire*, "to know," and religion from *religare*, "to link back"; the former is a manifestation of our yearning to understand the world and ourselves through systematized knowledge, and the latter of our yearning to reconnect with the spiritual source of our life and live in harmony with each other and with the larger order. Both science and religion are massive institutions, each employing millions of people and spending billions of dollars on projects that are all, in theory, intended to bring increased health, ease, security, understanding, meaning and happiness to our lives.

While few would argue that science and religion have not brought benefits to us, many would argue that they have strongly contributed to war, destruction, and misery as well—that they have exacerbated problems as well as solved them. Why is this? More specifically, why haven't the thousands seeking to improve and heal the world through scientific or spiritual development addressed the obviously violent and predatory mentality required by our food choices? Besides our universal resistance to admitting complicity in the cruelty of our meals, there is another factor operating: the reductionism promoted by many Western scientific and religious institutions that works to keep crucial connections invisible.

The revolution in human consciousness that apparently first began about ten thousand years ago in Iraq with the domestication and herding of large animals for food was a revolution of reductionism. Its distinguishing feature was the inner and outer act of reducing: reducing powerful wild animals to confinement and routinized slaughter, and reducing human respect for animals and nature in the process. Our forebears became predators of reduced prey—herded animals who were commodified and guarded and then stabbed and decapitated. They themselves became reduced and desensitized predators disposed to generating similarly reductionist scientific and religious institutions to validate their attitudes and behaviors.

Besides producing reductive scientific and religious systems, the old herding cultures produced reductive and predatory economic systems that increasingly viewed humans as economic units and led gradually to gross inequalities in the distribution of wealth. By the historic era three thousand years ago, we see in our most ancient writings such as Homer, the Old Testament, and Sumerian cuneiform writings a well-established economic system dominated by rich cattle-owning kings battling over lands for their livestock, with the masses of people reduced to mere resources who fought, produced, and consumed to benefit the wealthy elite. Early science was used to manipulate livestock bloodlines to maximize flesh, milk, and wool output, and religion was used to justify and even mandate the slaughter of animals for food. These are precisely the institutions we have inherited and that operate today and live in us because we continue to eat foods derived from reduced animals.

It's helpful to realize that conventional science and religion, while often feuding bitterly with each other, are in actuality strikingly similar in their underlying assumptions. They are two proud sons of the herding culture, and they both tend to reinforce the reductionist mentality required of those who inhabit their father's culture. This mentality is required to sustain the practice of enslaving and eating large animals, and to support an economic system based on exclusion and exploitation. It's instructive to see that while rare individuals have been able to transcend and uplift these scientific and religious institutions to a degree, the institutions themselves typically exert pressures that reinforce the reductionism required by the herding milieu. For example, though science and religion could be enormously enriched by the non-reductive feminine principle (Sophia), she is despised by the herding culture, and conventional science and religion typically view her with distrust, to their own disadvantage.

The father and his sons are successful in subjugating Sophia primarily because of the ongoing daily "sacrifice" of millions of animals for our dinner tables: the mass ritual that reduces our intelligence and suppresses our healing wisdom. As wisdom, Sophia is the ultimate goal of both science and religion, but in serving the authoritarian and reductive mentality of the herding culture, they have all but rejected her, with the tragic spiritual consequences we can see all around us.

Science and Slavery

"Converting living systems into machines for capital accumulation wouldn't be possible without the instrumentality of a reductionist science that achieves two things for you.

"On the one hand it kills your ethics of compassion because reductionism transforms a living system into inert parts that are put together from the outside—and that reductionism then creates the *ethical anesthesia* that basically says: 'You don't have to worry about the ethics of your relationship because this is just a bundle of matter which is in your hands to play around with.' It's as if you're playing with plasticine.

"And it also gives you the actual manipulative power to get more milk out of a cow, to produce more lean meat in the cows, to stock cows in smaller spaces, to slaughter them more quickly.

"These are the systems by which capital uses the reductionism of science for capital accumulation and appropriation of life from beings who have a right to their own life."

—Vandana Shiva, Ph.D.[1]

Rooted in the fallacious Cartesian split between mind and matter, conventional reductionist science flatly denies the existence of any reality beyond what can be physically quantified. This materialist mythos ignores spirituality and the mysterious adventure of consciousness, and tends to reduce both animals and humans to mere survival machines propelled by genetic and chemical forces. It intrinsically reinforces the delusion that beings struggle and compete in a universe that is devoid of any innate meaning or purpose. This has made reductionist science a potent tool of the wealthy elite and the military-industrial complex it controls.

In stripping away the inherent meaning and worth of animals and nature and reducing life to material processes, genetic programming, and operant conditioning, our own meaning, our worth, and our status are redefined in terms of how efficiently we serve the ends of the economic/political complex. Reductionist science cultivates the cold and calculating eye that validates reducing beings to numbers in the cost/benefit analyses carried out by industrial economists and military strategists. It has helped legitimize the herding culture's practice of commodifying animals and nature and, by extension, each other and ourselves.

Reductionist science serves the herding mentality faithfully. It has turned the pathological disconnectedness of masculine domination of nature, animals, and people into a reputable and prestigious art form. Today we can actually go to Dachau and stand in the same concrete buildings where Nazi scientists performed excruciating experiments on their fellow human creatures in the name of science. Just as ideas of supremacy justified the cruel Nazi experiments, they also justify the cruel experiments we perform by the untold thousands every day on defenseless animals. If we could gain admittance, we could go today to any state university or to thousands of private, military, or governmental research operations and witness cruel atrocities rationalized by the same argument of supremacy. We could also go, for example, to the School of the Americas in Fort Benning, Georgia, and see how the U.S. military trains military personnel from countries in Central and South America in the latest high-tech methods of torture, surveillance, and repression that help them to effectively dominate their people to further the interests of transnational corporations and the ruling elite.[2] Capital, cattle, riches, war, and exploitation of nature, animals, and people stand on the same foundation today as in the old herding cultures. They continue today in high-tech form aided by the reductive mythology of science.

There is perhaps nothing more terrifying than to be helpless and restrained, and to be looked at by a cold, disconnected eye that does not care about our experience of suffering. This is the eye of the herder toward his property animals, all of whom he will manipulate and kill for his own benefit; it is the eye of the soldier toward his enemies who threaten his rulers' cattle and capital interests; it is the eye of the scientist or research assistant deliberately subjecting sentient creatures to terribly painful experiments. This hard, unsympathetic eye is a deeply wounded parody of the true human eye that shines with lovingkindness, compassion, and a natural sense of caring and sympathy for all our fellow creatures on this earth. The hard eye is achieved only by rigorous practice—the practice that we are enlisted in practically from birth of disconnecting from the horror on our plates three times a day. We learn to cast this unsympathetic gaze on those outside our species, our race, our country, class, gender, tribe, religion, or sexual orientation, and particularly on pigs, cows, coyotes and other "food" or "nuisance" animals. We may look with softer eyes on certain species of "pet" animals, of course; it is fascinating and instructive, for example, to go to a science conference and hear from scientists themselves which animals they can vivisect without qualms. Some can work only on rats and mice, others can also work on cats, but not dogs or monkeys, others can "do" rabbits but not cats, and so forth. Where do we draw the line, and why? For most scientists, like most of us in this herding culture, animals raised for food fall far outside the circle of soft eyes. The more sensitive we become, the broader is our circle of compassion, and we feel qualms about harming a wider range of living beings because we find our eyes softening and caring even for little mice, birds, fish, shellfish, and insects. Scientific training, termed by Henryk Skolimowski "the yoga of objectivity,"[3] enforces a way of seeing that often tends to narrow our circle of compassion and to desensitize not only scientists but all of us.

Science has in some ways helped us appreciate "food" animals by demonstrating that, for example, fish have highly developed social awareness, feel pain, and quickly learn to avoid painful stimuli, and that pigs have intelligence that is surprisingly refined, surpassing dogs and approaching chimpanzees. However, its overall effect on animal welfare has been clearly negative. In fact there are still today many influential scientists who, while finally forced to admit that animals feel pain and are capable of suffering, nevertheless discount the pertinence and intensity of their suffering, much as scientists did with black people during the slavery era. Since the early days of the scientific revolution, scientists have used animals in painful experiments and have discounted the moral relevance of their pain. Descartes' well-known retort to his neighbors' complaints about the agonized howls of pain from dogs he was vivisecting still reverberates in the halls of science. He declared that animals, not possessing rational souls, were incapable of feeling pain, and the howls they made were merely like the creaking sounds of a turning mill wheel.[4] Such an attitude is the complete antithesis of the Golden Rule. By promoting illusions of objectivity, disconnectedness, reductionism, and materialism, and by encouraging researchers and the public to discount the suffering that sensitive creatures experience in its name and at the hands of our culture in general, science has done the herding mentality an enormous service, and the animals a monumental disservice. In this, it has done us human animals a disservice as well.

Besides contributing its disconnected reductive mythos to further

reinforce our culture's herding mythos, science has contributed technological devices that have allowed modern animal dominators to abuse
and enslave animals in ways never before conceivable. Modern factory
farms and slaughter plants are impossible without sophisticated
machinery, pesticides, drugs, hormones, confinement systems, electric
prods, and a host of other technological devices that inflict a living
nightmare onto creatures designed to run, fly, swim, play, and celebrate
their lives in the natural world. Unlike modern humans stuck in our
computer-adorned cubicles in high-rise office buildings, cows, chickens,
fish, and pigs have no way of beginning to make sense of the utterly foreign, frustrating, and terrifying artificiality into which we force them
their entire lives to satisfy our self-serving desires.

Reductionist science practically defines our culture and self-image
today, and though it has brought undeniable material progress and comfort, it has become a formidable force for our own enslavement as well.
Science is not just the source of technological devices that entertain and
comfort us, or that distract and addict us, or that pollute and potentially destroy our world. It also invents devices that can directly control us,
as it has done with animals. Some examples are hidden surveillance systems, electroshock belts, and computer microchips that can be embedded in our bodies to track us by GPS and, according to some sources,
potentially regulate us through stimulating painful muscle cramps, fear,
or mental confusion.[5] Microchips have already been tested and developed on animals, and versions of them are being widely implanted in
both wild and domestic animals and increasingly in humans.[6] According
to the *Los Angeles Times*, the microchips now being inserted into people with Alzheimer's and other medical conditions contain health
records and personal data and make people "scannable just like a jar of
peanut butter at the supermarket checkout line."[7] They can make us into
objects, easily trackable and controllable like the microchipped breeding sows[8] and dairy cows we use and eat ourselves.

On a deeper level, reductionist science enslaves us by legitimizing
only knowledge that is based on logical positivism and a fundamental
disconnection between the self and the world. Though there are a few
science popularizers who appear to the public to be more progressive,

holistic, and even spiritual, these people are typically rejected by the vast scientific enterprise that is founded on the principles of division, reduction, and analysis it inherited wholesale from its parent, the herding culture.[9] Its enemy is the enemy of the herding culture, the feminine principle that lives within all of us and manifests as a higher level of knowing than the separatistic rationality on which reductionist science relies. To the degree that science is disconnected from the compassionate, healing, interconnecting wisdom of intuition and the feminine principle, it tends to promote cruelty, destruction, slavery, and death.

Creating a science that authentically serves us rather than endangering, distracting, and controlling us requires a fundamental shift in our orientation away from the conventional reductive mentality that sees physical matter as primary and consciousness as merely emerging from it. When as a culture we stop seeing beings as things but as the conscious subjects of their lives, we will naturally create a more empowering science based on the primacy of consciousness and the interconnectedness of living beings. This is beginning to be seen in the work and writings of researchers and theorists like Rupert Sheldrake with his idea of morphogenetic fields, as well as Robert Jahn, Elizabeth Targ, Amit Goswami, Fred Alan Wolf, Vandana Shiva, Larry Dossey, Herbert Benson, Deepak Chopra, Fritjof Capra, and others who are attempting to reverse the reductionist mentality that pervades science. Some of these are exploring the role of thoughts, intentions, feelings, and prayer in healing, and some work to illuminate systemic interconnectivity and the essential power of consciousness in determining human experience of physical reality.[10] It's not surprising that these researchers, like Schweitzer, Einstein, and others, tend to question our culture's view and treatment of animals. Empowering approaches to science can also be seen in people working at grassroots levels with the Gandhian idea of appropriate technology: developing and using technologies that are cooperative and sustainable and do not enslave communities financially or politically to large-scale petroleum, agribusiness, chemical, or other interests. For these holistic approaches to science to catch on and become widely accepted, our culture must evolve beyond its current eating habits and the defining herding mentality that inevitably fosters a superficial and exploitive "predict and control" scientific reductionism.

Rational Nazi scientists worked on weapons of mass destruction and mass enslavement, as do armies of scientists today: can't we see that not only are their projects insane, but the way of thinking that underlies these projects is perverse? It could only be tolerated in a culture like ours, where people actually practice the same sorts of disconnections and cruelty on a daily basis. Until we stop reducing animals to food objects, reductionist science will wax stronger and more deadly because it is ultimately a reflection of ourselves. The entire outer world is a reflection of our inner reality, and war and distress in the world will cease as we eliminate war and distress within ourselves, our mental orientation, and our daily lives. The mental orientation of separation and reduction that underlies the conventional scientific method and that we were all saturated with as children continually blazes forth in our culture's meals, lives in our cultural attitudes, and manifests in the mirror of our world as the pain and struggle we experience and inflict on others.

Religious Reductionism

Conventional Western religion, like Western science, evolved within the same milieu of reducing and commodifying large animals and tends to be similarly reductionist in its essential orientation. The infinite divine mystery is typically reduced to a judgmental and often anthropomorphized authority figure; humans are reduced to self-centered, discrete temporal entities who may be chosen or saved or condemned to eternities of hell or heaven based on one fleeting lifetime; and animals, trees, ecosystems, and all of nature are reduced to being mere disposable props in this drama. Like science, the religious establishment has tended to reinforce the domination of animals, women, and nature, and to further the interests of the ruling elite. Like science, it tends toward being hierarchical, patriarchal, and exclusivist, and like science, it tells us to rely not on our own inner wisdom, but on its outside authority. Like reductionist science, which insists on the objectivist split between self and world, conventional Western religion insists on the primary dualism of Creator and creation, God and the world. This belief in a basic disconnection between the divine and all of us reinforces the illusion of separateness that is also propagated by reductionist science.

It is fascinating and instructive that while conventional science and religion fight endlessly with each other—bickering brothers sharing a common reductionist mythology—holistic science finds inspiring and helpful guidance and confirmation from progressive and non-Western religious traditions like liberation theology and many indigenous traditions, as well as Eastern traditions such as Taoism, Mahayana Buddhism, Sikhism, and Vedanta. These religious traditions tend to have evolved in cultures and subcultures in which animals were not systematically reduced to commodities.

The reductionist delusion of essential separateness is so ritualized in our daily meals that it inevitably thrusts itself into our religious lives. We are often told as children that we'll be excluded from heaven unless we subscribe to a set of exclusivist beliefs! Mainstream religious teachings typically tell us we are special if we agree to an exclusivist creed. They rarely question our violent food choices but rather encourage them by declaring that animals have no souls and that God gave us animals to eat—and they sponsor barbecues, pig roasts, fish fries, and turkey dinners in communities across America. It wasn't so long ago, when the fourth-century emperor Constantine made Christianity the Roman state religion, that its earlier vegetarian emphasis was completely repressed and actually became a heresy, with Constantine reportedly ordering his men to pour molten lead down the throats of any Christians who refused to eat animal flesh.[11] The original Christian teachings of mercy had to be repressed and twisted in order to be accepted by the dominant herding culture, and the enlightened teaching that *He who lives by the sword must die by the sword* became a bitter irony.

By interpreting the transcendent divine as masculine, conventional religion deifies the masculine the same way science does, and suppresses the feminine, which nurtures and connects. Even today, when there is virtually no theologian who would dare argue that the infinite Spirit that is referred to by the word God could be said to be more male than female, we still teach our children, as we were taught, that He is the Lord. In the old herding cultures, it was males who warred, herded, and raped, and it is basically the same today. By emphasizing the masculine nature of God, the herding cultures legitimized their ethos of domination, cruelty, and killing. In fact, as J. R. Hyland points out, the main form of worship in the old herding cultures was the sacrificial killing of animals to please the deity.[12] Underlying all this was the fundamental notion that "the Lord is my shepherd"—a terrifying idea when we contemplate the realities of the herding culture that propagated these teachings. The herder enslaved, castrated, and killed his sheep, goats, and cattle without mercy, and these creatures were, as they are today, powerless in his almighty hands.

The anxious preoccupation with being "saved" perhaps derives directly from this. Our ongoing failure to save the animals at our mercy may compel us into nervous concern about our own "salvation." Salvation from what, exactly? From the consequences of our actions, perhaps? Or more traditionally, from being damned to the fires of hell? Whence comes the power of this image? Could it be related to the untold centuries of herders gazing through flames into the charring bodies of animals they've condemned and killed as sacrificial offerings, and which they themselves will eat?

The Myth of Evil

The basic view promoted by conventional Western religion is of an unending battle between good and evil, with God as a male sky-dwelling deity on one side and Satan as a shadowy, malicious, bestial presence on the other. This devil is ironically represented as having the horns and hooves of a goat or cow—the very victims we relentlessly confine and attack for food! This evil or devil is certainly, on one level at least, the projection of our own shadow—the guilt, shame, and unexpressed grief we bear for the massive ongoing cruelty we engage in as eaters of animals in the herding culture's households. We repress our awareness of our cruelty and consequently find ourselves plagued by a dark and sinister presence. This is unavoidable, because the evil we see is our own denied and unadmitted cruelty, from which we can never distance ourselves. It emerges as devils, enemies, wars, and weapons of mass destruction. We are told we have to side with our shepherd king, who protects us but also controls us in his war with the enemy. Animals and the earth are seen as mere properties and stage for this cosmic battle, at best; at worst, animals and the earth (and women, and minorities) are seen as somehow in league with the dark, shadowy devil and therefore rightfully "subdued."

This lurking sense that we are basically evil, one of the characteristic traits of our Western culture, is a mainstay belief propagated by the religious establishment. It isn't necessary, though, and there is plenty in both the Old and New Testaments of the Bible to refute it. Matthew Fox argues, for example, in *Original Blessing*, that the doctrine of original sin—that we are by nature evil and depraved—is not founded upon either the core teachings of Jesus or the experience and writings of many of the recognized illumined Christian and Jewish sages and mystics.[13] These people have discovered the fundamental goodness of life and human nature and the "original blessing" at the heart of creation as an ongoing celebration and evolution of consciousness.

In the Eastern religious traditions, which tend to discourage meat eating and animal herding and are somewhat less dualistic than our Western traditions, this fundamentally positive orientation is well established. In Buddhism, for example, it is a core teaching that all sentient beings have "Buddha-nature," that is, that all beings are expressions of completely enlightened consciousness and can realize this directly through spiritual growth and understanding. This basic goodness is seen as our true nature and is the foundation of our spiritual practice. Many increasingly progressive strands within Western religious traditions similarly recognize that human nature, and all nature, is a reflection of divine love and is essentially good. Our spiritual path consists of contacting this inner light and purifying ourselves to be lambent vessels for its luminous presence.

The idea that we are fundamentally evil goes as completely against this universal idea of our original goodness as our ugly practice of confining and killing animals goes against our innate sense of kindness. The herding culture we were all born into carries an enormous reservoir of hidden guilt for the ferocious savagery it inflicts on animals for food, for the abuse and hardening of its boys, and for the violence it propagates against women and against rival herders and nations. This systematic cruelty and the repressed but healthy sense of compunction that naturally goes with it are the source of our cultural belief that people are inherently evil. The deep-seated sense of guilt, fear, and anxiety arising from this infects all of us unconsciously and causes us many problems, physically, mentally, and spiritually. Because of this, we find there is today a growing movement that urges freedom from guilt trips and judgment. We recognize that chronic guilt cripples us, depletes our energy, and keeps us trapped in old patterns, and we understandably want to be free of it—but we don't see that its source is in the ongoing cruelty of our daily meals. Thoughts and behavior produce after their kind.

We can thus see how difficult it is to effectively address and reduce the suffering caused to animals through vivisection, rodeos, circuses, canned hunts, dog fighting rings, and so forth while as a culture we still practice eating them. The desensitization inherent in reducing animals for food naturally expands to animals mistreated in non-food uses as well—but it doesn't just stop there, at the boundary of animals. This is why "man's inhumanity to man" is rooted in our inhumanity to animals.

Conventional religion, like science, accurately reflects the psychological trauma of the herding culture that birthed it and that still sustains it. Everything is justified by the culture's living mythology. As Joseph Campbell points out in *The Masks of God*, cultures dependent on animal flesh organize themselves around death because "the paramount object of experience is the beast, [k]illed and slaughtered. . . ."[14] This is true of our culture today, and the deaths of the millions of animals slaughtered daily ripple through all our religious institutions, which provide the mythos to justify it now as they did in the arid hills of the Mediterranean basin three thousand years ago.

Plant-based cultures, Campbell points out, organize themselves around life. The plant world provides "the food, clothing and shelter of people since time out of mind, but also our model of the wonder of life—in its cycle of growth and decay, blossom and seed, wherein death and life appear as transformations of a single, superordinated, indestructible force."[15] The revolution desperately needed today, if we are to survive, is a transformation of the basic orientation of the herding culture into which we were born: from a mythos of death and reductionism to a mythos of life and holism.

A transformation of science and religion and economics, releasing them from obsolete reductionism and orienting them toward furthering and celebrating universal compassion and the interconnectedness of all beings, is possible when we change our daily eating habits and the mentality of disconnectedness they require. Although we are products of the herding culture, we can heal it and ourselves through understanding. This understanding requires a change in our behavior because our behavior strongly conditions our consciousness. The science and religion and economics of holism, kindness, sustainability, and community begin with this.

As we cultivate awareness and question the death orientation that stares at us from our plates, we create a field of freedom and compassion, and as we move to plant-based meals, we can become agents of life, breathing a new spirit of protecting and including into our world that, by blessing the animals who are at our mercy, will bless us a hundredfold. This is a *radical* transformation because it goes, as the word radical implies, to the essential root of our unyielding dilemma, the commodification of animals for food.

CHAPTER TEN

THE DILEMMA OF WORK

⇌

"I am increasingly convinced that one of humankind's most grievous sins is our anthropocentrism. By cutting ourselves off from the rest of creation, we are left bereft of awe and wonder and therefore of reverence and gratitude. We violate our very beings, and we have nothing but trivia to teach our young."[1]
—MATTHEW FOX

"I think the person who takes a job in order to live—that is to say, for the money—has turned himself into a slave."
—JOSEPH CAMPBELL

"When a human kills an animal for food, he is neglecting his own hunger for justice. Man prays for mercy, but is unwilling to extend it to others."
—ISAAC BASHEVIS SINGER

Doing the Dirty Work

It is not only animals who suffer in factory farms and slaughterhouses. The people who must do the awful work of confining, mutilating, and killing farmed animals also suffer, as do their families. When we buy or order animal foods we directly instigate human violence, though it may be shielded from our physical view. As Emerson wryly pointed out, "You have just dined, and however scrupulously the slaughterhouse is concealed in the graceful distance of miles, there is complicity."[2] Instigating and eating violence, we sow the seeds of further violence, both in our actions and speech toward others and in others' actions and speech toward us. Perhaps "bad things happen to good people" because the good people are blindly complicit and have done bad things to others to which they are unfortunately indoctrinated to be oblivious.

Not a lot is written about the closed, cruel world of slaughterhouse life and of factory farm workers, but the research and writing that has been done is both disturbing and horrifying. *Slaughterhouse: The Shocking Story of Greed, Neglect, and Inhumane Treatment Inside the U.S. Meat Industry*, the result of Gail Eisnitz's interviews with slaughterhouse workers, is an excellent resource, as is *All Heaven in a Rage*, edited by Laura Moretti. *Fast Food Nation* by Eric Schlosser and *The Food Revolution* by John Robbins also discuss the subject. Video documentaries such as *Auction Block, Hope for the Hopeless, Meet Your Meat, Seven Minutes of Reality, A Day in the Life of a Massachusetts Slaughterhouse, A Cow at My Table, North Carolina Pig Farm Investigation, Victims of Indulgence, Peaceable Kingdom, Mad Cowboy*, and others listed in the resources section provide powerful glimpses into some of the worst ongoing nightmares on this planet.

According to Laura Moretti, it's not possible for us to grasp with our imagination the realities of slaughterhouse carnage:

> I realize it is incredibly easy to imagine the inside of a slaughterhouse and not be so affected by it—for the human grasp is limited. It can't hear the sound of a large animal pushed against its will into a kill chute, its frantic struggles, the reverberating pop of the captive-bolt pistol, the heavy thump to the floor, the kicking against metal, the groaning of the dying, the screech of pulleys and chains, the hydraulic release hiss, the splashing blood, like water from a garden hose hitting cement. It can't smell the stench of manure and sweat, blood and putrefying flesh and organs. It can't feel the absolute fear,

panic, terror. It can't know the absolute will of each and every life to desperately, frantically, vainly hold on.

The human mind can't imagine the inside of a slaughterhouse; it is something one can only experience—and it is utterly shocking.[3]

It is well documented that slaughterhouse and factory farm work is ugly and terribly stressful, emotionally, mentally, and physically. Slaughterhouse workers, perhaps the lowest caste in the U.S., have the highest rate of work-related injuries and one of the highest turnover rates.[4] Statistics aside, the mind-bending and heart-hardening actions that these brothers and sisters must do so that we can satisfy our desire for animal foods are excruciating to contemplate. With our dollars we communicate our desires to a vast and impersonal system that will fulfill those desires as cheaply as possible. This means high-speed production and a perverse philosophy of mechanization toward the animals who are imprisoned, "harvested," and disassembled. They are no longer sentient creatures but are categorized with fruits, machines, and other nonsentient things as unfeeling commodities, summed up by this advice to pork producers in a hog-farming journal, "Forget the pig is an animal. Treat him just like a machine in a factory."[5] Over and over, in the literature of animal "agriculture" and slaughterhouses, feedlots, stockyards, and transport operations, one hears workers and management repeating this, like a mantra: Don't think of it as an animal. Forget it has any feelings. And the workers use every type of denigrating language and categorization possible, referring to the chickens, pigs, turkeys, cows, and other animals they kill and mutilate as stupid, stubborn, ornery, or quite simply as "motherfuckers."[6]

What is the effect of all this upon the health and sensibilities of these workers? And upon their wives, husbands, and children? Violence, cruelty, and insensitivity breed more of the same; they are vibrations that affect consciousness, and it is not just the workers, but their families, friends, and ultimately all of us who are affected by what we force them to do by our market demand. As one former pig sticker (a slaughterhouse worker who stabbed pigs in the neck to bleed them to death) said, "You get just as sadistic as the company itself. When I was sticking

down there, I was a sadistic person."[7] Though slaughterhouse workers
are not literally forced to take these jobs, they are often desperate for
the money and cannot find other work; hence they keep the flesh, blood,
and body parts of enslaved animals flowing through the money chan-
nels into the millions of deadening centers throughout our society.

We should never imagine that animals go peacefully to their deaths.
They know what is coming, and can smell, hear, and often even see others being killed before them. They are filled with terror, and very often
with intense and overwhelming pain as they are boiled, skinned, or dismembered while still conscious. Since the workers at the Iowa Beef
Processing cattle slaughtering plant in Pasco, Washington, took undercover videos in 2001 of cows still fully conscious, blinking, kicking,
looking around, and having their skin torn off by workers forced to
keep the line moving, it is finally somewhat more generally known—
beyond the workers and management at these operations, who have
always known—that animal suffering is vast, intense, and systematically ignored for the benefit of profits and efficiency. This interview with a
livestock trucker from *A Cow at My Table* is instructive.

> Like this bull I had last year . . . he was just trying his hardest to get
> off the trailer. He had been prodded to death by three or four driv-
> ers . . . I just said, "Why don't you shoot the damn thing? What's
> going on? What about this Code of Ethics?" This one guy said, "I
> never shoot. Why would I shoot a cow that can come off and there's
> still good meat there?" When I first started, I talked to another truck-
> er about downers. He said, "You may as well not get upset. It's been
> going on for many years. . . . You'll get kind of bitter like I did. You
> just don't think about the animals. You just think that they aren't
> feeling or whatever."[8]

The vast majority of us who eat animal foods have never lifted the
curtain and taken a good, deep look at the horrendous brutality that
animals must endure for our tables, nor do we wish to do so. We are
rightly afraid that if we do, we won't be able to eat our usual meals with
a clear conscience, and knowing that, the industry keeps the conditions

on slaughterhouses, factory farms, and fishing operations well hidden, lobbying for laws to make it a crime for anyone to take pictures or video footage of the conditions in these places. Seeing the ugly truth behind the curtain helps to rid us of the illusion that our culture is based on kindness or caring. We see clearly the hidden dark side of our society, the vicious and unrelenting cruelty that permeates the foundations of our culture, and we begin to understand. It is our ongoing refusal to look behind the curtain that keeps the cultural chains and illusions firmly in place.

To meet the enormous demand for animal flesh, the huge transnational corporations that now dominate the meat, dairy, and egg industries, like Cargill, ConAgra, Tyson, Perdue, Swift, and Smithfield, construct ever larger animal prisons and slaughterhouses. At the slaughterhouses, some of which run twenty-four hours a day, living animals are forced into a line and disassembled, and the various parts of their bodies come out at the other end, all shipped for profit to a diversity of destinations: flesh and organs for human food; skin for clothing, jewelry, furniture, and accessories; blood for fertilizer; bones and connective tissue for beauty creams, soaps, glue, and gelatin; some organs for the pharmaceutical industry; offal and scraps for the renderer to be cooked and made into livestock feed, pet food, and other products. The faster the disassembly lines run, the more profit is made in a given time. Workers are constantly pushed to work much more rapidly than they should, and this causes improper stunning of the animals and increased cruelty and danger because many animals are skinned, scalded, and disemboweled while still conscious and struggling.

Most people do not realize that, as discussed earlier, the animals are not actually killed before their throats are cut. Their hearts must be pumping when the large arteries in their necks are cut, so that the blood is actively pumped out of their bodies; otherwise the flesh is soggy with too much blood. Therefore, they are simply stunned, not killed, prior to being bled. If they are properly stunned, the animals bleed to death. How long does it take to bleed to death? From twenty seconds to several minutes, which could feel like an awfully long time, especially if an animal is *not* properly stunned, which occurs all too often.

The stunning methods used today are crude and extremely cruel, because they frequently do not work. Cows are typically stunned with a captive bolt pistol that slams a rod of steel through their foreheads and into their brains as they enter the line. There is only one stun man, and if the cow suddenly moves, the bolt may miss its mark, sometimes hitting the animal in the eye. There is often no time to fire a second bolt, because to slow down the line or to hire a second stun man as a back-up would cost money. So some cows, still conscious, move down the line where other workers have to bleed, skin, and dismember them. These workers cannot send the cows back to get stunned, so their job is made even more horrifying, and extremely dangerous as well, by the conscious animals' pain and fear. Many worker injuries are caused by desperately kicking animals on the line. Though it was quickly hushed up, when workers at the cattle-slaughtering operation in Washington took their own undercover videos, *The Washington Post* investigated.

> It takes twenty-five minutes to turn a live steer into steak at the modern slaughterhouse where Roman Moreno works. For twenty years, his post was "second-legger," a job that entails cutting hocks off carcasses as they whirl past at a rate of 309 an hour.
>
> The cattle were supposed to be dead before they got to Moreno. But too often they weren't.
>
> "They blink. They make noises," he said softly. "The head moves, the eyes are wide and looking around."
>
> Still Moreno would cut. On bad days, he says, dozens of animals reached his station clearly alive and conscious. Some would survive as far as the tail cutter, the belly ripper, the hide puller. "They die," said Moreno, "piece by piece."[9]

Pigs are stunned either by a bolt to the brain or by electric shocks on their backs. Again, there is only one stunner. When shocking is the chosen method, management often keeps the voltage lower than it should be for proper stunning, since more flesh ("meat") may be damaged if higher voltages are used. Thus, the "stickers" who cut the throats of stunned pigs find themselves every day or every night facing live, desperate animals.

Sooner or later many of the workers get severely cut by the long, razor-sharp knives they use against the struggling animals.

Slaughterhouse workers must shackle chickens and turkeys by the ankles and hang them upside down on a conveyor line that passes their heads through a "bath" of electrically charged brine. The shock, which is extremely painful, immobilizes the birds but does not stun them, so they are fully conscious when they hit the next station on the conveyor: the knives, wielded by workers or by a machine, that cut their throat arteries. Often the birds manage to pull away from the water and may then, in their panicked flailing, miss the knives, so they are still conscious when they hit the next station on the fast-moving disassembly line: the huge vat of filthy water where their bodies are boiled, dead or alive.

Due to slaughter industry deregulation over the last fifteen years, there is virtually no government oversight to protect animals used for food. The consequent climate of speed and inhumane treatment harms workers as well, making "meat packing . . . the most dangerous factory job in America."[10] According to worker affidavits, for example, workers are not allowed to leave the line for many hours and therefore are sometimes forced to urinate or defecate on the slaughter plant floor or in their clothes.[11] Eisnitz writes,

> Over the course of my investigation I'd heard about workers being crushed by cattle; burned by chemicals; stabbed; breaking bones; and suffering miscarriages and fainting from the heat, fast pace, and fumes. . . . As line speeds have as much as tripled in the last fifteen years, cumulative trauma disorders have increased nearly 1,000 percent.[12]

Workers are our human brothers and sisters who administer corporate cruelty around the clock. Profits are prioritized rather than "humane killing"—if such a thing exists. The Humane Slaughter Act, for example, which carries no penalties and has proven to be completely inadequate to protect farmed animals, doesn't even include chickens, turkeys, fish, and other non-mammalian animals. It does nothing to prohibit the many cruelties at slaughter plants, such as dragging non-ambulatory pigs and cows by the legs or necks, cutting and tearing animals who arrive frozen to the sides of the livestock trucks, and hanging conscious and panicked animals on the line to endure being skinned and boiled alive. Since it's very conservatively estimated that at least five to ten percent of the land animals slaughtered are not stunned properly, a staggering 500 million to one billion mammals and birds per year are skinned, dismembered, or boiled while still conscious—in the United States alone.[13] This is a terrible load for workers to bear emotionally, on top of the already grisly work they do. It's a load not just for the workers, however. We are all responsible. (In fact, in courts of law, the one who wills the death of another and pays an assassin is more heavily accountable than the assassin.)

Of course, it's not just at slaughter plants that animals suffer at our hands. The workers on the factory farms where animals are imprisoned for their eggs, flesh, and milk enforce an almost unbelievably cruel system. In fact, if we took our most celebrated scientists and asked them to devise a system, simply as a scientific experiment, that maximized terror, pain, cruelty, and misery, it seems they would be hard pressed to devise anything more effective than the one that has evolved through corporate domination of the lucrative business of supplying the body parts of hapless animals to millions of people who have been indoctrinated to eat them.

On factory farms, workers have to imprison animals in unimaginably toxic and restrictive environments, and mutilate them as well, without anesthesia. The Animal Welfare Act, which protects dogs, cats, parakeets, and other animals from abuse by humans, specifically omits *all* animals who are raised for food from its provisions. Any practice, no matter how cruel, that is considered standard in the industry is allowed, so chopping off the beaks and bills of chickens and ducks, for example, or starving chickens to force a molt, or mutilating, shocking, confining, and crowding animals is permitted by the government because these have become accepted industry practices. Baby pigs scream loudly with the torment of having their ears "notched" for identification, patterns of flesh cut away, and their tails "docked" (cut off) and teeth painfully clipped, so that under the stress of overcrowding they cannot bite each other's tails or damage each other. It is also common practice to break the pigs' noses, according to the logic that this makes overcrowded boars less likely to fight! Calves endure the agony of being branded with hot irons and of having their young horns either cut off, which often causes profuse bleeding, or burned off with acid or hot irons. Sheep undergo the excruciating process of mulesing—having the flesh around their rumps cut away to reduce fly infestation—and the shearing itself is often a brutal process, resulting in painful cuts and rough handling that sometimes kills the sheep. They are, of course, sent to slaughter anyway when their wool production declines. Young male sheep, pigs, and cows are virtually always castrated as well, and anesthesia is never used as they are cut and their testicles ripped out.

Geese and ducks are debilled as chickens are debeaked, and are force-fed to produce foie gras, an expensive delicacy that is the product of an unnaturally enlarged and traumatized liver. It is often called the cruelest food in the world, and for this reason its production has been outlawed in South Africa, Israel, and seven European countries.[14] The bird's liver is forcibly enlarged by inserting a metal pipe down the throat and pressure-driving much larger quantities of corn into his or her stomach than it can manage. This often causes "blowout" or rupture of the animal's internal organs. When the duck or goose's liver is inflated to ten times its natural size, he or she is killed so the diseased liver can be eaten.

It is hard for us to imagine the trauma factory farm workers inflict, and on an enormous scale, with billions of creatures involved. Most of us have had the experience of receiving pain at the hands of doctors or dentists, yet the hands that administer the pain are, we feel, ultimately well-intentioned. The fact that they are doing these painful things for our own good makes the infliction of pain tolerable and gives it a meaningful context. To imagine those same hands performing painful procedures on our bodies with the sense that these hands do not care at all about our good, but are causing us pain simply because it profits them or they enjoy doing so, is horrifying in the extreme, particularly if we are powerless in their hands. When we put animals in this position by purchasing their flesh, fluids and eggs, we must bear responsibility not only for their suffering but for the hardening of the human hands and hearts that inflict this suffering.

Factory farms, like slaughterhouses, are brutal places, concentration camps for animals, in which all manner of atrocities are inflicted on the defenseless inmates. The conditions in these places bring out the worst in people. Undercover video footage shows that workers routinely terrorize animals with kicks, shocks, shouts, stabs, clubbings, and draggings. They have been documented playing sadistic games like forcing dry ice into the rectums of live chickens to make the birds explode, drop-kicking them like footballs, blowing them up with firecrackers, or squeezing birds with such force they spray feces over other birds.[15] People who are not naturally sadistic may become that way, and people who have been abused as children and perversely enjoy causing pain to others may well be attracted to working in slaughterhouses and factory farms, where there is an unending flow of defenseless victims they can torture, beat, and abuse. For example, some slaughterhouse and stockyard workers use extremely painful electric prods to keep disabled or downed cows, pigs, and sheep moving into the disassembly line. Being touched by an electric prod is not like getting a mildly disturbing shock. The animals experience thousands of powerful volts of pure pain, more comparable to being stabbed with a knife. Workers have been seen and even videotaped sticking these prods into animals' mouths and anuses, and stabbing animals with knives in their anuses and eyes. On pig factory farms, it is standard practice to weed out pigs whose size and weight are below the standards that make it profitable to continue feeding them. Workers kill these animals on the spot using a method known in the industry as "PACing." PAC stands for "Pound Against Concrete"; the workers grab the pigs by their hind feet and slam them on the floor.

In *Slaughterhouse*, Gail Eisnitz relates dozens of recorded conversations with signed affidavits from slaughterhouse workers describing the routine cruelties they perform when forced by high line speeds to "process" animals still conscious and active after they've passed the stunner. According to one sticker,

Down in the blood pit they say that the smell of blood makes you aggressive. And it does. You get an attitude that if that hog kicks at me, I'm going to get even. You're already going to kill the hog, but that's not enough. It has to suffer. When you get a live one you think, Oh good, I'm going to beat this sucker.

Another thing that happens is that you don't care about people's pain anymore. I used to be very sensitive about people's problems—willing to listen. After a while, you become desensitized. . . .

It's the same thing with an animal who pisses you off, except it *is* in the stick pit, you *are* going to kill it. Only you don't just kill it, you go in hard, push hard, blow the windpipe, make it drown in its own blood. Split its nose. A live hog would be running around the pit. It would just be looking up at me and I'd be sticking, and I would just take my knife and—eerk—cut its eye out while it was just sitting there. And this hog would just scream.[16]

This worker, and others, told even more cruel and gruesome stories, but ended by saying, "It's not anything anyone should be proud of. It happened. It was my way of taking out frustration."

Another worker describes the psychological hardening that inevitably occurs.

The worst thing, worse than the physical danger, is the emotional toll. If you work in that stick pit for any period of time, you develop an attitude that lets you kill things but doesn't let you care. You may look a hog in the eye that's walking around down in the blood pit with you and think, God, that really isn't a bad-looking animal. You may want to pet it. Pigs down on the kill floor have come up and nuzzled me like a puppy. Two minutes later I had to kill them—beat them to death with a pipe. I can't care. . . . I was killing things. My attitude was, it's only an animal. Kill it. Sometimes I'd look at people that way, too. I've had ideas of hanging my foreman upside down on the line and sticking him.[17]

How do people who spend their days PACing animals, electro-prodding them, bashing their noses, killing, beating, stabbing, and cutting them, treat their girlfriends, spouses, and children? How do these people cope with the violence they endure around them and administer to weaker and defenseless creatures?

The Living Roots of Our Work

The herding culture into which we've all been born forces boys to learn to be tough and to disconnect from their natural feelings of gentleness and compassion. The work of herding that evolved between four thousand and ten thousand years ago is the work of harsh and relentless domination of powerful animals. It requires men capable of performing cruel mutilation, confinement, manipulation, and killing—both of the herd animals, who have become valuable commodities, and of other, potentially predatory animals. Besides this, herders are engaged against other herders for precious land and water for their animals. By owning animals, the old emergent herding cultures, which form the historic foundation and the living core of our culture today, distanced themselves from the natural world and entered into an adversarial relationship with it. These ancient cultures have so much power over us today because we engage in the same core behavior: confining animals and eating foods sourced from these animals.

Although we have perhaps made some progress in our treatment of each other over the centuries, our continuing practice of enslaving, torturing, and killing animals has always worked against our being able to make substantial progress. Though we decry the enslaving, exploiting, torturing, and killing of other people in certain circumstances, on a larger scale we still rationalize and justify it, and it remains undeniably widespread today.

In *Eternal Treblinka,* historian Charles Patterson shows how the parallels between the ways that the old herding cultures abused both animals and humans have continued into the present day (see Chapter 2). Focusing on the rational, democratic culture that became Nazi Germany, he points out the startling similarities between our domination of other people and our domination of animals for food. Adolf Hitler kept on his office wall a framed picture of Henry Ford, the consummate capitalist and racist supremacist whose assembly lines inspired Hitler's mass extermination mechanism. Ford, in turn, got his assembly line idea from the disassembly lines in the old Chicago slaughterhouses. In Nazi Germany, Jews, communists, homosexuals, the mentally ill, and other "vermin" were treated as food animals, transported from stockyards on cattle cars to concentration camps like modern factory farms, where they might be vivisected before being sent into the same sort of final tunnel that awaits every animal slaughtered for food. Ironically, the term "holocaust" originally meant "whole burning" and referred to the killing and sacrificing of animals as burnt offerings.

The same underlying dynamic is still in place today. We universally condemn supremacism, elitism, and exclusivism for destroying peace and social justice, yet we unquestioningly and even proudly adopt precisely these attitudes when it comes to animals. The lesson is plain: when we harden ourselves to the suffering we inflict on animals in our own interest, and justify it by proclaiming our superiority or specialness, it is but a short and unavoidable step to justifying and inflicting the same kind of suffering on other humans in our own interest while likewise proclaiming our supremacy or specialness. The unremitting conflict and oppression of history are inevitable by-products of confining and killing animals for food, as is the male role model of macho toughness that is required of both the professional animal killer (herder) and the soldier. If we desire to eat animal foods, this suffering is the price we must pay.

Work as Joy, Work as Burden

The progressive voices of the left, while often criticizing conventional science and religion, and even questioning our rampant exploitation of nature and domination of the feminine, have so far almost completely failed to see the connection between the core ritual of our herding culture—eating animals—and our destructive values and institutions. Whether we're of the right, left, or in between, we all agree to ignore this basic causal root of our problems. For example, in his book *The Reinvention of Work*, progressive theologian and priest Matthew Fox probes deeply into the values and beliefs that underlie our experience of work and our attitudes toward it. Drawing upon a wide range of scriptures including the Bible, the Bhagavad-Gita, and the Tao Te Ching, as well as writings by illumined poets and saints like Kabir, Rumi, Rilke, St. Francis, Hildegard of Bingen, Meister Eckhart and the more modern voices of Thomas Berry, E. F. Schumacher, and Theodore Roszak, he passionately argues that work is fundamentally spiritual. If we look around us, he says, to the cosmos, to our earth, and to nature and animals, we find an infinity of action unfolding continually, with every part playing its assigned and vital role. Every part, every cell, plant, animal, planet, and star, has a function to fulfill in the larger unfolding, and this is its work. Fox argues that to do this work is to participate in the becoming of the infinite universe, and that this is thus both sacred and ecstatic. "[A]ll of creation," he writes, "exists because of the 'sheer joy' of God. The work of creation was a work of joy whose whole purpose was to bring more joy into existence. This not only gives us permission to find joy in work but charges us with a responsibility to do so. Joy is an essential source of motivation in our work."[18]

Fox recognizes, however, that there is a big problem with work for us humans, noting that over one billion of us are actually unemployed. If we look about us in nature, we see that every being is working and fulfilling its purpose, and it is only humans who are unemployed, underemployed, overworked, or unable or unwilling to work. We are the only species to enslave other species for food, to drink milk as adults, and to view work as disagreeable and try to avoid it. Why is this? Predictably, Fox blames our dissatisfaction with work on the disconnection from nature and spirituality caused by the scientific and industrial revolutions and urges us to become more creative, more loving, and more joyful in our work, to care more for the earth and each other, and to "reinvent" work as the joy it is meant to be as the expression of our heart's purpose.

What he does *not* articulate is that the fundamental and defining work of our herding culture is the brutal confining, mutilating, and killing of sensitive creatures. This is hardly a motivation for joy in working! This is the obvious but unrecognized and unarticulated inconsistency at the root of our dilemmas. Thousands of us starve to death daily, millions of us labor like slaves for pennies a day in toxic factories producing consumerist junk, millions more of us work as soldiers and agents of violence and fear—and it's rooted in our plates.

The commodifying, confining, and killing of animals is a complete perversion of the word "work" as defined by Fox. Until our defining work is transformed from killing animals for food to protecting and caring for life, we will never "reinvent" work in our culture. We will only make technological progress that gives us the means to exploit animals, nature, and each other more efficiently and cruelly, and to eat more animal flesh, eggs, and dairy products than ever in recorded history.

World peace and harmony require those of us in positions of power and affluence in the global village to stop dominating people, animals, and nature through our craving for animal foods. It's easy to forget that if we're reading these words we are actually among the richest and most powerful people on this planet. Because of our relative wealth and power, our example, our voice, and our lifestyle can impact many people, either positively or negatively. We are thus obliged to honor this responsibility to our brothers and sisters.

Resurrecting Work

Because of the fundamentally violent nature of its defining work—herding and killing animals—our culture has a basic distaste for work itself. We all hear that working less is better than working more, and not working at all is best of all. The story we all learned in Genesis, of being cast out of the garden, is significant, for it was then that God punished us with enforced hard labor while we live on this earth. This metaphor, part of the herding mythos, is revealing, for it depicts work as a distasteful burden and attributes it to a divine edict that came with being thrown out of the garden. In the garden, we ate a completely plant-based diet, and there was no concept of work as a separate activity. We lived in harmony with animals, the earth, and each other, not killing them for food or competing with each other. Our work was our life, and it was joy, and all was "very good." There was no work as separate activity, nor any concept of being saved, for we had not committed the original sin of seeing others as objects to be manipulated, used, and killed.

Many other world mythologies also talk about a lost golden age of innocence and peace. Perhaps these stories, as Eisler and others suggest, are reminiscences of the ancient partnership cultures described by contemporary anthropologists, before the hunting of large animals, herding, and the domination of animals and women. Returning to the garden of abundance, innocence, and natural blessedness has always been seen as the goal of religious yearning in the West, yet to actually accomplish this we must unseat the basic mythos of domination and exclusion that our culture propagates. In its heart of hearts, our culture longs to transcend itself, as we ourselves do, and to return, spiral-like, to a time of connectedness, mercy, and creative joy. The seeds of this yearning are planted in our culture's heart and in our spiritual essence.

The fall from grace, innocence, freedom, and mercy began when we ate of the fruit of the illusion of dualistic separatism and stopped showing mercy to those at our mercy. The fall came when we began commodifying animals. We can resurrect our work from defiling slavery to joyous participation. The path simply requires that we give the same opportunities to the animals who are at our mercy: release them from slavery and grant them freedom to once again fully participate in the unfolding of their unique purpose and consciousness. What we would wish for ourselves we must first give to others: this is, it seems, an everlasting spiritual principle.

To resurrect work from the depths of the trivialization, dissatisfaction, and exploitation into which it has fallen, we'll need a cultural shift far more radical than any currently proposed by the left or the right. We'll need a positive transformation of our relationship to those at our mercy, which means shifting from animal foods to plant foods, and from a mythos of death and domination to a mythos of life and co-creative participation. Anything less is mere irony and hypocrisy.

As individuals, as a culture, and as a human family, we pay a remarkably steep price for work that is demeaning or destructive to others or ourselves. When we work primarily for money, we transgress against our spiritual purpose, and sell our life energy and time, which is unfathomably precious. Spiritual traditions and teachings have all emphasized that each one of us has a unique purpose and mission in this life to unfold and fulfill, and that this is our work. Our work has to do with purifying and awakening our consciousness, contributing creatively to our community, and being the voice and hands that confer blessings on others. As we discover our calling, and live it as fully as we can, we discover joy and meaning, and our life becomes precious and filled with blessings. Evolving and growing as individuals, we can authentically contribute to the evolution of our species, and there is enormous satisfaction in these efforts.

If we fail to spend our time and energy in this activity, we become deeply frustrated and dissatisfied, no matter how wealthy or powerful we may be, and this frustration, pooling, collecting, and fermenting, becomes bombs and bullets, toxic dumps and cancers, roving gangs and terrorists. Work, like birth and meals, is sacred, a sacrament, and by desecrating work with competitiveness, killing, cruelty, and exploitation, our herding culture has sown seeds that can only bear misery for everyone.

In the current modern incarnation of the old viciously dominating herding culture—displaying its values now in amplified, high-tech form as fast food chains, megacities, giant hog farms, floating slaughterhouses, nuclear warheads, and rampant injustice, inequality, and exploitation—the resurrection of work means first and foremost understanding the roots of domination in the commodification of animals for food. The key to reclaiming our birthright and harmony, hidden in the most obvious of places—our plates—requires (as appropriate to mythic wisdom) that for us to be free, we must first free those whom we chain. To reclaim our purpose, we must restore the purposes we have stolen from others. As we remove the violence from our daily meals, we will naturally increase our ability to heal our divisions, nurture our creativity and joy, restore beauty and gentleness, and be role models of sensitivity and compassion for our children. As we look more deeply at our food, the healing of our children can begin, and our work can be resurrected as an instrument for blessing and bringing joy and caring to our world.

CHAPTER ELEVEN

PROFITING FROM DESTRUCTION

"The worst sin toward our fellow creatures is not to hate them, but to be indifferent to them. That is the essence of inhumanity."
—George Bernard Shaw

"The impact of countless hooves and mouths over the years has done more to alter the type of vegetation and land forms of the West than all the water projects, strip mines, power plants, freeways, and subdivision developments combined."
—Philip Fradkin in *Audubon*, National Audubon Society

"Pigs and cows and chickens and people are all competing for grain."
—Margaret Mead

The Industrialization of Farming

It would be difficult to conceive of a more wasteful, toxic, inhumane, disease-promoting, and destructive food production system than our farmed animal industry. Besides being outrageously inhumane to the animals imprisoned for food—and to the wild animals whose habitats are destroyed and who are poisoned, trapped, and shot by ranchers, agribusiness farmers, government agencies, and the fishing industry as pests and competitors—the farmed animal industry also extravagantly wastes water, petroleum, land, and chemicals; destroys forests and fisheries; severely pollutes land, water and air; and, at enormous expense, floods our markets with products that are toxic in the extreme to our own health.

It would not be possible for us to eat the high quantities of inexpensive animal foods that we do today without a massive infusion of fossil fuels into our food production system. If we look at the sharply ascending human population growth curve of the last hundred years, we see that it precisely matches the energy growth curve that has allowed us to create enormous amounts of food. Excess food has fueled the population explosion of humans—and of confined cows, pigs, chickens, fish, and other animals raised to be slaughtered for food.

In the 1950s and '60s our nation's agriculture became industrialized, a process that was euphemized as the "Green Revolution." This current food production system is based on cheap and abundant oil and natural gas. Industrial agriculture relies on natural gas to create the twelve million tons of nitrogen fertilizer used annually in the U.S., which represents an energy equivalent of over 100 million barrels of diesel fuel.[1] It also requires millions of barrels of petroleum to manufacture the 1.3 million tons of pesticides used every year[2] (over eighty percent of which is applied to the four crops—corn, soybeans, wheat, and cotton—that are the major constituents of livestock feed);[3] to pump the trillions of gallons of irrigation water these crops require; to power the farm machinery that has virtually replaced human labor; to transport and house billions of animals annually; and to run the stockyards, slaughter plants, rendering operations, and refrigerated product transportation systems. Cheap oil is also a prerequisite of the so-called "Blue Revolution," the explosion of factory fish farming. The fish in aquaculture operations consume both grain and other fish, and the immense fishing fleets currently over-exploiting planetary fish stocks also require unsustainably large amounts of cheap diesel fuel. The foundation of agriculture has switched from soil to oil, and though this has allowed more people to eat more animal foods than ever in history, the price we and others pay for this is staggering. Now that we are entering a new period of declining fossil fuel production, bitter and violent conflicts for the precious oil demanded by our omnivorous eating habits loom larger every day.

Eating Soil, Water, and Fossil Fuels

The major environmental problem with eating animal foods is that these animals, whose populations are vast, must eat, and eat *a lot*. Eighty percent of grain grown in the U.S. and about half the fish hauled in are wasted to grow billions of animals big and fat enough to be profitably slaughtered, or to produce dairy products and eggs at the high levels demanded by consumers. And over ninety percent of the protein in this grain turns into the methane, ammonia, urea, and manure that pollute our air and water. A conservative estimate is that the amount of land, grain, water, petroleum, and pollution required to feed one of us the Standard American Diet could feed fifteen of us eating a plant-based diet.[4] Understanding the implications of this is crucial to our survival, because our industrialized animal-based agriculture is disastrously depleting the three essentials on which it depends: soil, water, and fossil fuels.

Most of us have little comprehension of the enormous amount of land devoted to growing grain to feed imprisoned pigs, cows, sheep, birds, and fish. Already, over 521,000 square miles of U.S. forest have been cleared to graze livestock and to grow grain to feed them. This amounts to more land than the states of Texas, California, and Oregon combined, yet it grows daily, with about 6,000 square miles cleared every year. This amounts to about 10,000 acres per day, seven acres every minute.[5] This ongoing deforestation, which is *seven times* the amount of deforestation caused by building roads, homes, parking lots, and shopping centers,[6] means loss of wildlife habitat, loss of genetic diversity, loss of topsoil, degradation of streams and rivers, and increased pollution. Forests create topsoil, generate oxygen, clean the air, help bring needed rain, and provide habitat for thousands of species of animals and plants.

Besides the obliteration of vast areas of forest, animal agriculture is responsible for the destruction and degradation of even larger areas—of virtually all our prairie grasslands and much of the arid regions of the

West. These complex and beautiful ecosystems once supported a wide variety of plant and animal species, now lost because the lands have been converted to monocropped fields of feed grain or used to graze cattle. Using forest, prairie, and arid lands for animal agriculture destroys complex interconnected ecosystems so that only one desired species can survive on the land. Ranchers and agribusiness farmers see most species besides their livestock and feed grains as pests to be exterminated. The annihilation and disruption of forests, prairie grasslands, and arid regions to graze and grow feed for slaughter-bound animals is not only a destruction of biological diversity and intelligence but has other serious repercussions as well.

Few of us are aware of the tremendous strain imposed on our water supplies by animal agriculture. Agriculture consumes fully eighty-five percent of all U.S. freshwater resources,[7] mainly to produce animal foods. A day's production of food for one omnivore human requires more than four thousand gallons of water, compared with less than three hundred gallons for a vegan;[8] this fact represents enormous environmental damage, especially in the lands west of the Mississippi, where precious aquifers are being depleted and rivers and streams diverted into irrigation canals, causing death and suffering to birds, fish, and other wildlife in order to provide the massive quantities of irrigation water required to grow livestock feed grains.

Forty percent of irrigation water comes from underground aquifers that take centuries to replenish.[9] In fact, the great Ogallala aquifer that underlies much of central North America, which took millennia to form and was the largest in the world, is being rapidly and recklessly depleted, over thirteen trillion gallons of water pumped out annually to irrigate the immense expanses of land that grow livestock feed.[10] Meanwhile, people are being told to conserve water by using low-flow showerheads and toilets. University of California soil and water specialists have estimated that while the purchase of one pound of California lettuce, tomatoes, potatoes, or wheat requires only about 24 gallons of water, the purchase of one pound of California beef requires over 5,200 gallons of water. John Robbins points out that this is more than would be used in a year of daily showers![11] Much of this water goes to irrigate grain fields devoted to livestock feed, pumped by petroleum from faraway rivers and aquifers, with dams, canals, and pumping stations paid for by taxpayers rather than by the animal agribusinesses that profit from them. Marc Reisner, author of *Cadillac Desert*, concludes, "The West's water crisis— and many of its environmental problems as well—can be summed up, implausible as this may seem, in a single word: livestock."[12]

Animal foods also require immense quantities of petroleum to produce. For example, while it takes only two calories of fossil fuel to produce one calorie of protein from soybeans, and three calories for wheat and corn, it takes fifty-four calories of petroleum to produce one calorie of protein from beef![13] Animal agriculture contributes disproportionately to our consumption of petroleum and thus to air and water pollution, global warming, and the wars driven by conflict over dwindling petroleum reserves.

How is it possible that it could take *twenty-seven times* as much petroleum to supply people with hamburgers as it does to provide soy burgers, and what are the implications of this? Soil used for agriculture tends to become deficient in nitrogen because plants pull it out of the ground to synthesize protein. Traditional solutions were to spread manure or guano to re-enrich the soil, to plant legumes and rotate crops, and to allow the land to lie fallow and replenish itself. In 1909 two German chemists devised a method for fixing atmospheric nitrogen in making ammonia that allowed later scientists to invent methods of producing inorganic nitrogen fertilizer from natural gas cheaply and in immense quantities. This relatively sudden availability of nitrogen enabled the huge increase in food production that has driven the population explosion of both humans and farmed animals over the last century.[14] It is this same artificial fertilizer that causes nitrogen "nutrient-rich" runoff into streams and rivers, which is one of our most significant water pollution problems, causing excess algae growth, depleting oxygen, and killing fish.

Besides the natural gas for fertilizer, our agricultural system needs petroleum to produce the enormous quantities of hydrocarbon-based insecticides and herbicides that have increased thirty-three-fold over the past twenty years.[15] Meanwhile, every year more crops are lost to pests because of monocropping and the abandonment of traditional soil-regenerating practices. When large tracts of land are used to grow only one crop, the fields strongly attract "pest" species that feed on that specific crop. Because of the lack of variety in the plant and insect population of the area, few birds and other predators come there to feed, and the pests become immune to the ever-increasing levels of pesticides directed at them. The same crop is planted in the same soil season after season, compounding the profusion of pesticide-resistant organisms. According to Worldwatch Institute, there are now about a thousand major agricultural pests that are immune to pesticides.[16] Dousing our food fields with poison is part of a cancer-causing battle against nature's persistent resistance to the industrialized methods agribusiness prefers, which turn millions of acres of monocropped lands into toxic killing fields for wildlife.

Modern intensive agriculture also inevitably destroys topsoil, which requires centuries to build up—approximately five hundred years for one inch.[17] Because of the harshness of industrial agriculture, cropland soils are eroding at thirty times the formation rate, and every year more than two million acres are lost to erosion and to salinization from chronic irrigation.[18] At this point, the soil of large-scale monocropping operations is depleted of minerals and nutrients, and is little more than a lifeless medium into which agribusiness pours inorganic nitrogen fertilizer in order to produce high-yield crops—primarily livestock feed—of questionable nutritive value.

This intensive agriculture is unsustainable. The more it damages land and water supplies and drains aquifers, the more fossil fuel input it requires to irrigate, replace nutrients, provide pest protection, and simply hold crop production constant. Unless we switch from eating resource-gobbling animal foods, we will have to face the consequences of our limited and declining supply of fossil fuels.

Richard Heinberg makes clear in his book *The Party's Over: Oil, War and the Fate of Industrial Societies* that leading petroleum experts believe that worldwide production of petroleum is currently peaking, and we are now entering a period of declining production as existing reserves are being rapidly depleted.[19] Four gallons of petroleum are extracted for every gallon that is discovered, and advances in geo-chemistry and seismic technology have made it clear that undiscovered petroleum reserves are small and rapidly disappearing.[20] We continue to escalate consumption and to ignore the severe consequences because we have so much practice three times daily in ignoring conse-quences. Petroleum expert C. J. Campbell has said, "The warning sig-nals have been flying for a long time. They have been plain to see. But the world turned a blind eye, and failed to read the message. Our lack of preparedness is itself amazing, given the importance of oil to our lives."[21] It's less amazing when we realize that our ability to block feedback is an integral aspect of the mentality of domination and dis-connectedness that eating animal foods requires. We are unfortunate-ly only too willing to cooperate with the military-industrial-meat com-plex by unconsciously suppressing any healthy feedback that might threaten our eating habits.

The collision of soaring demand for fossil fuels with their permanent-ly diminishing availability will cause unremitting upward price pressure as demands continue to expand and conflicts over limited oil escalate. With the coming unavoidable decline in fossil fuel availability, the days of cheap animal foods are numbered. We may begin to recognize that eating animal foods is an unacceptable waste of our limited petroleum supplies. Already people are getting outraged about the petroleum wast-ed by large SUVs that are inefficient compared to economy cars by a fac-tor of perhaps three to one. Will we get similarly outraged at people eat-ing beef, chicken, fish, eggs, and dairy products, which are inefficient compared to plant foods by factors that far exceed those of the biggest SUVs—factors of 10, 15, and 25 to one? It's easier to see the gallons of fossil fuel poured directly into our cars than it is to see the gallons of fos-sil fuel poured into our cheese, eggs, fish sticks, hot dogs, and steaks.

The Toxins in Animal Agriculture

The vast, monocropped fields devoted to feeding the animals we eat cover millions of acres of land and are heavily doused with toxic pesti-cides and fertilizers. Two of these crops, corn and soybeans, are now genetically modified and have become the main components of animal feed, with *over half* of all U.S. farmland devoted to just these two feed crops alone.[22] They're genetically engineered to be herbicide-resistant so that agribusinesses typically spray two to five times more toxic chemicals on these fields than on non-GMO crops, killing wildlife and polluting water at ever-higher levels.

These toxic fields are the foundation of the dairy products and eggs we eat, as well as the beef, poultry, pork, and many fish, like factory-farmed catfish, trout, and tilapia. The carcinogenic residues of the chemical fertilizers and pesticides used on these fields contaminate our rivers and oceans. They concentrate in the animal foods we eat and in our own flesh and milk as well. In addition, the manure that is used to "enrich" animal feed concentrates toxins to an even greater extent than the plant foods that the animals are forced to eat.

Fungicides, insecticides, herbicides, and chemical fertilizer residues concentrate in livestock excrement. Anyone building a house knows how strict most communities are about human sewage disposal, and yet disposal of livestock sewage is virtually unregulated. The ten billion land animals confined and killed every year excrete massive quantities of feces and urine, not just equal to what we humans produce, or even two or three times greater, but according to a study by the U.S. Senate, 130 times greater.[23] This farm animal waste can be hundreds of times more concentrated than untreated human sewage.[24] It is more highly toxic because of its high bacteria, chemical, and drug residues. For example, the high levels of antibiotics running into streams from livestock manure have been shown to contribute to more dangerous antibiotic-resistant bacteria in rivers.[25] The dairies in central California create more sewage than a city of twenty million people, and just one mega pig factory farm creates more sewage than New York City![26] Farmed animal waste disposal is much less regulated than human waste disposal because animal agriculture industries are supported in their resistance of regulations by their friends in governmental agencies and politicians beholden to them for campaign contributions. This unregulated toxic waste pollutes groundwater, rivers, lakes, and oceans.[27] When gigantic open lagoons of pig excrement spill, the resulting outbreaks of pfisteria can kill millions of fish and seriously harm human swimmers in downstream rivers and bays. According to the Environmental Protection Agency, more than thirty-five thousand miles of rivers were polluted by large-scale feedlots in the past decade.[28] When factory farms pollute groundwater, it is typically public money, rather than industry funds, that is used to clean up or contain the pollution.[29]

Livestock excrement causes horrific air pollution as well, as those who are unfortunate enough to live near these operations attest. The stench causes mental stress and respiratory ailments, and when the manure dries, it can blow for miles around. Livestock also emit large quantities of methane gas, which is a major factor in global warming because it retains heat more strongly than carbon dioxide. Grilling animal flesh creates more air pollution: researchers have discovered that much of the smog haze over cities is formed not just by cars but by the smoke and fat particles of thousands of fast-food restaurants and kitchens grilling meat.[30]

Healing the Earth and the Economy

We don't seem to realize that our economy would be far healthier if we switched to eating plant-based meals. If we all ate a plant-based diet, we could feed ourselves on a small fraction of the land and grains that eating an animal-based diet requires. For example, researchers estimate that 2.5 acres of land can meet the food energy needs of twenty-two people eating potatoes, nineteen people eating corn, twenty-three people eating cabbage, fifteen people eating wheat, or two people eating chicken or dairy products, and only one person eating beef or eggs.[31] Everyone on earth could be fed easily because we currently grow more than enough grain to feed ten billion people;[32] our current practice of feeding this grain to untold billions of animals and eating them forces over a billion of us to endure chronic malnutrition and starvation while another billion suffer from the obesity, diabetes, heart disease, and cancer linked with eating diets high in animal foods.

The drugs we take to combat these diseases are discharged through the urine, flow into the water and become yet another major stream that adds to the pollution of our earth. This is an especially serious problem surrounding some of the larger cities of the industrialized world.

Toxins—like other negative consequences of animal foods—don't just disappear once we swallow them. They are excreted right into our ecosystems, although large traces accumulate in the fatty tissues of our bodies as well. Thus, by eating a more plant-based diet we could reduce our pollution of the earth, and our own bodies could become less polluted and diseased, saving us from the vicious cycle of dousing the earth and ourselves with increasingly toxic chemicals, which is part of our unwinnable war against nature.

Switching to a plant-based diet, we could reduce petroleum usage and imports enormously, and slash the amount of hydrocarbons and carbon dioxide that contribute to air pollution and global warming.[33] We could save hundreds of billions of dollars per year in medical, drug, and insurance expenses, which would boost personal savings and thus reinvigorate the economy, providing fresh funds for creative projects and environmental restoration. Desolate monocropped fields devoted to livestock feed could be planted with trees, bringing back forests, streams, and wildlife. Marine ecosystems could rebuild, rain forests could begin healing, and with our demand for resources of all kinds dramatically reduced, environmental and military tension could ease. Grain that is now fed to the livestock of the world's wealthy could feed the starving poor.

If we ceased the practice that creates the spiritual, psychological, social, and economic force behind human war and violence, the military budget, which saps economic vitality, could be reduced considerably. U.S. military spending is obscene, with over half of the entire federal discretionary budget going to the military. It's well known that military spending, when compared with spending on education, environmental restoration, human services, health care, construction, and so forth, creates the fewest number of jobs and results in non-consumable products, like bombs, mines, weapons, and weapons tests, that also create enormous pollution and destruction.

The Consequences of Evading Consequences

Much has been written on the disastrous environmental impact of confining animals for food, including *Diet for a Small Planet*, *Diet for a New America*, *Mad Cowboy*, *Vegan: The New Ethics of Eating*, *The*

Food Revolution, and many other books and articles. The information is available, and any of us who are interested can do the research and discover that a diet based on animal foods is a primary driving force behind the most serious environmental problems we face: the ongoing extinction of species, rain forest destruction, air and water pollution, loss of water resources, global warming, dependence on foreign oil, proliferation of disease, topsoil loss, drought, forest fires, desertification, habitat destruction, and even war and terrorism. This information is not publicized, however, and our understanding of it is suppressed, because eating animal foods is the elephant in our living room that we all pretend not to see—unrecognized behavior that destroys our family but is taboo to confront or discuss.

Our institutions reflect the mentality required by our omnivorism. Part of the problem is that the toxins used in industrial agriculture are highly profitable for the wealthy and privileged elite that dominates our cultural conversations through its power over the media, government, and education. The military-industrial-meat-medical-media complex has and offers no incentive to reduce animal food consumption. Poisoning the earth with massive doses of toxic chemicals and petroleum-based fertilizers is highly profitable for the petroleum and chemical industries. These toxins cause cancer, which is highly profitable to the chemical-pharmaceutical-medical complex. While the world's rich omnivores waste precious supplies of grain, petroleum, water, and land feeding and eating fattened animals, the world's poor have little grain to eat or clean water to drink, and their chronic hunger, thirst, and misery create conditions for war, terrorism, and drug addiction, which are extremely profitable industries as well. The richest fifth of the world's population gets obesity, heart disease, and diabetes, also highly profitable for industry. The transnational corporations profit from animal food consumption, as do the big banks, which have made the loans that have built the whole complex and demand a healthy return on their investments. The system spreads relentlessly and globally, and while corporate and bank returns may be healthy, people, animals, and ecosystems throughout the world fall ill and are exploited and destroyed.

With its immense financial resources and legendary influence at all levels of government, animal agribusiness receives billions of dollars in subsidies, price supports, income assistance, emergency assistance, commodity loans, direct payments, allotments, tax breaks, rail and feed subsidies, grazing privileges, the dairy export incentive program, and other governmental services every year. Without this aid, the industry could never survive in its present form; the cheapest hamburger meat would cost at least thirty-five dollars per pound without taxpayer-funded irrigation systems, subsidies, remediation allowances, and countless other government handouts.[34] The 2002 Farm Bill, for example, provoked outrage among Central and South American countries because the unprecedented amount of federal money it gave to U.S. agribusiness—$182 *billion*—enabled U.S. meat, dairy, egg, and grain producers to flood Latin American markets with low-priced products that put local farmers out of business there.

The research presented in Marion Nestle's *Food Politics* details how the animal food industry maintains an iron grip on governmental agencies and policies, and how our food production system is designed to maximize profits for the relatively few large corporations that dominate it. She writes, for example,

> My job was to manage the editorial production of the first—and as yet only—Surgeon General's Report on Nutrition and Health. . . . My first day on the job, I was given the rules: No matter what the research indicated, the report could not recommend "eat less meat" as a way to reduce intake of saturated fat, nor could it suggest restrictions on intake of any other category of food. In the industry-friendly climate of the Reagan administration, the producers of foods that might be affected by such advice would complain to their beneficiaries in Congress, and the report would never be published.[35]

We should have no illusions that governmental agencies and authorities will work to protect consumer, environmental, or animal interests, because, as numerous journalists and researchers have discovered and pointed out (though seldom in mainstream media), they cater to the wealthy and powerful industries and corporations that apply constant direct pressure on them. These industries also provide new government personnel through the "revolving door" between jobs in industry and jobs in the government agencies that serve those industries. Just as the Department of Defense is run by people from the weapons industries, the Department of Agriculture is run by former ranchers, executives, and lawyers for the meat, dairy, and egg industries. It is in the interest of the animal food industries that consumers be kept as unaware as possible of the abysmal conditions in which the animals must live, as well as the horrendous effects of these foods on human health and on our ecosystems.

The production and selling of our animal-based diet disproportionately benefits a small elite at the expense of imprisoned animals, sick and starving people, and future generations. This elite, an inevitable result of our culture's mentality of domination and exclusion, controls agribusiness, industry, and the governmental, media, military, educational, medical, and financial institutions. These institutions promote eating animals because the slavery of animals is fundamental to this elite's power structure, as it has been since its rise to power with the herding of animals roughly eight thousand years ago. It is still maintained in the traditional ways, by controlling the concentration of money and political power and thereby managing thought through manipulation of education, religion, government, and other social institutions.

It is no accident that we find transnational corporations increasingly intruding in and controlling our public and private lives. Corporations are manifestations of our desire to evade responsibility (euphemized as "limiting liability") and they are rooted in the violence on our plates, for through our daily meals, we kill, confine, and abuse animals in ways for which we cannot bear to be responsible. This psychological woundedness and disconnectedness, gathering cultural momentum over centuries and combined with the mentality of domination and commodification of living beings required by our meals, eventually incarnated as corporations and became the transnational behemoths that bestride us and our world today. Over the past one and a half centuries, they have grown enormously and have succeeded in casting off the legal limitations that were imposed on them in earlier generations.[36] They are now recognized by our courts as legal persons, but they lack flesh, blood, and spirit. Abstract instruments merely, they exist solely to maximize their power and their investors' wealth. They don't die but instead grow ever stronger and more virulent. They are our creations and are reflections of us, and yet they pressure us to serve their interests at the expense of our families, our relationships, our communities, our earth, and ourselves. The more corporations can "externalize" costs, passing them to workers, animals, future generations, governments, communities, and others, the more profitable they can be.

Our animal-based meals are also the source of the complacency and sense of disempowerment that permit the environmental and social holocaust that our media prevent us from seeing and comprehending. Eating animal foods diminishes our sensitivity, paralyzing us by reducing our ability to respond—our response-ability. Eating the violence on our plates requires an evasion of responsibility so that we come to believe our actions don't make much difference. This erroneous belief is actually rooted in our semi-conscious understanding that with every meal we cause exactly the kind of suffering and pollution that we would naturally want to prevent. The social and economic system I've described requires a large population of reliably sick, desensitized and distracted people. Encouraging the continued eating of the flesh, fluids, and eggs of mistreated animals is a fundamental way to assure this, and to assure profitability, the god enshrined on the highest corporate altar.

One way this is done is through increasing corporate control of medicine and science. Today, the medical-pharmaceutical industry's emphasis is on genetics. As corporations pave their way into university research facilities with much-needed funding, we see that academic assumptions are following corporate money lines. Researchers are encouraged by grant money, prestige, and peer pressure to view disease and health in terms of genetics, because this is a profitable view for the pharmaceutical industry—and is in alignment with the mechanistic and reductionist mentality that underlies conventional science.

If diseases are seen as being the result of our thinking, our lifestyle, our eating habits, our feelings, our actions, and our ability to respond to our life's calling, and as messages, teachings, and opportunities for us on our spiritual path, then we are empowered to respond to them creatively and directly, and to become more healthy by taking responsibility for the health of our inner and outer environment. This would all be very bad for corporate control and profits. If we can be convinced that our diseases are due to mere "genetic predisposition" over which we have no control, then the corporations have us right where they want us: at their mercy. And they have no mercy.

The gene theories have appeal because they release us from responsibility for our inner attitudes and outer actions and place us securely in the hands of the corporations that profit from our forsaking our ultimate responsibility for our health. Not only profit-intensive for the medical industry and for the banks and financial institutions supporting them, prescription drugs also disempower us, fog our thinking, numb our feelings, and weaken our natural recuperative powers. According to the pharmaceutical industry, in 2001 3.2 *billion* prescriptions were filled in the U.S., with *46 percent* of adults taking at least one prescription drug on a daily basis—and these drug sales are increasing about twenty-five percent every year![37] Side effects of pharmaceuticals continue to be a top killer, and virtually all of these drugs are potentially addicting. From 1962 to 1988, for example, street drug addiction increased thirty percent, while addiction to prescription drugs increased three hundred percent.[38] Why do we hear so much about the former and so little about the latter, and why is our war on drugs focused only on those drugs that don't directly contribute to corporate profits? Trying to evade consequences has further consequences.

A plant-based diet cannot be patented, so it is of absolutely no interest to the pharmaceutical complex. It is an enormous threat, in fact, and huge campaigns are waged to keep us distracted and believing that complex carbohydrates are bad for us while animal protein is absolutely necessary, and that science can save us from diabetes, cancer, and the other diseases brought on by our callous domination of animals for food. Billions are spent searching for drugs and other material means to cure what is actually an ethical and spiritual disease. Sowing disease and death in animals at our mercy, we reap the same in ourselves. Much of medical research today is actually an apparently desperate quest to find ways to continue eating animal foods and to escape the consequences of our cruel and unnatural practices. Do we *really* want to be successful in this?

We become free as we stop cooperating with the system of domination that would like to feed us its blood foods. If the blood of animals is on our hands, we are—perhaps unwittingly—enslaved. The powerful elite that controls the military-industrial-meat-medical-media complex strives to pull the strings of control ever tighter, and with awareness we can see it all around us. Violence only begets further violence. We are called to retaliate with love, directed at those who are most vulnerable and abused—food animals—and spread the word.

Our lives flow from our beliefs, and our beliefs are conditioned by our daily actions. As we act, so we build our character and so we become. By consciously making our meals celebrations of peace, compassion, and freedom, we can sow seeds in the most powerful way possible to contribute to the healing of our world.

CHAPTER TWELVE

SOME OBJECTIONS ANSWERED

"We must fight against the spirit of unconscious cruelty with which we
treat the animals. Animals suffer as much as we do. . . . It is our duty to
make the whole world recognize it."
—ALBERT SCHWEITZER

"Animals of the world exist for their own reasons. They were not made for
humans any more than blacks were made for whites or women for men."
—ALICE WALKER

"And now a third, a Brazen people rise,
Unlike the former, men of monstrous size.
On the crude flesh of beasts, they feed alone,
Savage their nature, and their hearts of stone."
—HESIOD, 8th Century B.C.E.

Nurturing Objections

The ideas presented in this book, though not complicated or particularly difficult to understand, have long been invisible and almost impossible to articulate because they directly contradict the hidden assumptions
of our herding culture. Their ramifications, if contemplated, discussed,
and acted upon, are enormously subversive to the status quo. Even

other subversive social theories that are rarely seen in schools or the media—such as Marxism—don't begin to address the deeper issue we are discussing: the mentality of domination and exclusion that necessarily flows from commodifying animals and eating animal foods, and that gives rise to competition, repression of the feminine principle, and the exploitation of the lower classes by the wealthier cattle- (capital-) owning classes. Marx's "Workers of the world, unite!" never questioned the underlying ethic of dominating animals and nature, and hence was not truly revolutionary. It operated within the human supremacist framework and never challenged the mentality that sees living beings as commodities. Veganism is a call for us to unite in seeing that as long as we oppress other living beings, we will inevitably create and live in a culture of oppression. Class struggle is a result of the herding culture's mentality of domination and exclusion, and is just part of the misery that is inevitably connected with eating animal foods.

The vegan commitment to consciously minimize our cruelty to all animals is so revolutionary in its implications that it is often summarily dismissed because it triggers cognitive dissonance and deep anxiety. We have been so ingrained with the herding mentality since birth that even those of us who consider ourselves to be quite progressive aren't typically prepared to question the exploitation of animals and humans that we cause by our food choices. Like a ball being held under water, our natural compassion wants to come bobbing up to the surface, so we must continually work to keep it repressed. The way we keep the ball of kindness and intelligence submerged is not only by practicing disconnecting but also by the practice of nurturing some culturally induced objections to eating a plant-based diet, which we repeat to ourselves if the ball starts rising.

Animals as Ethically Trivial

One of these basic objections is that compassion for animals gives them more importance than they merit. With this objection, the dominant herding paradigm trivializes animals, scoffing at vegans for caring about them while their fellow human beings suffer from poverty, the breakdown of the family, war, drug addiction, terrorism, pollution, and so forth. This objection is merely a restatement of the herding culture's fundamental supremacist orientation that legitimizes the domination of animals. It is based in an attitude that animals don't matter, that their suffering at our hands is not an issue, and that they are somehow superfluous or expendable. If we can get our minds and hearts somehow outside the box constructed by our culturally defining core practice of enslaving and killing animals for food, which traps our thinking and feeling within the narrow confines of the dominator herding mentality, we will begin to see, feel, and understand what animals actually are.

We will see that, like us, animals are expressions of infinite, universal love-intelligence; that, like us, they yearn for satisfaction of their drives and desires, and avoid pain and suffering; that, like us, they are profoundly mysterious. If we've learned anything at all about animals, it is that we can in no way make them fit into the categories of our limited understanding. When we look at animals in nature it is possible to see competition, struggle, and violence, as many scientists are trained to do, and yet it is also possible to see cooperation and mutual aid, as Kropotkin[1] and other scientists have discovered. Further, it is possible to see celebration, joy, humor, love, caring, and the wondrous interplay and expression of an absolutely infinite complexity of life forms. There is deep truth in the old saying that we see things not as they are but as we are.

We have not begun to scratch the surface of understanding animals. How can we know what it is to swim as whales, at home in the ocean depths and migrating thousands of miles, speaking in underwater songs and breathing together in conscious harmony, or to fly in a flock of sandpipers, whirling in an effortless synchronicity, fifty birds as one, or to burrow as prairie dogs, creating complex underground communities with virtually endless chambers, passageways, and interactions? Our knowledge and understanding of nonhuman animals is polluted far more than we acknowledge by our belief in our own superiority, our unrecognized cultural programming, and our separation from nature. Our theories about animals will be seen in the future as quaint balderdash, as we now view the medieval theories of healing through bleeding and leeches and of an earth-centered solar system.

Our understanding is so contaminated by our mentality of objectification that we are killing off animals and destroying species and natural communities at a rate unparalleled in history. When we look deeply we see that understanding brings and awakens love, and that love brings and awakens understanding. If our so-called understanding of animals does not ignite within us a loving urge to allow them to fulfill their lives and purposes, to honor, respect and appreciate them, then it is not true understanding. Our science is in many ways incapable of this authentic understanding, and, because it is also often a vehicle of corporate power, it is best not to rely on it too heavily in our quest for wisdom or healing.

The Myth of Human Predation

A second objection to veganism raised by the herding culture is that eating animal foods must be natural and right because we've been doing it for such a long time. The first response to this objection is to question its basic validity. We know as individuals that it is often counterproductive and crippling if we carry into adulthood the same strategies and beliefs we used as children. The fact that we've been doing something a long time hardly makes it right or appropriate. The same defense of human slavery was used here in the nineteenth century. How will we progress or evolve if we continue to justify outmoded behavior and obsolete beliefs by giving them validity they don't deserve? War, genocide, murder, rape, and human exploitation have been going on a long time as well, but we would never dare to use their longevity to justify them. That we would do so to justify the enslavement, exploitation, murder, rape, and extinction of animals is telling, but completely specious. It undermines our healthy yearning to grow in wisdom and to strive to build a society that is more free, peaceful, and sustainable.

The second response to this objection is to question its veracity. What is a "long time"? The ten thousand years we've been herding and commodifying animals and the twenty to sixty thousand years we've been hunting large animals[2] are very short compared to the three hundred thousand years *homo sapiens* has been here and the seven to ten million years that hominids have been here. Our closest living relatives, supposedly sharing ninety-five to ninety-eight percent of our DNA, are gorillas, bonobos, and chimpanzees. The powerful and gentle gorillas eat a totally plant-based diet, as do bonobos, and chimpanzees eat a primarily plant-based diet. Our own ancient forebears were probably similar, given our physiology, and according to fossil evidence of such early humans as *Australopithecus*, plant foods made up virtually all of their diet.[3] The problem has been that our culture has fostered its own "man the predator" mythology, based on and justifying our eating of animals, propagating the erroneous notion that, as Swiss zoologist C. Guggisberg wrote in 1970, "man has been a predator and ruthless killer for as long as he has existed."[4] This same lie, that "man is a beast of prey" (Oswald Spengler), has been repeated so much that we believe it and perpetuate it. Jim Mason explains:

> Deeply ingrained in our culture, then, are some very strong values that favor killing and consuming animals for food. How could they *not* have affected studies of human diet, food collection, and evolution?
>
> Surely our own culture's meat-eater values have been a factor in the exaggeration of the hunter role in human evolution in the same way that its patriarchal values have been a factor in the exaggeration of the male role in evolution. Indeed, both of these cultural biases worked well together in promoting the man-the-mighty-hunter model of human evolution. Hunting, as men's work, was highly valued by anthropology's mostly male investigators. And since hunting provided meat, it was doubly valued by meat-eating investigators.
>
> The hunter-creation myth also helps a meat-eating society with a very troublesome problem. People, generally, are more than a little uncomfortable with killing animals for food. Most would probably not be willing to kill an animal themselves, except in dire circumstances. Even northern hunting peoples surrounded their hunting and butchering activities with ritual—much of it, as we shall see, to ease anxiety and discomfort.[5]

Anthropologists Donna Hart and Robert W. Sussman, in their recent groundbreaking synthesis of fossil evidence and primatology, explain that early humans did not have teeth that could eat meat and were not predatory hunters. They argue that the views of "man the hunter" and of our ancestors as "bloodthirsty brutes" are based on three things: "perverted Western views of modern humans, the Christian concept of original sin, and ... just plain sloppy science" (ellipses in original).[6]

We must question our culture's underlying assumptions, and understand how these assumptions perpetuate themselves. No one knows exactly why we humans began killing and eating animals. According to Plutarch, writing nearly two thousand years ago,

> The primitive people who first ate meat likely did so out of extreme privation. People in those days were reduced to eating mud, bark, grass sprouts, and roots. Finding acorns and buckeyes would have been cause for celebration. If these people could only speak to us today they would undoubtedly tell us how fortunate we are to have such an abundance of delicious vegetable foods at our finger-tips; and how fortunate that we can fill our stomachs without polluting ourselves with flesh. They would be perplexed by the lust that leads people to eat meat in these times of plenty. They would ask, "Don't you think the good earth can sustain you? Aren't you ashamed to mix the wholesome produce of the earth with blood and flesh?"[7]

Today there are masses of conflicting theories as to why we began flesh-eating, and they are all, to some degree, warped by being products of the herding culture itself. Many attribute it partially to our early migrations out of the tropical and subtropical regions into the cooler temperate regions where plant foods weren't so easily available. Many of the theories are skewed by the invisible assumptions of male researchers who assume that men have always dominated women, hunted large animals, and warred with each other. Even when these theories are shown to be inaccurate, they tend to live on because they fit nicely with the herding culture's overall paradigm, and they serve the interests of other writers who have similar erroneous theories.

A good example is Peter D'Adamo and his popular *Eat Right for Your Type* books, which encourage eating animal foods based on blood type. D'Adamo claims that type O people are best suited to eating animal flesh, because type O is allegedly the oldest blood type.[8] His books are based on completely outdated anthropological research that postulated the earliest humans (allegedly blood type O) were more carnivorous. D'Adamo ignores the more recent research that shows the early "hunter-gatherers" were much more gatherers than hunters. The mass culture, raised on the stereotype of macho cavemen dragging women around by the hair and eating mastodons for lunch, eagerly believes D'Adamo because his books argue that most people, being of the "older" blood types, "need" meat and just won't do well on a vegan diet. The theory has obvious mass appeal, since forty to sixty percent of our population is blood-type O, but is grossly inaccurate: there are many happy, healthy type O vegans, and blood type has nothing to do with the basic herbivore design of our bodies or with the cruelty inflicted on animals for food. Because it dovetails so well with our herding culture's basic view of reality, though, the books sell well and provide some of us an erroneous justification to continue our omnivorous mealtime traditions. The same could be said for the "high-protein" and "low-carbohydrate" diets that are so predictably popular, as well as the "high-iron" or "high-calcium" diets that promote eating animal foods. It's well established that plant-based diets give us ample calcium, iron, and protein, without the damaging effects of the cruelty, adrenalin, cholesterol, saturated fat, and toxins endemic to animal foods.

Confronted with the problems that characterize our herding culture, we are perhaps like the metaphorical man wounded by an arrow that the Buddha discussed with his students. He said that the man would be foolish if he tried to discover who shot the arrow, why he shot it, where he was when he shot it, and so forth, before having the arrow removed and the wound treated, lest he bleed to death attempting to get his questions answered. We, likewise, can all remove the arrow and treat the wound of eating animal foods right now. We don't need to know the whole history. We can easily see it is cruel and that it is unnecessary; whatever people have done in the past, we are not obligated to imitate them if it is based on delusion. Perhaps in the past people thought they needed to enslave animals and people to survive, and that the cruelty involved in it was somehow allowed them. It's obviously not necessary for us today, as we can plainly see by walking into any grocery store, and the sooner we can awaken from the thrall of the obsolete mythos that we are predatory by nature, the sooner we'll be able to evolve spiritually and discover and fulfill our purpose on this earth.

We're in an auspicious position today, because the industrialized nations of the world, which eat the highest percentage of animal foods and are generally in the north, have food distribution systems that bring plant-based foods to all their inhabitants, regardless of their climate and topography. Fruits, vegetables, grains, legumes, and even soy milk, tofu, tempeh, and so forth, are available in markets everywhere. There are very few people today who must eat animal foods for geographic reasons. It is the height of irony that eating a diet based on animal foods, which are complicated, wasteful, cruel, and expensive to produce, is seen as simple in our culture, and that eating a vegan diet based on plant foods, which are simple, efficient, inexpensive, and free of cruelty to produce, is seen as complicated and difficult. Nevertheless, the truth is slowly coming to light, and the pressures within the old paradigm are building as more of us refuse to see animals as objects to be eaten or used for our purposes.

The Justification of Science

A third objection is that science uses animals in experiments, and if science, which has brought us the technological progress we value so highly, doesn't question dominating animals, who are we to do so? We can see, though, that scientific theories always reflect the fundamental orientation of the mainstream culture, and that science and culture echo and reproduce each other. As Thomas Kuhn demonstrated in his classic work, *The Structure of Scientific Revolutions*, scientific paradigms, like cultural paradigms, resist change. The history of science shows not so much a gradual accumulation of objectively true knowledge (which can hardly be said to exist because of the way context determines meaning and truth) but a series of shifts in the discipline's underlying paradigms.

Paradigms are the internal patterns through which we structure knowledge and experience and make sense of the world, and these paradigms are learned. In school, while we are learning content on the surface level (e.g., facts and ideas about biology, history, or mathematics), we are also learning on a paradigmatic level through the form of the educational process itself. It is invisible learning, conveyed through educational structures like giving tests, having students compete with each other, dividing knowledge into discrete subjects, using animals for dissection, giving teachers authority over students, and so forth. It is through this paradigmatic learning that the culture reproduces itself. The fundamental paradigm of our culture and science toward nature, which is of quantification and commodification, is learned in this way, though it is being increasingly challenged by paradigms of a higher order, like the vegan and spiritual paradigms of compassion for all beings and the interconnectedness of all life. We are now beginning to see the tension between these paradigms reflected in all our cultural institutions.

Kuhn emphasized that theories and findings that challenge the prevailing scientific paradigms typically come from researchers who are either young or from outside disciplines, and who are thus more free to think outside the conventional paradigmatic boxes. The response from those within the dominant paradigm is first to ignore and deny the new paradigm, and then, if it gets stronger, to ridicule and attack it. Eventually, if the new paradigm continues to gain credence over time, it may overturn and replace the dominant paradigm. With regard to eating, as the pressure continues to build, coming primarily from people who are either young or from outside (home-leavers), the dominant paradigm can no longer just ignore the vegan paradigm.

Science, a stalwart defender of the dominant herding paradigm, could be a potent tool for unseating it. Openly and fairly applied and publicized, science easily and clearly demonstrates that plant-based diets are far healthier and more sustainable than animal-based diets, and that animals experience a full range of feelings, including physical and psychological anguish when confined and treated cruelly. However, the old paradigm is protected by those who control funding to scientific institutions. Scientific studies tend to "prove" conclusions that support the corporate agenda. With corporations now providing massive research funding to universities, and with the government's industry-serving orientation, it is easy for the country's two largest industries—food and medicine—to produce a steady stream of well-publicized articles, books, public relations pieces, and scientific studies all distracting attention from the role of animal foods in disease etiology, or proclaiming that animal foods contain vital nutrients. Behind these two huge industries lurks the banking industry, which has invested billions of dollars to finance the high-tech meat-medical complex, and requires a reliable and ample flood of demand for both animal foods and for medical treatment. Veganism is profoundly dangerous to both of these, and to this economic empire's status quo. There is thus enormous pressure within the research community to resist movement toward the evolution of higher awareness and compassion that is embodied in vegan ideals.

Rather than relying on science to validate veganism and our basic herbivore physiology, we may do better by calling attention to universal truths: animals are undeniably capable of suffering; our physical bodies are strongly affected by thoughts, feelings, and aspirations; and we cannot reap happiness for ourselves by sowing seeds of misery for others. Nor may we be free while unnaturally enslaving others. We are all connected. These are knowings of the heart and veganism is, ultimately, a choice to listen to the wisdom in our heart as it opens to understanding the interconnectedness and essential unity of all life.

Deepening our understanding of these truths will give science the guidance it so desperately needs. Einstein was both correct and prescient when he wrote, "It has become appallingly obvious that our technology has exceeded our humanity." Disconnected from the direct intuitive knowing of our interconnectedness with others, science can amplify our mental delusion of separateness and bring us quickly to self-destruction. We should by now be aware that conventional science is in actuality its own mythology with a set of value-laden underlying assumptions that are taken on faith like any religion, and that it is easily prostituted, as other religions have been, by those with money and influence.

The Justification of Religion

Our religious institutions often preach that we're spiritual beings and animals are not, that we have souls and they don't, that it's all right to eat them because we've been given dominion over them. While these objections reflect the orientation of the herding culture in which they originated, biblical scholars point out that the Hebrew word translated as "dominion" in Genesis has the connotation of stewardship and would certainly never imply or condone the extremes of exploitation, confinement, neglect, and torture to which animals are routinely subjected today for our use. The Bible has been interpreted in a wide variety of ways, and the religious institutions that are seen as our culture's primary vehicles for moral and ethical guidance, have, like science, almost unquestioningly adopted the herding paradigm that considers animals mere property objects.

However, as soon as we look beyond the shallow doctrines, we find that there have been strong voices resisting the oppression of animals from within the Jewish and Christian traditions since the beginning, from the later Hebrew prophets like Isaiah and Hosea to Jesus and his Jewish disciples; to the early church fathers like St. Jerome, Clement, Tertullian, St. John Chrysostom, and St. Benedict; to the later voices of John Wesley (founder of Methodism), William Metcalf (Protestant minister and writer of the first book on vegetarianism published in the United States), Ellen White (a founder of the Seventh-Day Adventist Church), and Charles and Myrtle Fillmore (co-founders of the Unity School of Practical Christianity); as well as the voices of prominent Jewish rabbis and writers like Shlomo Goren, Moses Maimonides, Rabbi Abraham Isaac Kook, and Isaac Bashevis Singer.[9]

The vegan ideals of mercy and justice for animals have been articulated for centuries, often from within the religious establishment, and it is fascinating and instructive to see how these voices have been almost completely silenced or marginalized by the herding culture. It seems to be an unconscious reflex action. For example, if we read Jesus' teachings, we find a passionate exhortation to mercy and love, yet the possibility that the historical Jesus may have been a vegan is a radical idea for most Christians. Nevertheless, Jesus' exhortation that we love one another and not do to others what we wouldn't want done to us is the essence of the vegan ethic, which is a boundless compassion that includes all who can suffer by our actions.

In light of this, it is intriguing that Keith Akers argues convincingly in *The Lost Religion of Jesus* that Jesus and his earliest followers were ethical vegetarians committed above all to nonviolence and the spiritual harmony of simple living. Drawing entirely on the earliest written source materials by and about the early followers of Jesus, who were Jewish people known as Ebionites, Akers' careful scholarship reveals how Jesus' original message was tampered with and suppressed. He shows how, through the schisms and pressures within the early church, Jesus' followers were clearly recognized by their contemporaries as ethical vegetarians opposed to the ongoing sacrifice of animals in the temple in Jerusalem.

Jesus' message was intolerably radical, for it was the revolutionary vegan message of mercy and love for all creatures that strikes directly at the mentality of domination and exclusion that underlies both the herding culture we live in today and the culture of Jesus' time. Jesus questioned the foundation of war and oppression, which was then, as it is now, the killing and eating of animals. Back then it was animal sacrifice performed by priests at the Temple, in Jerusalem, which was the main source of wealth and prestige for the Jewish religious power structure as well as being the source of meat for the populace. Jesus' confrontation at the Temple, in which he drove out those selling animals for slaughter, was a bold attack on the fundamental herding paradigm of viewing animals merely as property, sacrifice objects, and food. Akers writes, "We must remember that the temple was more like a butcher shop than like any modern-day church or synagogue. 'Cleansing the temple' was an act of animal liberation."[10] As Akers, J. R. Hyland, and others have written, it was for this flagrantly revolutionary act that Jesus had to be crucified by the herding culture's power elite.

Akers argues that the reason the early church was so plagued by schisms was that Paul and others wanted to take the church in a direction almost completely opposite from what Jesus' teachings actually were. (Paul in particular was antagonistic toward the veganism that was apparently a core tenet of Jesus' teaching.) Akers explains many passages in Acts, such as conflicts between Paul and James, the brother of Jesus, in the light of the earliest writings attributed to Clement, Epiphanius,

Tertullian, and Origen, that point to the understanding that Jesus, James, Peter, and the direct disciples were ethical vegetarians, whereas Paul, Barnabas, and others who came later were not. Through a detailed historical analysis, Akers shows just how Paul's non-vegetarian movement was eventually able, often through brutal means, to eclipse the original thrust of Jesus' teachings regarding nonviolence, and why the original Christians, the vegetarian Ebionites, were unable to survive.

In religion, as for science and society, major paradigmatic inconsistencies cannot be tolerated. The dominant paradigm of the parent culture is exploitation, symbolized and articulated in sacrificing animals, and for Jesus to be widely recognized as Lord and Savior by the people of that culture, his opposition to animal sacrifice had to be hidden and denied. Why, then, was his revolutionary opposition to war, to religious elitism, to seeking personal gain at others' expense, to nationalism, racism, and many of the other fundamental characteristics of the parent culture preserved and canonized? His opposition to killing animals is drastically more radical, practical, and threatening to the established order, because it questions our meals, the intimate landscape of our daily lives. We don't, after all, declare war three times a day. This same pattern of denial continues today. As mentioned earlier, the passionate teachings of Unity's co-founders, Charles and Myrtle Fillmore, advocating the vegan ethic of kindness to animals have been virtually completely repressed and forgotten in less than seventy years! While Unity ministers and congregants avidly and respectfully discuss the Fillmores' books and teachings on prayer, metaphysics, and Christian healing, their teachings on veganism are ignored or passed off as just one of their "quirks."

An interesting objection to adopting a plant-based way of eating that many Christians rely on is the saying by Jesus that "Not that which goeth into the mouth defileth a man; but that which cometh out of the mouth, this defileth a man" (Matthew 15:11).[11] This is often interpreted as giving us permission to eat anything we like and instructing us instead to be mindful of our speech. By now it should be clear that this objection misses the point entirely. When we order a chicken or a cheeseburger at a deli, restaurant, or market, *that* is the moment that we engage in violence and cause "murders," "thefts,"[12] and suffering to defenseless animals and disadvantaged people. At that moment we are like the general who gives an order to kill someone in a faraway country; though he never sees the blood or hears the scream, he is nevertheless responsible for the killing.

There are many Buddhists who use a somewhat similar justification for eating animal foods. Although Gautama Buddha clearly forbade the eating of animal flesh, there are Buddhists who say that he allowed us to eat animals who were not killed specifically for us. The chicken in the market or the cheeseburger in the restaurant was not ordered specifically for us; it's already there. This obviously does not apply to our situation, however, for as soon as we order the chicken or cheeseburger, the inventory in the market or restaurant is depleted and the next morning, because of our purchase, an order will be placed for another dead chicken or another cheeseburger, and animals will be transported and killed to provide it—specifically because of us.

Another standard "religious" objection to being concerned about the animals we harm for food is to deny them the souls we grant ourselves. The mentality of domination is invariably a mentality of exclusion and, like the consumption of animals, reaches even into the New Age movement. A good example is Gary Zukav's *Seat of the Soul*, a best-selling book esteemed by people who consider themselves progressive, open-minded, and spiritually aware. Not surprisingly, in the chapter entitled "Souls," we find Zukav's proclamation that only humans have individual souls, and that every animal is simply part of what he refers to as the "group soul" of its species. "Each human being has a soul. The journey toward individual soulhood is what distinguishes the human kingdom from the animal kingdom. Animals do not have individual souls. They have group souls. Each cat is a part of the group soul of cat, and so on."[13] He also says that there is a hierarchy within the group souls of animals, and that dolphins and apes are higher than dogs, which are higher than horses, and so forth. He offers no evidence, though, for his hypotheses.[14]

This book appears to be another wave in the sea of literature our culture has produced that tries to justify our abuse of animals on spiritual grounds. Readers of Zukav's book are no doubt comforted knowing that the chicken, fish, cow, or pig they are eating was not really an individual with a soul, but just an expression of its species' "group soul." It's ironic that while the book purports to elucidate spirituality and raise consciousness, it may actually do the opposite, reducing its readers' sensibilities and blinding them to the reality of the suffering that individual animals experience because we reduce them to objects, mere fractions of a hypothetical "group soul."

It harks back to the era of slavery in the United States, when religious leaders, Bibles in hand, used similar wording to proclaim that black people had no individual souls, that they were more like animals than soul-endowed white people.[15] It harks back also to Thomas Aquinas who, a thousand years ago, proclaimed that neither animals nor women had souls. Though blacks and women were eventually granted souls, it appears that those in power decide who have souls, for their own purposes.

Voltaire wisely said, "If we believe absurdities, we will commit atrocities." Culture is the product of conversations, and our conversations are still dominated by the ideas and assumptions of the exploitive herding paradigm we were all fed as children. To stop the atrocities, we must awaken from the absurd belief that animals are insentient, trivial, soulless property objects and challenge our religious institutions to extend ethical protection to animals. This of course will mean challenging the meals at the center of social and religious life and the atrocities "hidden in plain sight" within those meals. These words by Swami Prabhupada reveal an alternative to our culture's dominant paradigm.

Prabhupada: Some people say, "We believe that animals have no soul." That is not correct. They believe animals have no soul because they want to eat the animals, but actually animals do have a soul.

Reporter: How do you know that the animal has a soul?

Prabhupada: You can know, also. Here is the scientific proof. The animal is eating, you are eating; the animal is sleeping, you are sleeping; the animal is defending, you are defending; the animal is having sex, you are having sex; the animals have children, you have children; you have a living place, they have a living place. If the animal's body is cut, there is blood; if your body is cut, there is blood. So all these similarities are there. Now why do you deny this one similarity, the presence of the soul? That is not logical. You have studied logic? In logic there is something called analogy. Analogy means drawing a conclusion by finding many points of similarity. If there are so many points of similarity between human beings and animals, why deny one similarity? That is not logic. That is not science.[16]

And Schopenhauer, in criticizing how some Christians treat animals, wrote, "Shame on such a morality that fails to recognize the eternal essence that exists in every living thing, and shines forth with inscrutable significance from all eyes that see the sun."[17]

Whether or not we believe that animals have souls, the knowledge that they can suffer as we do compels religious persons to refrain from causing them to suffer. As guardians and vehicles of our spiritual impulses and teachings, our religious institutions have a profound obligation to speak on behalf of all beings who are voiceless and vulnerable, and to the degree they fail in this obligation, they betray their mission and become enablers of terror and oppression. Failing to act to protect life is itself an action, a turning away. By looking the other way and ignoring the plight of defenseless animals, religious institutions have supported our culture's inhumane agenda of reducing animals to objects. Willfully neglecting to defend innocent lives from cruelty is immoral action, and by its failures religion has forfeited its mandate and dissipated its credibility as an authentic moral or spiritual authority.

Religion's turning away has allowed the atrocities to continue and legitimized the turning away of the general population. This turning away is the paradigmatic learning that our culture specializes in, particularly with regard to the plight of the animals we eat and use; it is the everyday teaching of not seeing, not caring, disconnecting, and ignoring. This learning to look the other way brings spiritual death in everyone who practices it. In encouraging it, religious institutions show how far they have strayed from the passionate mercy and all-seeing kindness taught and lived by those whose spiritual evolution and illumination inspired the institutions themselves. Spiritual teachings of our interconnectedness and the vegan ethic of universal compassion, besides being vital and transformative, are in profound alignment with the core instruction of the world's religions, which is to love others. They are dangerous to the status quo, subverting the prevailing paradigm that justifies turning away, self-aggrandizement, and violence.

As omnivores, we may resent vegans for reminding us of the suffering we cause, for we'd rather be comfortable and keep all the ugliness hidden, but our comfort has nothing to do with justice or with authentic inner peace. It is the comfort of blocking out and disconnecting, and it comes with a terrible price. We may rationalize our meals by saying that we always thank the animal's spirit for offering her body to nourish us. If someone were to lock us up, torture us, steal our children, and then stab us to death, would we acquiesce as long as they thanked our spirit? Disconnecting and desensitizing in comfort is not the same as inner peace, which is the fruit of awareness and of living in alignment with the understanding that comes from this awareness.

If we believe absurdities, we will commit atrocities, and we pass it on to our children, generation upon generation. Our violent actions speak so much more loudly than our peaceful words, and this is the unyielding dilemma of the herding culture we call home. The only way to solve this dilemma is to evolve cognitively and ethically to a higher level where our actions do not belie our words and force us into unconsciousness and denial, but rather align with and reinforce our words and the universal spiritual teachings that instruct us to love one another, and to have mercy on the weak and vulnerable rather than exploiting and dominating them. All of us are celebrations of infinite mysterious Spirit, deserving of honor and respect. If our religions don't emphasize this and include all of us, it's time to replace them with spiritual teachings and traditions that do.

Other Objections

There are a number of other objections to veganism that our minds may use to keep us confined by justifying the incarceration and abuse of other beings. As with enslaving and killing innocent humans, there are no valid justifications for enslaving and killing innocent animals, but our minds, having been indoctrinated by the herding culture, may still resist with some of these gems: plants feel pain too; vegetarianism is also violent, because the big grain-harvesting combines kill little mice and voles; what would we do with all the cows if nobody ate them?; animals eat other animals so why can't we?; I don't like to be so strict and narrow-minded; I just like to eat normally; I wouldn't want to be "holier than thou" like most vegans/vegetarians are; I don't like somebody telling me what to eat.

For many people, such arguments justify the continued commodifying, confining, mutilating, killing, and eating of animals for food, so some response is needed. First, as for the plants, mice, and voles, if we truly care about them so much, we need only recall that eighty percent of all grain grown in the U.S. is fed to animals to produce flesh, eggs, and dairy foods; switching to a plant-based diet actually saves plants as well as the small creatures who live in the fields.[18] Hundreds of millions of acres of verdant forests and wildlife habitat have been and continue to be destroyed in order to grow the corn, soybeans, and other plants we feed the billions of animals we eat every year. Millions of acres of tropical rain forests are being devastated to provide cheap beef for American fast food outlets as well. If we really care about plants and animals, going vegan is an excellent way to help ecosystems, habitats, and animal populations recover. Second, as we gradually stop breeding cows, the prairies, mountains, and arid regions of our country, which have been ravaged by cattle, especially in the West,[19] will slowly be able to recover, and streams, aquifers, flora, birds, fish, prairie dogs, elk, coyotes, antelope, and other native wildlife will be able to repopulate, bringing stressed and depleted ecosystems back to life and into celebration again.

Third, while it is true that some animals eat other animals, animals with herbivore physiologies don't (except if forced by humans to do so), nor do they drink the milk intended for other species. It's telling that we use this rationalization in this case, but not in relation to other animal behaviors that we prefer not to emulate, such as the practice by the males of some animal species of killing and eating their own young. The range of animal behaviors is huge and mysterious, and we could justify almost any conceivable human behavior by finding it in some animals, but we certainly wouldn't do so. As for the other objections, if every time we wanted to eat some animal flesh, we had to hold the terrified animal in our hands, look her in the eye, and stab her with a knife, we would find these rationalizations evaporating quickly. Finally, the last objection is especially ironic; we've all been told what to eat our entire lives, and that's the only reason we eat animal foods.

This brings us to another common objection to switching to plant-based meals: that it is just too difficult, inconvenient, or unappetizing to do so. This nearly universal objection of the herding paradigm ignores the difficulty and inconvenience (to put it mildly) we impose on animals, starving and disadvantaged people, and future generations by eating animal foods. It also ignores the connections between eating animal foods and the intractable problems of pollution, terrorism, drug addiction, chronic disease, and so forth that were discussed earlier. Slave owners used the same objection to justify commodifying human beings and, short of a war, were unwilling to give up the convenience of enslaving people. Just how difficult, inconvenient, and unappetizing must the suffering we sow and reap today become before it motivates us to transform our paradigm and change our behavior?

A more serious objection to veganism is the reverse of the previous one. The objection says that we can't expect to effect impressive positive changes in our individual and collective lives by adopting this simpler, tastier, more affordable diet. This objection is influenced by our culture's mentality of violence, which assumes that peace, joy, harmony, and fulfillment are difficult to attain. Of course they are difficult to attain when we are practicing daily food rituals that force us to view beings as objects, kill them relentlessly, and divide and numb ourselves to keep the whole affair hidden from ourselves. However, we will find that as we begin to view animals as unique beings with interests, feelings, drives, and purposes, and as our behavior changes to reflect this view, then harmony, peace, and joy easily and naturally begin unfolding in our lives. Practicing nonviolence in our daily lives, we can discover the easy equanimity that shines as the foundation of our being.

While becoming a vegan may appear easy enough, why then is it not more common in our culture, especially among the millions of us who consider ourselves deeply committed to spiritual growth, social justice, world peace, religious freedom, and raising consciousness? Taking responsibility for the violence we are causing others and ourselves through our actions, words, and thoughts is never as easy as blaming others for the violence in our world. Judging by the generally small numbers who have actually gone vegan in our culture, it appears that this commitment requires a certain breakthrough that has been generally elusive because of the mentality of domination and exclusion we've all been steeped in since birth. There is something about veganism that is not easy, but the difficulty is not inherent in veganism, but in our culture.

Of itself, veganism is not a panacea, but it effectively removes a basic hindrance to our happiness, freedom, and unfoldment. As a living and ongoing expression of nonviolence, it is an enormously powerful agent of transformation in our individual lives, especially since our culture opposes it so vehemently. Living a consequent vegan life naturally encourages us to awaken from the consensus trance that brings unquestioning conformity and allows cruelty and slavery to continue. Refusing to see animals as commodities, we are able to see through countless other pretenses. And, as transformative as this is for an individual to experience, it would be infinitely more transformative for our culture to do so, and to evolve beyond the obsolete orientation that sees animals as mere food commodities.

It is like being in a boat tied to a dock with a length of rope. As we take off to cross to the other shore, we find that we make satisfying progress for a while, until the rope runs out. After that, we continue running the engine, but we can no longer make any real progress, though we do create a lot of smoke, waves, and commotion, and move perhaps from side to side or in circles. Until we realize that there's a rope holding us back and untie it, we'll be unable to make significant progress in our quest for the other shore. The boat of course represents our life, the other shore the fulfillment of our spiritual, creative, and intellectual potential, and the rope our culturally induced practice of buying, abusing, killing, and eating animals. When we untie the rope, we are free to go out across the waters and we may eventually reach the other shore. If we are eating animal foods, however, there is an invisible barrier hindering our progress because the disconnectedness and unconscious cruelty required to do so will keep us confined to the shallows of our potential.

As our culture moves toward a vegan orientation, we will see enormous healing and liberating forces unleashed. Indeed, imagining our culture as a vegan culture is truly imagining an almost completely different culture. This ever-present potential beckons to us. Every one of us, as representatives of our culture, is an essential part of this fundamental transformation and awakening. It is exciting to contemplate educational, economic, governmental, religious, medical, and other institutions based on honoring and protecting the rights and interests of both animals and humans. When as a culture we stop commodifying creatures, a new world of kindness, fairness, cooperation, peace, and freedom will naturally unfold in human relations as well.

Changing our individual daily food choices to reflect a consciousness of mercy will transform our lives and move our culture in a positive direction far more than any other change we can contemplate. Following right behind this change in our individual food choices is the necessity of practicing mindfulness and nonviolence in all our relations in order to bring our mind and heart into alignment with the truth of our interconnectedness, and to allow us to enter the present moment more deeply and experience directly the mystery, joy, and beauty of being.

CHAPTER THIRTEEN

EVOLVE OR DISSOLVE

＞～＜

"If you have men who will exclude any of God's creatures from the shelter of compassion and pity, then you have men who will deal likewise with their fellow men."
—St. Francis of Assisi

"Without love the acquisition of knowledge only increases confusion and leads to self-destruction."
—Krishnamurti

"The only real valuable thing is intuition."
—Albert Einstein

The Two Limited Perspectives

Looking from a variety of perspectives at our animal-based meals, we discover that eating animals has consequences far beyond what we would at first suspect. Like a little boy caught tormenting frogs, our culture mumbles, "It's no big deal," and looks away. And yet the repercussions of our animal-based diet are a very big deal indeed, not only for the unfortunate creatures in our hands, but for us as well. Our actions reinforce attitudes, in us and in others, that amplify the ripples of those actions until they become the devastating waves of insensitivity, conflict, injustice, brutality, disease, and exploitation that rock our world today.

Even those who acknowledge that our treatment of animals is indeed a great evil may feel that it is, like the other evils in our world, simply a product of human limitations, such as ignorance, pride, selfishness, fear, and so forth. According to this view, the horror we inflict on animals is a problem, but not a fundamental *cause* of our problems—and, because it's a problem for animals, who are less important than us humans, it's a lesser problem.

Only by going beyond "it's no big deal" and "it's just a problem like our other problems" will we be able to step outside our conditioning and see the full import of our relentless abuse of animals, recognizing it as the motivating, hidden fury behind our global crisis.

The Cycle of Violence

There is much talk today about stopping the cycle of violence, which is typically understood as the "hurt people hurt people" syndrome. Children who are violated and abused will, when they become adults, tend to violate and abuse their children in a self-perpetuating cycle of violence that rolls through generations. We address it by trying to stop the child abuse, and fail to see the deeper dynamic. This human cycle of violence will not stop until we stop the *underlying* violence, the remorseless violence we commit against animals for food. We teach this behavior and this insensitivity to all our children in a subtle, unintentional, but powerful form of culturally approved child abuse. Our actions condition our consciousness; therefore forcing our children to eat animal foods wounds them deeply. It requires them to disconnect from the food on their plates, from their feelings, from animals and nature, and sets up conditions of disease and psychological armoring. The wounds persist and are passed on to the next generation.

Compelling our children to eat animal foods gives birth to the "hurt people hurt people" syndrome. Hurt people hurt animals without compunction in daily food rituals. We will always be violent toward each other as long as we are violent toward animals—how could we not be? We carry the violence in our stomachs, in our blood, and in our consciousness. Covering it up and ignoring it doesn't make it disappear. The more we pretend and hide it, the more, like a shadow, it clings to us and haunts us. The human cycle of violence is the ongoing projection of this shadow.

The Shadow

In Jungian terms, our culture's enormous, intractable, overriding shadow is the cruelty and violence toward animals it requires, practices, eats, and meticulously hides and denies. As mentioned in Chapter 1, according to Jungian theory, the shadow archetype represents those aspects of ourselves that we refuse to acknowledge, the part of ourselves that we have disowned. To itself, the shadow is what the self is not, and in this case it is our own cruelty and violence that we deny and repress. We tell ourselves that we are good, just, upright, kind and gentle people. We just happen to enjoy eating animals, which is okay because they were put here for us to use and we need the protein. Yet the extreme cruelty and violence underlying our meals is undeniable, and so our collective shadow looms larger and more menacing the more we deny its existence, sabotaging our efforts to grow spiritually and to collectively evolve a more awakened culture.

As Jungian psychotherapy emphasizes, the shadow *will* be heard! This is why we eventually do to ourselves what we do to animals. The shadow is a vital and undeniable force that cannot, in the end, be repressed. The tremendous psychological forces required to confine, mutilate, and kill millions of animals every day, and to keep the whole bloody slaughter repressed and invisible, work in two ways. One way is to numb, desensitize, and armor us, which decreases our intelligence and ability to make connections. The other is to force us to act out exactly what we are repressing. This is done through projection. We create an acceptable target to loathe for being violent, cruel, and tyrannical—the very qualities that we refuse to acknowledge in ourselves—and then we attack it. With this understanding of the immense violence toward animals that we keep hidden and the implacable shadow this creates, the existence of 50,000 nuclear warheads[1] becomes comprehensible. Our "never-ending" war against terrorism becomes not just comprehensible but inevitable, as does our appalling destruction of ecosystems, the rampant exploitation of the world's poor, and the suicide, addiction, and disease that ravage countless human lives.

The shadow is the self that does the dirty work for us so we can remain good and acceptable in our own eyes. The more we repress and disconnect, the more inner disturbance we will carry that we must project on an outer evil force, an enemy or scapegoat of some kind, against whom we can direct our denied violence. We will see these enemies as the essence of evil and despise them, for they represent aspects of our self that we cannot face. In our quest to eliminate them we are driven to build the most hideous weapons imaginable, developing them throughout the centuries so that today we have the capacity to destroy all of humanity hundreds of times over. This is not just something in our past, like the generations of inquisitions, crusades, and wars. We eat more animals, project more enemies, and create more weapons than ever before. Every minute, our slaughterhouses kill 20,000 land animals and the Pentagon spends $760,000.[2] This huge expenditure on maintaining and developing systems to harm and destroy other people is a particularly egregious manifestation of the tragic suppression of intelligence caused by eating animal foods. The 2004 U.S. military budget of $400 billion, spent by just five percent of the world's population, is over forty percent of the entire world's annual military budget of $950 billion. These are enormous resources to be squandering on death and violence. It's estimated that an annual expenditure of just $237.5 billion for ten years would enable us to provide global health care; eliminate starvation and malnutrition; provide clean water and shelter for everyone; remove land mines; eliminate nuclear weapons; stop deforestation; prevent global warming, ozone depletion and acid rain; retire the paralyzing debt of developing nations; prevent soil erosion; produce safe, clean energy; stop overpopulation; and eliminate illiteracy![3] Yet we lack the will and understanding to use our resources constructively. Instead, we frenetically expand our bloated arsenal of biological weapons, chemical weapons, nuclear weapons, psychological weapons, and secret high-tech weapons. The disconnect between those who use these weapons and their intended victims also characterizes our cruel slaughter and abuse of animals.

The bomb pilots, generals, and politicians who make the decisions and administer the weapons never actually see the horror and agony the weapons cause. As a culture we've learned well how to dissociate from the violence we inflict on others because we all practice it when we eat animal foods: somewhere, because of our decision, an abused and terrified creature is attacked and stabbed to death. In war and in food production, we use similar euphemisms, like "harvesting" animals, or "collateral damage," and we shield ourselves from the carnage of either the slaughterhouses or the bombed villages and cities. Turning away from our violence against animals, we naturally sanitize and gloss over our war violence against other humans as well. We are shown by our mass media complex the evil enemies who require us to do all the bombing and killing, and we not only agree to it; we are unconsciously instigating and demanding it through the denial and projection of the immense shadow we create through our eating habits.

Every day, we cause over thirty million birds and mammals and forty-five million fish to be fatally attacked so we can eat them,[4] and it's universally considered to be good food for good people. With these meals, we feed our shadow, which grows strong and bold as it gorges itself on our repressed grief, guilt, and revulsion. Strangely enough, the larger and more powerful the shadow becomes, the harder it is to see, though it is literally not just under our noses, but actually *in* our noses and all our cells. It is well known in psychotherapy that it's liberating but difficult to see our own shadow archetypes and how they operate. We instinctively resist it, which is why the undercover videos of animal abuse on factory farms and slaughterhouses are mostly watched by vegans who never eat animal foods. The shadow is by definition what we are actively repressing, so it's inevitable that we avoid experiences that might trigger its coming into consciousness. Even Jungian scholars who spend their time writing about the shadow fail to see the greatest shadow of all, the shadow that springs from our abuse of animals, because they're typically eating and exploiting animals like everyone else. We become spiritually and psychologically free only as we are able to see and integrate the shadow aspects of ourselves, and this will only be possible when we stop eating animal foods, relaxing and releasing the irresistible need to block our awareness. In unchaining animals, we unchain ourselves.

Ends and Means

All sentient beings have interests, and we have created complex social and legal systems to ensure that our interests are not violated, though our ability to ensure this is strongly determined by our race, class, gender, and other factors of privilege. To be physically confined, to be subjected to painful or damaging attacks, to be starved or stolen from, or killed, or forced to perform degrading, unnatural actions all violate our interests, and anyone who does this to us will face legal and social consequences. Yet we act in precisely these ways against animals on an unimaginably massive scale with impunity. We want our interests protected, but we don't care about theirs. This is our unconfronted shadow and the real cause of the cycle of violence beyond which we must evolve or perish. Our perishing, though tragic, would be an enormous blessing for most of the animals of this earth. That deeply disturbing thought should motivate us to examine ourselves and change.

We will only survive and thrive if we recognize the central power of our meals to shape our consciousness. Food is eaten and becomes the physical vehicle of consciousness, and consciousness chooses what to incorporate into itself from itself. Do we cultivate and eat fear or love? Terrorized animals or nurtured plants? We cannot build a tower of love with bricks of cruelty.

Mahatma Gandhi and other spiritually mature people have emphasized that the means we use and the ends we attain are one and the same. They can never be different. The devoted peace activist A. J. Muste once said, "There is no way to peace. Peace is the way." The path of spiritual evolution is the path of focusing on this moment, and *being* the evolution and positive transformation we long to see in the world. To live in peace we must be peace. To experience the sweetness of being loved, we must be loving.

All of us can prove this in our own lives. Our love, to actually *be* love, must be acted upon and lived. Developing our capacity for love is not only the means of evolution; it is the end as well, and when we fully embody love, we will know the truth of our oneness with all life. This makes us free. Love brings freedom, joy, power, grace, peace, and the blessed fulfillment of selfless service. Our true nature, our future self, beckons irresistibly as an inner calling to awaken our capacity for love, which is understanding. With love and understanding awakening in us, compassion expands to include ever-larger circles of beings. Compassion may be seen as the highest form of love, for it is the love of the divine whole for all its parts and is reflected in the love of the parts for each other. It includes the urge to act to relieve the suffering of apparent others, and this urge requires us to evolve greater wisdom and inner freedom to relieve suffering more effectively. Compassion is thus both the fruit of evolution and the driving force behind it. Love yearns for greater love.

Evolution is the essence of life. All being is evolving, growing, transforming, and so the urge to evolve permeates our being. We thrive on opportunities to grow emotionally, artistically, intellectually, and spiritually. Our life is precious because it is such an opportunity. Our lives have meaning to the degree we answer the universal and undeniable call to evolve, the call to love.

Evolution implies not only change but transformation. In world mythology, when heroes refuse the call to leave home to take the evolutionary journey, they become sick. For us as a culture it is the same. We must shake the old stagnation and comfortable disconnections out of our minds and bodies, embrace the evolutionary urge within us to awaken compassion and intuitive wisdom, and live our lives in accord with the truth that we are connected intimately with all living beings. Achieving this transformation means living the truth of love and authentically comprehending our interconnectedness, and not merely talking about it. It means changing our thinking and our behavior—how we view animals and what we eat. As we recognize our shadow and become free of it, compassion returns and we naturally stop feeding it with our diet of hidden terror.

The Intuitive Imperative

The lesson is quite basic. If we can't stop the cruelty of eating animal foods, how can we presume to develop the sensitivity, the spiritual consciousness, the joy, peace, and creative freedom that are our potential? Our evolution requires that we develop our intuition, the higher, post-rational knowing that sees and makes wholes from parts, and that lifts us out of the prison box of self-preoccupation. Intuition is direct knowing, unmediated by the illusion of an essentially separate self, and it is knowing that brings healing, for it sees the larger wholes that the self, through logical analysis alone, can never see. Analysis and rationality rely on dividing and comparing, and are helpful tools only when subordinated to the wisdom and compassion inherent in the direct knowing of intuition. Without intuition, rationality and analysis become profoundly irrational; they become tools of exploitation and conflict, agents of confused self-destruction. Lacking intuition's guiding sense of compassion and interconnectedness, they easily serve the hysterical fear, aggression, and scapegoating projection that invariably arise when we commodify and eat animals.

Not surprisingly, rationality and analysis are prized in our academic and educational institutions while intuition is ignored and repressed. Intuition liberates, connects, illumines—and threatens our herding culture's underlying paradigm of violent oppression of animals and of the feminine. Intuition sees the shadow clearly, and disarms it by embracing it and not feeding it. It sees the animal hidden in the hot dog, ice cream, and omelette, feels her misery and fear, and embraces her with love. Intuition opens the door to healing. It never sees any living being as an object to be used but sees all beings as unique and complete expressions of an infinite universal presence, to be honored, respected, learned from, and celebrated. Intuition is Sophia, the beloved wisdom we yearn for and seek.

The evolutionary imperative is an intuitive imperative. Intuition is the fruit of spiritual ripening, and it is cultivated by practicing compassion, which is the sacred masculine. The ability to leave our self-preoccupied perspective and see things from the perspective of others gives rise to compassion. Through this we learn to leave the imprisoning illusion of being an isolated object, and enter into the ecstatic knowing of the interconnectedness of all life. This can bring the understanding that life is consciousness and that consciousness is, in essence, eternally free, complete, radiant, and serene. Our true nature is thus undefiled and resplendent.

We are not predatory by nature, but we've been taught that we are, in the most potent way possible: we've been raised from birth to eat like predators. We've thus been initiated into a predatory culture and been forced to see ourselves at the deepest levels as predators. Farming animals is simply a refined and perverse form of predation in which the animals are confined before being attacked and killed. It doesn't stop with animals, however. As we all know in our bones, there is a predatory quality to our economic system, and competition underlies all our institutions. We prey upon each other. It may not be obvious from within our planet's dominant society, but our culture and our corporations and other institutions act in ways that can only be described as predatory vis-à-vis those who are less industrialized, less wealthy, and less able to protect themselves. As we prey upon and "harvest" animals, we use and prey upon people, employing euphemisms according to the situation as "foreign aid," "privatization," "advertising," "spreading the gospel," "capitalism," "education," "free trade," "lending," "fighting terrorism," "development," and countless other agreeable expressions. The tender loving heart of our true nonpredatory nature is troubled by all this, but it shines unceasingly, and though it's perhaps covered over by our conditioning, it nevertheless inspires the selfless giving, compassion, and enlightenment that our spiritual traditions expound.

Some Traditions of Intuition and Compassion

Although our religious institutions have generally mirrored the prevailing cultural paradigm that sees animals as commodities and have thus offered them little real relief in their suffering, there are nevertheless many spiritual teachings and traditions existing within the world's religions that exhort us to abandon the predatory mentality and to cultivate compassion for animals. These spiritual traditions also fundamentally agree in their emphasis on intuition, or direct inner knowing, as an essential element of spiritual discipline and practice. This is true not only with regard to Eastern traditions such as the various forms of Buddhist, Hindu, Jain, and Taoist practice, but also in the more esoteric Western traditions, such as those of the Sufis, cabalists, Christian mystics, and others. These traditions typically encourage their adherents to cultivate intuition, recognizing that through compassion inspired by intuitive revelation we develop spiritually and attain wisdom, inner peace, and freedom.

The spiritual traditions also fundamentally agree that intuition is fostered by a twofold discipline. One aspect is consciously cultivating compassion as the primary motivation in our outer lives and living this as ethical conduct. The other is practicing mindfulness, awareness, and silent receptivity in our inner lives. The two are seen to reinforce each other and lead to spiritual wisdom.

The first universal aspect of spiritual cultivation is compassion and its reflection—ethical behavior. Religions are fundamentally concerned with the ethics of human conduct. This is because they are repositories of the spiritual impulse, which at its core connects us not only with the infinite mystery that is our source, but also with all the apparently other manifestations of this source, our "neighbors"—the human family and all living beings. Authentic spiritual teachings must necessarily teach an ethics of loving-kindness, because this reflects our interconnectedness and the truth that what we give out comes back to us. It leads to the harmony in relationships that is necessary not just for social progress, but also for our individual inner peace and spiritual progress.

Compassion and ethical conduct are essential to the second universal aspect of spiritual cultivation, inner silence and mindfulness. We won't be able to approach the state of relaxed, awake, and fully aware receptivity that authentic living depends upon if we are armoring ourselves due to acting in ways that are harmful to others. If we abuse others, and then sit quietly to reflect, meditate, pray, become open, or deepen our experience of inner serenity, we will find our mind invariably disturbed and plagued with relentless self-oriented thinking. This inner agitation, the price we pay for harming others, impedes our unfolding intuition, which is born from inner stillness and compassion.

We can see that in general, the more a culture oppresses animals, the greater its inner agitation and numbness, and the more extroverted and dominating it tends to be. This is related to the scarcity of meditation in Western cultures, where people are uncomfortable with sitting still. Quiet, open contemplation would allow the repressed guilt and violence of the animal cruelty in meals to emerge to be healed and released. Instead, the very activities that would be most beneficial to people of our herding culture are the activities that are the most studiously avoided. We have become a culture that craves noise, distraction, busyness, and entertainment at all costs. This allows our eaten violence to remain buried, blocked, denied, and righteously projected.

Spiritual traditions universally recognize that we humans yearn to enter states of awareness that are more luminous and serene, where our usual anxious and compulsive thinking diminishes and recedes into the background. This yearning has given rise to a wide range of meditation practices that help people enter the present moment more deeply and perhaps experience the transcendent reality that we might call God or the Absolute. In this experience the walls that usually separate us from others and the world begin to dissolve and we can see directly that we are not essentially separate from others, that the same light that shines in us shines in everyone. This unmediated intuitive knowing reinforces and deepens our sense of compassion.

The connection between intuition and compassion has been universally recognized in both Eastern and Western spiritual traditions, and it extends not just to other humans but to animals as well. In the Buddhist tradition, for example, intuitive wisdom is the sacred feminine and compassion is the sacred masculine, and they give rise to each other and nurture each other within all of us as our true nature and potential. It's well known, therefore, that monks and nuns are to refrain from eating animal flesh, particularly during meditation retreats. This is basically true in the Hindu, Jain, Sikh, Baha'i, and Taoist traditions also. The Catholic monastic traditions that are the most contemplative, such as the Cistercians and Trappists, tend to require monks to abstain from animal flesh, especially during periods of extended prayer and purification.

An Example: Samadhi and Shojin

Meditation is not an exotic or specific activity. It's a fundamental human potential and simply refers to a mind that is present, open, relaxed, and aware. It can be induced and developed by all kinds of things, such as chanting, singing, sitting quietly and attending to our breathing, mindfully walking in nature, dancing, whirling, playing music, running, repeating a prayer, gardening, and so forth. Activities that we love tend naturally to bring our mind more fully into the present moment and thus can be meditative practices.

An example of the connection between meditative practice and compassion toward animals may be seen in the concepts of *samadhi* and *shojin* in the Zen tradition. Although this is an example from a specific tradition, the underlying principles are universal and can be applied to all of us, whatever our religious inclinations may be. Samadhi refers to deep meditative stillness, in which the mind transcends its usual conflicted, anxious, busy, and noisy condition, quiets down, and becomes clear, bright, free, relaxed, and serenely poised in the present moment. Shojin is "religious abstention from animal foods" and is based on the core religious teaching of *ahimsa*, or harmlessness, the practice of refraining from causing harm to other sentient beings. Shojin and samadhi are seen to work together, with shojin purifying the body-mind and allowing, though certainly not guaranteeing, access to the spiritually enriching experience of samadhi.

In some Zen Buddhist traditions it is taught that there are two types of samadhi. "Absolute samadhi" refers to an inner state of one-pointed, relaxed and bright awareness in which the body is still, typically seated. The mind is totally absorbed in the present moment, and the usual inner dialogue has ceased. In "positive samadhi," which is based on the experience of absolute samadhi, we are functioning in the world, walking, gardening, cooking, cleaning, and so forth, with a mind that is fully present to the experiences arising every moment. This is similar to the practice of mindfulness, and to the Taoist practice of *wu wei*, or "non-action," in which the illusion of a separate doer dissolves in the immediacy of fulfilling the potential of the present moment. In Christian terms, this may be similar to "practicing the Presence" and to the practice recommended in the admonition to "pray without ceasing," whereas absolute samadhi may be akin to a state of profound at-one-ment with the divine.

Both absolute and positive samadhi are universal human potentials that transcend the particularities of tradition and labeling. They heal the mind and body at a deep level and reconnect us with our true nature. Because of the fear, shame, and woundedness we have all experienced, however, they seem to be difficult to attain and practice, and to require an enormous ongoing commitment to diligent inner cultivation. Entering the inner stillness of samadhi requires patiently returning our attention to the present moment, and requires that our mind be undisturbed by our outer actions. This is why the spirit of shojin, which sees animals as subjects and not as commodities to be used or eaten, is so essential on the path of spiritual evolution. The spirit of shojin is compassion and allowing others to be free, and the practice of shojin in turn liberates us from the inner mental states that accompany eating animal foods. These mental states—agitation, worry, fear, panic, despair, sadness, grief, nervousness, aggressiveness, anger, disconnectedness, despair, dullness, fogginess, and stupor—are unavoidable if we are omnivores, brought into us as vibrational frequencies with the foods we are eating, and generated within us by our own undeniably violent and harmful food choices and the psychological blocking these actions demand. These negative mental states generally make meditation a negative experience and ensure that it will not truly quiet our mind or help us reach higher levels of spiritual illumination. First we must purify our actions and stop harming vulnerable creatures. This requires mindfulness, the ancient spirit of shojin that is the foundation of veganism.

To be effective, to tame the mind, this spirit of nonviolence and compassion must be actually lived; otherwise our mind will be too disturbed to enter the inner peace of samadhi. This stillness and serenity of mind lies at the heart of spiritual life, whatever religion or non-religion we may hold to, and it requires the inner purity of a clear conscience. It allows the old inner wall, splitting "me" here from "the world" out there, to dissolve. With this, a deeper understanding of the infinite interconnectedness of all life can blossom.

Shojin and veganism are vital because they foster the inner peace required for spiritual maturity. They are forms of inner and outer training and discipline that lay the foundation for the meditative exploration that opens us to the truth of interbeing. This is why shojin is so essential to samadhi, and why veganism and nonviolence are essential for deep prayer, meditation, and spiritual awakening. Outer compassion and inner stillness feed each other. Shojin and veganism are essential to our spiritual health because they remove a fundamental hindrance on our path.

Though veganism is often denigrated and opposed by our mainstream Western religious institutions, its spirit actually underlies them, as Steven Rosen, Norm Phelps, Keith Akers, J. R. Hyland, Andrew Linzey, Tony Campolo, Steven Webb, and many others have pointed out. Rosen reports, for example, that Mohammed is acknowledged to have eaten a strictly vegetarian diet, and that there are numerous passages in the Koran and in Mohammed's teachings that urge or require refraining from cruelty to camels, cows, birds, and other animals.[6]

Many writers have approached this subject from the Judeo-Christian perspective and concluded that there is a strong mandate, from both the teachings in the Bible and related commentaries and from the practices and lives of influential Jews and Christians, to extend vegan compassion to nonhuman animals. For example, Norm Phelps points out in *The Dominion of Love* that both the Old and New Testaments of the Bible contain what he calls two Prime Directives.[7] These two fundamental spiritual teachings, to love God and to love our neighbor, are the essence of the Judeo-Christian spiritual tradition. Because God is the infinite whole in which we all have our being, and because there is no way to extend our love to God concretely since God transcends us completely, it follows that loving God means loving and caring for God's creation. This leads directly to the second Prime Directive, to love our neighbor. There is no reason, biblical or otherwise, to exclude animals from our neighborhood, because they are our neighbors on this earth and we know they suffer and feel emotions. Loving God concretely thus means loving and caring for God's creation and all our neighbors in this world, and loving God abstractly means opening through the inner silent receptivity (samadhi) of meditation and prayer to a direct experience of God's presence through which we can *be* God's loving hands and voice in the world. The core biblical teachings can thus be seen to point insistently to compassion for all creatures, and toward a vegan ethic of responsibility and caring for all creation.

Is Shamanism an Answer?

Human welfare, animal welfare, and environmental welfare are completely and inextricably interconnected. Our dilemmas can be resolved to the degree we evolve into a living understanding of this, awakening a sense of universal compassion as articulated by Pythagoras, Jesus, Buddha, Plotinus, Gandhi, Schweitzer, and countless others. The shamanic traditions, while containing many valuable teachings and in some ways revealing a more multidimensional view of the world and of human potentials than that of conventional Western science and religion, are nevertheless products of hunting and herding cultures. While they typically seem to view animals with less disdain than in our culture, they also seem to treat animals as food and ritual objects. They often rely on plants to induce the altered states of consciousness that are central to the shaman's ability to walk between worlds, perform extraordinary feats, and heal.

It seems enormously ironic, but it appears that cultures that eat animals and use them for clothing, entertainment, and ritual sacrifice, whether they are industrialized herding cultures or the more indigenous shamanic cultures, use plant foods as drugs to escape ordinary reality. Obvious examples of this are the use of heroin and other opium products, psilocybin and other mushrooms, ayahuasca, peyote, marijuana, tobacco, cocaine, and alcoholic products from the fermentation of fruits and grains. There are many others as well. Users of these plant-based substances have forgotten that the mind is the source of its experiences. Visions and altered states of consciousness that are induced by relying on plants can also be attained directly.

Our mistreatment of animals is a spiritual problem. It reflects a misunderstanding that reduces beings to things. The shamanic traditions, though born in cultures less overtly exploitive than ours has become, still view animals as objects to be used and killed for food, apparel, healing ceremonies, and other uses. They may perhaps be able to teach us about respecting animals more than we currently do, and about not taking more from the earth than we need, but, at the risk of overgeneralizing a vast subject, shamanic traditions seem to tend toward parochialism, in being devoted primarily to the welfare of a particular tribe or group of people, and to humans more than nonhumans. Motivated by "noble savage" stereotypes and disillusionment with modern culture, we may want to revert to what must seem like the good old days of more primitive life, before factory farms, zoos, mechanized production, nuclear weapons, and so forth.

However, the way out is not to go back, but to go through. We must go forward. For one thing, primitive cultures are often not as we would romanticize them, and some American Indian cultures, for example, practiced cannibalism, genocidal warfare on other tribes, and horrific ritual torture on captives from other tribes. For another, shamanic traditions may be co-opted by the animal abuse industries, as we see beef producers linking eating meat to romanticized images of the plains Indians, and the Japanese whaling industry using the whaling by Makah Indians of the Pacific Northwest to undermine the global whaling moratorium and justify their whaling practices.[8]

This is not to say that the shamanic traditions didn't serve their people well, or that they don't have profound truths to teach us today. If the American Indian sentiment of concern for "all my relations" is taken to its spiritual and practical limits, in some ways it approaches the noble Bodhisattva ideal of Mahayana Buddhism, which is to dedicate one's life to be of benefit and service to all sentient beings by realizing complete spiritual enlightenment. Both bring universal compassion into the heart of our motivation on the spiritual path.

However, attending an American Indian gathering today, we would find dead animals being served as food, likely from the same producers as those served at a Christian or Jewish function—and we would find the participants at any of these events prepared to vehemently justify their meals.

The Vegan Imperative

We can see that the essential teachings of the world's major religions support the cultural and spiritual transformation that veganism calls for. All the world's major religions have their own form of the Golden Rule that teaches kindness to others as the essence of their message. They all recognize animals as sentient and vulnerable to us, and include them within the moral sphere of our behavior. There are also strong voices in all the traditions emphasizing that our kindness to other beings should be based on compassion. This is more than merely being open to the suffering of others; it also explicitly includes the urge to *act* to relieve their suffering. We are thus responsible not just to refrain from harming animals and humans, but also to do what we can to stop others from harming them, and to create conditions that educate, inspire, and help others to live in ways that show kindness and respect for all life. This is the high purpose to which the core teachings of the world's wisdom traditions call us. It is an evolutionary imperative, a spiritual imperative, an imperative of compassion, and, in reality, a vegan imperative. The motivation behind vegan living is this universal spiritual principle of compassion that has been articulated both secularly and through the world's religious traditions; the difference lies in veganism's insistence that this compassion be actually practiced. The words of Donald Watson, who created the term "vegan" in 1944, reveal this practical orientation and bear repeating:

> Veganism denotes a philosophy and way of living which seeks to exclude, as far as is possible and practicable, all forms of exploitation of, and cruelty to, animals for food, clothing, or any other purpose; and by extension promotes the development and use of animal-free alternatives for the benefit of humans, animals, and the environment.

Buckminster Fuller often emphasized that the way of cultural transformation is not so much in fighting against destructive attitudes and practices, but in recognizing them as being obsolete and offering positive, higher-level alternatives. The competitive, violent, commodifying mentality of the ancient herding cultures is, in our age of nuclear weapons and global interconnectedness, profoundly obsolete, as is eating the animal foods of these old cultures, which are unhealthy in the extreme both to our body-minds and to our precious planetary ecology. Eating animal foods is an indefensible holdover from another era beyond which we must evolve, and with the ever-increasing profusion of vegan and vegetarian cookbooks and vegan foods like soy milk, soy ice cream, rice syrup, tofu, veggie burgers, and so forth, as well as fresh organically grown vegetables, legumes, fruits, grains, nuts, pastas, and cereals, we see alternatives proliferating. Books, videos, websites, vegetarian/vegan restaurants and menu options, animal rights groups, and vegan organizations are also multiplying as we respond to the vegan imperative.

Seeing the role of our systemic violence against animals in creating our problems, we can begin to comprehend and solve them. To truly solve a problem, we must rise to a higher level and, in fact, transcend it with our understanding. As long as we abuse and commodify animals, we chain ourselves to the same deluded evolutionary levels as our problems and thus continually re-experience them as violence, stress, bondage, and disease.

The Emotional Miseducation of Boys

For example, a best-selling book entitled *Raising Cain: Protecting the Emotional Life of Boys*, written by two experienced psychologists, contains a wealth of understanding about the enormous suffering boys experience in our culture, but it does not and cannot begin to address the underlying causes of this suffering rooted in our socially approved brutalization of animals for food. The authors, Kindlon and Thompson, build a powerful case that boys in our culture are emotionally damaged by our culture's male stereotypes of toughness, and that these wounds not only cause them misery but warp them for life and cause enormous suffering to females as well.

The two authors blame the culturally imposed image of stoic, unfeeling masculinity as the fundamental cause of boys' pain and stress. They document and discuss how boys are taught to disconnect from their feelings by cultural forces on every side: their parents, their teachers, cultural institutions, the media, and each other. They call the culture of adolescent boys "the culture of cruelty" and write powerfully about the emotional devastation caused by the psychological and physical cruelty and teasing that boys inflict on each other.

The book offers poignant glimpses into the rage, pain, despair, shame, hopelessness, depression, numbness, and embattled solitude that boys experience, making the connections between these inner emotional torments and the outer problems of adolescent suicide (the third leading cause of death), drinking, drugs, illicit sex, violence, and cruelty. As a solution, it emphasizes that we need to "provide boys models of male heroism that go beyond the muscular, the self-absorbed, and the simplistically heroic,"[9] that we need to be more understanding of boys, use less harsh discipline, and encourage them to express and connect with their feelings.

Yet *Raising Cain* makes a contribution that is acceptable to the herding culture in which we live, for it never makes the connection with the real source of the "emotional miseducation" of boys, which is our cultural practice of eating cruelly confined and slaughtered animals. Ironically, in order to build rapport with boys they work with, the two researchers often have lunch with them and may take them out for hamburgers.[10] Neither these omnivores nor their omnivorous culture, it seems, can begin to make the deeper connections between the violence we impose on animals and the "emotional miseducation" of our youth, particularly boys. Nor do they recognize the more obvious surface connections, for example that boys are generally pushed to eat animal flesh—and thus to identify themselves as predatory and privileged—more than girls are. Boys are also more commonly hardened by being encouraged to deceive and attack animals through hunting and fishing activities. Even if they could see these connections, though, the authors probably knew better than write about them in a book that they and their publishers hoped would make the best-seller list. It seems that the shadow of animal food cruelty is too enormous and dangerous to be faced directly by the mass consciousness of our culture, though in order to evolve as a culture, this is precisely what we are called to do.

The entire testimony of Kindlon and Thompson in *Raising Cain* reflects profound and obvious evidence that the herding culture mentality of domination, exclusion, and cruelty to animals that forces boys to disconnect from their feelings is alive and well today, so that like their fathers and their fathers before them, boys can grow up to kill competing herders, vie for power through the accumulation of livestock/capital and, at the end of the day, eat the flesh and/or secretions of their confined and killed animals as a ritual celebration. What drives this entire heartless enterprise, generation after generation, so that we are powerless not just to challenge it but even to recognize and discuss it intelligently? The cruelty we routinely inflict on animals haunts our boys and the cycle continues, ravaging the earth, the generations, and the landscape of our feelings.

The Birth of Post-Rational Consciousness

We have looked from many perspectives at our ongoing practice of eating animals and have seen how it creates an internal mental climate of distractedness and disconnectedness that reduces our inherent intelligence and ability to make meaningful connections while numbing and paralyzing us emotionally. The resulting cycle of violence keeps us confined to patterns of competition and acquisition that drive the same commodifying and destructive elitist economic system that began emerging ten thousand years ago with the herding culture. Even though many people and traditions have urged us to practice compassion and develop direct intuitive knowing, we have remained mired in omnivorism, self-preoccupation, and disconnected analytical thinking. This has allowed us to develop technologically but has blocked our emotional and spiritual progress with painful results for us, for our children, and for our children's children.

Pre-rational processes may be called instinctual, and many of us enjoy believing we've progressed beyond instinct—and thus beyond animals—in our development and use of the complex symbolic languages that give us the ability to think conceptually. Matthew Scully points out in his book, *Dominion*, that some scientists and theorists, such as Stephen Budiansky, John Kennedy, and Peter Carruthers, claim that our human language gives us the ability to think, and that without language and thus thinking, we would not be conscious.[11] We have to wonder how they would construe this statement by Albert Einstein:

The interaction of images is the source of thought. The words of the language as they are written or spoken do not seem to play any role in my mechanism of thought. The physical entities which seem to serve as elements of thought are . . . clear images which can be voluntarily reproduced or combined.[12]

We can argue that animals are largely unconscious, decreeing that because animals seem to lack the complex language that allows them to formulate thoughts in words as we do, their experience of suffering must therefore be less significant or intense for them. This same thinking, however, could be used to justify harming human infants and senile elderly people. If anything, beings who lack the ability to analyze their circumstances may suffer at our hands more intensely than we would because they are unable to put the distance of internal dialogue between themselves and their suffering. As long as we remain imprisoned in the maze of self-oriented thinking, we can easily justify our cruelty to others, excuse our hard eyes and supremacist position, discount the suffering we impose on others, and continue on, rationalizing our actions and blocking awareness of the reality of our feelings and of our fundamental oneness with other beings.

Spiritual health requires introspection and that we practice quieting the disturbed waves of our compulsive verbal thought processes in order to contact directly the deeper reality of being that shines always in our heart. Without this inner practice and its twin practice of compassionate behavior toward others, our mind runs along, acting out its preprogrammed thinking, unable to stop or even witness its basic self-centered delusion. We mistake this state for being "conscious," whereas it is actually profoundly unconscious. Yet we condescendingly proclaim that since we can "think" (compulsively chatter to ourselves) we are conscious, and since animals can't they must be unconscious.

By ceasing to eat animal foods and thus causing misery to our neighbors, and by practicing meditation and quiet reflection, which can eventually extract our consciousness out of the brambles of compulsive thinking, we can begin to understand what consciousness actually is. We will see that to the degree we can be open to the present moment and dwell in inner spacious silence, beyond the ceaseless internal dialogue of the busy mind, we can experience the radiant, joy-filled serenity of pure consciousness. Post-rational intuitive knowing can be born as a sense of being connected with all beings. No longer being merely a parade of conditioned thoughts revolving around a sense of being a separate self, we can sense more deeply into the nature of being and begin to *know* outside the limitations of linear thinking. With this comes an under-standing that our essential nature is not evil, confined, selfish, or petty, but is eternal, free, pure, and is of the essence of love. When we lower our vibration from this clear state and begin verbal thinking again, we see that the mind busy with conditioned thinking can never attain the understanding that pours in when the mind is able to be still.

So what are we, and what are animals? Our concepts only reveal our impeding conditioning. We are neighbors, mysteries, and we are all manifestations of the eternal light of the infinite consciousness that has birthed and maintains what we call the universe. The intuitive knowing that would reveal this to us, though, is mostly unavailable because as a culture we are outer-directed and fail to cultivate the inner resources and discipline that would allow us to access this deeper wisdom. Our minds and consciousness are almost completely unexplored territory because we have been raised in a herding culture that is fundamentally uncomfortable with introspection. Our science blatantly ignores con-sciousness as an unapproachable, unquantifiable and unopenable "black box" and distracts us with focusing solely on measurable phe-nomena. Our religions discourage meditation and reduce prayer to a dualistic caricature of asking and beseeching an outside, enigmatic, and projected male entity.

Because of our herding orientation and our unassuaged guilt com-plex due to the misery in our daily meals, we have warped our sacred connection with the infinite loving source of our life to an ultimate irony: comparing ourselves to sheep, we beg our shepherd for mercy, but since we show no mercy, we fear deep down we'll not be shown mercy either and live in dread of our inevitable death. We bargain and may proclaim overconfidently that we're saved and our sins are forgiv-en (no matter what atrocities we mete out to animals and people out-side our in-group), or we may reject the whole conventional religious dogma as so much absurd pablum and rely on the shallow materialism of science. However it happens, our spiritual impulse is inevitably repressed and distorted by the guilt, violence, and reductionism that herding and eating animals requires.

For all our scientific and theological theorizing, we know little of human consciousness, because as a culture of omnivores we are uncomfortable with ourselves. We have lost touch with our innate urge to learn to remain quiet and undisturbed long enough to become open to the greater light and higher wisdom that lie beyond the narrow margins of conceptual thinking. Entering the joy, peace, and wonder of the present moment requires an inner stillness that allows us to experience directly. This is a practice that benefits both others and us. Clear awareness requires us to cease from harmful actions that keep our minds agitated, and to practice inner silence.

As an improvisational pianist, I can attest from personal experience that thinking stops the flow of musical creativity. It is when I'm able to be more fully conscious, beyond thought, in the present moment, and allow the music to pour through that the most creative and inspired music arises. People now call this being in "the zone" and it is seen as a requirement for "peak performance." Compulsive verbal thinking turns off the flow of the zone and constricts consciousness. Perhaps animals are always in the zone. As Joseph Campbell once said, watching birds speeding through webs of branches and never even grazing a wing tip, animals may dwell in a realm beyond mistakes, totally present to life in ways our concept-crowded thinking cannot fully understand.

By living the truth of compassion in our meals and daily lives, we can create a field of peace, love, and freedom that can radiate into our world and bless others by silently and subtly encouraging the same in them. We may discover that we can "think" with our hearts, without words, and we may learn to appreciate the consciousness of animals and begin to humbly explore their mysteries. There is perhaps much we can learn from animals. Not only do they have many powers completely unexplainable by contemporary science, but they are fellow pilgrims with us on this earth who contribute their presence to our lives and enrich our living world in countless essential ways. In fact, without the humble earthworms, bees, and ants whom we relentlessly kill and dominate, the living ecosystems of our earth would break down and collapse—something we *certainly* cannot say about ourselves!

Who are we? What is our proper role on this earth? I submit we can only begin to discover these answers if we first take the vegan imperative seriously and live compassionately toward other creatures. Then peace with each other will at least be possible, as well as a deeper understanding of the mysteries of healing, freedom, and love.

CHAPTER FOURTEEN

JOURNEY OF TRANSFORMATION

"First, live a compassionate life. Then you will know."
—Buddha

"By having reverence for life, we enter into a spiritual relation
with the world."
—Albert Schweitzer

"There are a thousand hacking at the branches of evil to one who
is striking at the roots."
—Henry David Thoreau, *Walden*

The Jeweled Web of Journeys

How can we best contribute to our culture's awakening and evolution to greater intelligence, compassion, peace, and fulfillment? We each have a unique piece of the puzzle to contribute, which emerges out of responding to the dreams, aspirations, and yearnings in our heart that develop through the course of our particular life journey. When we develop a sense of the wonder and potential of our unique life, we feel the same toward others. This emerges as respect and understanding for them and the urge to cooperate with and support them. This is a basic expression of our innate sanity. Because we value our life, we value the lives of others and naturally yearn to live to benefit them. If we feel our life to be a distasteful burden, we will most likely have a low opinion of the worth of the lives of others. We can reverse this by switching to a more compassionate diet and by contemplating and affirming the preciousness of our life—of all life. The urge of compassion will grow as we cultivate our sense of connectedness with everything. As we become freer and more grateful for our life, we naturally become a force for positive change in the world.

To better understand the unique nature and power of our journey, it may be helpful to examine our lives in order to discover the hidden seeds from our past that are now pushing, like living green shoots, into our consciousness. Small unrecognized seeds, when recognized and honored, can grow into strong and beautiful trees in the garden of our lives. I offer this chapter as a modest example of this process and encourage everyone to look into the soil of their own garden for the hidden seeds that may already be sprouting into beautiful and beneficent plants. In particular, by further discovering the seeds of veganism within us, we can nurture them and develop our understanding of our unique contribution to the healing of our world. We will touch many, for our journeys are all connected.

In the Avatamsaka tradition of Mahayana Buddhism, there is a central teaching metaphor that is referred to as the teaching of the jeweled web. It is not only a teaching but also an image to be meditated upon for greater insight into the truth of being. The universe is likened to an infinite web, and at every node of this vast web there is a jewel. Every *dharma* in the universe—every being, thing, or event—is one of these jewels. Thus every being, thing, and event is connected to every other being, thing, and event throughout infinite space and time. Not only that, but if we look deeply into any one jewel in this vast web, we can see reflected in this jewel *all* of the other jewels in the cosmic net! Each and every individual dharma contains *all* others, and if we truly know one, we know all of them. The ancient teaching that emerges from and sustains this metaphor of the jeweled web is known as the teaching of the conditioned arising and mutual interpenetration and interdependence of all phenomena. Everything is dependent upon everything else;

nothing is ever separate, and each particle contains the entire universe. We are all profoundly and radically related!

We can see that our stories and journeys are also intimately inter-connected and that each journey, though unique, miraculously contains all the other journeys of all beings. We learn from each other, though at the deepest levels we see that there are, ultimately, no others. We all share the same source, and the walls that we build to separate us are illusory. As we evolve and as the imaginary walls dissolve, compassion and freedom increase along with our deepening understanding of the interbeing of all life. This teaching of the profound interconnectedness of all life is not unique to Buddhism but has been intuited for centuries by people from many traditions and cultures. A universal teaching that is inseparable from this understanding of interbeing is mindfulness, cultivating our ability to be fully present in our actions and to see the connections between our actions and their effects. Mindfulness brings freedom and insight by increasing our awareness. The more aware and mindful we are, the more free we become.

In terms of food, in order to understand the rippling web of suffering that we as a culture create, perpetuate, and magnify through our daily sacred acts of eating, and the web of interconnection in which freedom, compassion, and love can grow and illuminate our world, we must go on a journey. A journey undertaken with mindfulness is a pilgrimage, because it has a spiritual purpose: to increase our awareness and our ability to love and understand. Our culture is in the halting first steps of a journey of transformation in which we all participate and to which we all contribute by our own journeys. It necessarily unfolds in time, but the gestalt it points to is our living, breathing situation—our shared life today. It is our pilgrimage together, and for this, mindfulness is essential.

Seeds of Inspiration

My journey toward questioning the pervasive abuse of animals for food began in a seemingly unlikely way, for I was born and raised in a family and neighborhood with no interest in plant-based eating at all. Consequently, for the first twenty-two years of my life I, like most

Americans, ate large quantities of animal flesh, eggs, and dairy products. I did, however, encounter seeds of inspiration that lay dormant at first but later began to sprout vigorously. Though these seeds pertain to one unique journey, they may illumine half-hidden seeds that are sending forth new shoots of understanding for others.

For me, one seed was being born and raised in the town of Concord, Massachusetts, the home of two of the so-called revolutions that the United States has experienced: the political revolution of the 1760s and '70s, and the literary revolution of the 1840s and '50s. Being born and raised in Concord gave me a sense of intimate connectedness with these two revolutions and of being their descendant, with an urge to question them, understand what motivated them, and carry them on myself. I believe these two revolutions have contributed to the emerging vegan revolution, which is a cultural revolution of profound significance that can heal our culture at the deepest level.

The political revolution culminated in the beginning of the Revolutionary War at the Old North Bridge in Concord on April 19, 1775. The farmers and villagers living in Concord and the other towns surrounding Boston provided some of the strongest resistance to British imperialist rule and fought the unjust economic domination imposed by the British East India Company and other British multinational corporate forces that were being militarily and politically supported and legitimized by the British government at that time. This eighteenth-century revolution led eventually to independence from the British Empire and birthed the epic American experiment in democracy, equality, cultural pluralism, and individual freedom that continues to attract and inspire people all over the world.

It is remarkable that the literary and philosophical revolution of the following century was also based in Concord. It sprang from the lives and writings of the American transcendentalists living there—Ralph Waldo Emerson, Henry David Thoreau, Bronson Alcott, Louisa May Alcott, William Ellery Channing, Nathaniel Hawthorne—and many others, like Walt Whitman, who were inspired by the transcendentalists and journeyed to visit them. We recognize these leading thinkers today for the deep questioning of traditional values that they introduced and for the artistic, literary, and spiritual inspiration they provided. Emerson's philosophical writings, like "Nature"; his oratorical contributions, like the "Harvard Divinity School Address"; and his poetry, which pioneered bringing Eastern philosophical ideas for the first time to the United States, made him something of a living legend, a magnet that attracted writers and thinkers from many directions and whose influence is still strongly alive today, urging respect and love for nature, self-exploration, and appreciation of the essentially spiritual nature of all manifestation. He emphasized that true wisdom *transcends* materialistic knowledge, and that the natural world is also a manifestation of the divine. Whitman wrote: "I was simmering, simmering. Emerson brought me to a boil."

Thoreau was strongly influenced by Emerson (and vice versa), and in some ways has eclipsed his teacher and mentor in influence. His radical experiment, to live in solitude at Concord's Walden Pond and "to suck out the marrow of life," continues to inspire spiritual seekers and in a powerful way pioneered the planting of introspective inner listening in the excessively extroverted American cultural soil. The Concord philosophers saw clearly that an internal element was missing from their culture, which was overly focused on external conquest and success. Thoreau had the largest library of books on Eastern philosophy in the United States at the time, and his book *Civil Disobedience* (still one of the primary source documents of nonviolent resistance and an enduring revelation of the power and responsibility of individuals to actively oppose unjust governmental policies) deeply influenced Tolstoy, Gandhi, King, and the lives of countless people.

Bronson Alcott's radically progressive ideas regarding the education of children are being rediscovered and finally appreciated today. He was an ethical vegetarian and a prime moving force behind the formation of Fruitlands, an unlikely experiment in vegetarian community living in the countryside outside Concord. The Concord transcendentalists were the first Americans to explore and weave into Western thought many of the noble and subtle ideas from Taoist, Buddhist, Jain, and Vedantist writings, and to build progressive bridges that included honoring nature, emphasizing the essential goodness and vast potential of human nature, and exploring lifestyles of nonviolence, simplicity, and inner contemplation.

The American roots of deeply questioning food and developing the philosophical foundation for a more compassionate relationship with animals can be traced to the progressive writers clustered around Emerson in Concord in the mid-nineteenth century. Thoreau wrote, "I have no doubt that it is a part of the destiny of the human race in its gradual improvement, to leave off eating animals as surely as the savage tribes have left off eating each other when they came into contact with the more civilized." Emerson's "You have just dined, and however scrupulously the slaughterhouse is concealed in the graceful distance of miles, there is complicity," shows the esteemed Concord sage's ability to make the connections that elude most. Bronson Alcott's daughter, Louisa May, wrote, "Vegetable diet and sweet repose. Animal food and nightmare. Pluck your body from the orchard; do not snatch it from the shambles [slaughterhouse]. Without flesh diet there could be no blood-shedding war." She makes explicit the connection between the violence inherent in eating animals, nightmares, and the nightmare of human violence turned against ourselves.

Perhaps as a child, wandering through the forests and along the streets of Concord and along the shore of Walden Pond, where I learned to swim, I sensed the noble and courageous thoughts of these spiritual pioneers. Though there seemed to be little in the outer world to encourage questioning the cruel food customs I was born into, perhaps the thoughts and feelings of these luminaries filtered through the inner worlds that I was exploring along with the outer world. I am sure that all of us have such memories of seed experiences, perhaps only dimly recognized, that are now unfolding in consciousness. We learn from each other and plant seeds in each other. Through examples, actions, words, expressions, writings, and gestures, we touch each other, sometimes deeply. As sensitive children, we can be blessed or wounded enormously.

Several other seeds stand out in shaping my journey. One was growing up with a noble and gentle German shepherd. Our family got Bismarck as a puppy when I, the oldest of three children, was about a year old. He was my loyal friend until he passed away in my teens, which was a sad loss for our entire family. He always accompanied us on our frequent camping and hiking expeditions in the mountains of New Hampshire and Vermont. My parents disliked animal cruelty and killing, so we never included hunting or fishing in our regular outings into nature. Besides instilling in me a loving appreciation of the outdoors from an early age, my father taught me to play the piano and to explore the mysterious power of music to relax, uplift, and express deep feelings. He was a semi-professional pianist, and his love for music and harmony was an abiding inspiration. I will always remember how he taught my brother and me to sing in harmony up in the mountains.

Being born into a newspaper family was another significant seed in my life journey. Around the time I was born my parents bought a tiny weekly newspaper in the Concord area. I grew up in the midst of a swirling world of linotype machines and printing presses, promotions, weekly deadlines, and an unending parade of local politicians and merchants. My father's stream of editorials and stories, my mother's painting and graphics, and the constant growth of the little newspaper were the hub of our family's life. The newspaper, *The Beacon*, thrived and expanded, and my father was able to purchase or start newspapers in other towns in the Concord area as well. By the time I reached high school, we had a chain of thirteen newspapers with several hundred employees, housed in a large new building in the neighboring town of Acton. I saw firsthand the fabled power of the press and how senators, congressional representatives, and local politicians all came to my father hoping for his backing, and how the local merchants required advertising. I saw also how our newspaper needed the merchants as well and would zealously defend them. Through our immediate involvement in the town meetings, issues, and local politics, I felt as though I had an insider's view on all that was happening in our community.

Another seed was the sense pervading our lives that we were true Americans. My father was patriotic in the extreme and loved to quote Patrick Henry and fly the flag. My mother's relatives came over as Pilgrims on the *Mayflower* in 1620, and our Tuttle ancestors came from England as Puritans on the *Planter* in 1630. Every April 19, when thousands of people gathered at the Old North Bridge in Concord to celebrate and reenact "the shot heard 'round the world," the beginning of the Revolutionary War in Concord, my father dressed as one of the Minutemen and marched the six miles from Acton to Concord, retracing the original line of march and reenacting the historic battle. Growing up conscious of being descended from the Pilgrims and Founding Fathers, I felt especially connected to the American Dream. I relished and valued the ideals that the United States is supposed to stand for, and the idea of revolution. The Pilgrims and Puritans, like Emerson and Thoreau, valued simplicity, community, and viewing life essentially as a spiritual quest. When these seeds began to sprout, they transformed my view, as I began to see life more as a pilgrimage and to focus less on acquiring and competing and more on the purpose of the pilgrimage. I also began to see that such a view would be considered somewhat subversive.

The Organic Dairy at Camp Challenge

Another seed experience from my childhood that stands out vividly, and that I am grateful for having helped awaken my heart, is witnessing the killing of a cow on an idyllic Vermont dairy farm. I was about twelve years old, and attending a summer camp in the Green Mountains called Camp Challenge. The philosophy and practice of the camp was to challenge boys in positive ways, and I have many memories of these challenges: difficult whitewater canoe expeditions, five-day forays in the steep mountains, living outdoors for weeks at a time and cooking all our meals on campfires, washing in the icy brook, and even doing a two-day solo in the wilderness equipped with only three matches, a knife, and a hook and fish line.

The camp was affiliated with an organic farm in the valley below us where we would sometimes work baling or weeding. At one point all of us boys went down there and were told to catch one of the hens that roamed freely. We were shown how to put her head between two nails in a board on the ground and hold her with one hand while we chopped off her head with a hatchet held in the other hand. I was glad I was one of the few who made a clean cut with the first blow and watched the headless chicken, like the other unfortunate creatures, run around the barnyard spouting blood till she expired. We all learned how to dip the corpses in scalding water, pluck and eviscerate them, and we all ate chicken for many days afterward. I was a bit uncomfortable with the whole thing, but I was a well-trained omnivore, and by age twelve I knew I had to be tough and that certain animals were put here for humans to eat. We had to eat them or we would be unhealthy.

A few weeks later, we all went down to the farm again. There were horses and cows and fields of beans and wheat under a beautiful blue sky, and we were brought to the barn where a cow was standing alone, in the middle of the wooden floor. She was one of the dairy cows, and Tom (the owner-director of the camp and the farm, a handsome Dartmouth-educated outdoorsman we all admired enormously) informed us that she could not give enough milk and we would there-fore be using her for meat. He held a rifle in his hand and pointed to a precise spot on her head where the bullet would have to hit so that she would fall. He asked if one of the older boys would like to try making the shot. One boy raised his hand, took the rifle, aimed, and fired a bul-let into her head at point-blank range while we all stood and watched. The cow jolted but continued standing. Tom gave the rifle to another of the older boys who wanted to try, and he also fired a bullet into her head. Again she jolted upon the impact but continued to stand there, blinking.

Then Tom took the rifle, aimed, and fired. I was astounded as the cow instantly crashed to the floor, feces and urine gushing from her rear near where I stood. Tom immediately grabbed a long knife, jumped astride her prostrate body, and with a great strong stroke, cut her head almost completely off. I was amazed at how far the blood shot out of her open neck, propelled by her still-beating heart, long red liquid arcs flying far through the air and splattering all around us as her body con-vulsed on the blood-soaked floor. We all watched silently as she finally stopped moving and bleeding, and many of us had to wipe our blood-spattered arms and legs. While I stood in shock and horror at what I had just witnessed, Tom wiped his brow and calmly explained that the meat would be no good if her heart didn't pump the blood out of her flesh; it would be soggy and useless. We spent the next hour or so disemboweling her body, pulling out all the different organs, identifying them and holding them. I noticed how the pools of blood coagulated into large globs of red jelly on the wooden floor. Tom at one point called us over to show us a part of her anatomy he held in his hand. She apparently had something wrong with her ovaries and he was showing us the defect, telling us that was why she had to be killed. We all finally got the large edible parts into the back of a truck to be taken to a butcher; we would eat her flesh for the rest of the month. Some of the boys took souvenirs: teats, tail, eyes, brain.

The following summer I again attended Camp Challenge, and though I enjoyed the hiking, canoeing, and outdoor living, I was a bit anxious when, a few weeks into the session, Tom again told everyone to walk down to the organic dairy farm. Again, there was a cow singled out, standing in front of the barn on that gorgeous summer day. It would be her last day, and she looked very uncomfortable. Tom said he didn't want to do it in the barn this year; we would bring her up to a flat grassy area a few hundred yards away. We put a rope around her neck and tried to pull her along with us as we walked up the little hill. She didn't want to go, and resisted strongly. The harder we pulled, the more strongly she resisted. I was surprised at her strength. There were probably thirty or so kids pulling on that rope and we could hardly get her to move at all. Seeing we wouldn't be successful that way, Tom got a heavy chain, tied it around her neck, and attached it to the back of his four-wheel drive truck. We all rode in the back or walked along as the truck pulled her, still strongly resisting, up the hill. Then an incredible thing happened. We were getting close to the flat area, the cow still resisting with all her strength, the wheels steadily turning, when suddenly the chain snapped, the truck lurched forward, and we in the truck all fell down! The cow stood there in the road, her head at an oblique angle, looking up at us. As I saw her standing there, mute, and yet expressing herself so profoundly, I wished we could just leave her alone and let her live. Still, I believed she was our *food*—this was her only purpose. The tension between seeing her as a being and seeing her as meat was intense. I don't remember much of what happened after that, except that we did somehow get her up to the flat spot and proceeded to shoot

her, bleed her, disembowel her, send her to the butcher, and eat her during the following weeks. When we did it this time, though, I wasn't
shocked, because I'd seen it before. I had lost my feelings.

Seeds of Understanding

For nine more years, I continued, undaunted, to eat the flesh, milk, and
eggs of animals. I simply did not know one could survive without doing
so, and I had never met anyone who ate a plant-based diet. When I went
away to Colby College in Maine and heard of vegetarianism, something
inside me was kindled, but the programming of my inherited
omnivorism was still far too strong to have me question my fundamental eating habits.

Then, while at Colby in 1974, my junior year, I heard of The Farm
in Tennessee, a relatively newly formed spiritual community of about
eight hundred people, mainly from San Francisco. The more I read
about The Farm, the more intrigued I became, and one of the things that
intrigued me most about The Farm was that everyone there was a vegetarian. It was a vegan community, actually (though that word was not
yet in commom usage), for they were vegetarian not for health reasons,
but for ethical and spiritual reasons, and they ate no animal products
whatsoever, not even eggs, dairy products, or honey. I had yet knowingly even to meet a vegetarian in my life at that point, but I saw in the
books published by The Farm pictures of happy, healthy-looking and
highly creative people living with a mission to demonstrate a more sustainable and harmonious way of living. I did my senior thesis in
Organizational Behavior on The Farm, examining the theory and practice of a community based on cooperation rather than competition,
sharing rather than owning, and compassion rather than oppression. It
was an eye- and heart-opening project for me to study their way of living. Success was measured in terms of spiritual values rather than material values, emphasizing quality of life and service to humanity and to
all life rather than the accumulation of wealth and things. Their purpose
was clearly stated: "We're here to help save the world!"

In my last two years at Colby I felt a major shift happening within
me. I hungered for a deeper connection with nature and with spiritual-

ity, and began exploring meditation and both Eastern and Western spiritual traditions. One book from the late nineteenth century stood out: *Cosmic Consciousness* by R. M. Bucke. In this book, which had a profound impact on me, the author introduced the idea that while most people operate with what he termed self consciousness—an unsatisfactory state of self-preoccupation—certain people had attained what he termed cosmic consciousness. Bucke maintained that this higher level of consciousness, which is marked by moral elevation, intellectual illumination, spiritual wisdom, and loss of the fear of death, is the next stage of human evolution. When I read these words, the world of careers that awaited after graduation looked like a bleak and unfulfilling distraction from the real goal of living, which had to be to reach a higher level of consciousness than the narrow pursuit of self-interest I saw around me. When I talked about these ideas with my brother, he responded with whole-hearted agreement. Together we formulated a plan of action.

Leaving Home

In the late summer after graduating from Colby in 1975, my brother Ed and I, aged twenty and twenty-two, decided to go on a spiritual pilgrimage. With small backpacks and large yearnings, we left our parents' home in Massachusetts. I longed to go deeper spiritually, to discover directly the truth of myself, and to understand this life on earth more fully by consciously seeking an escape from the prison of self-consciousness through spiritual discipline.

We discovered a book about the life and teachings of Ramana Maharshi (1879–1950), a sage from South India who recommended meditating continually on the question "Who am I?" as a way of achieving spiritual understanding. This practice is based on the understanding that what we are is not merely a physical body, or feelings, thoughts, or beliefs, and that it is possible to directly experience the truth that we are, which transcends conditioning, delusion, and physical death. We need only inquire as deeply and authentically as possible into this question of who or what we actually are.

This was my focus as we traveled across the countryside, going west—perhaps, we thought, to California. After a few weeks we had gotten as far as Buffalo, and I was feeling the effect of the new experience of meditation and self-inquiry. The deeper I was able to go with this inquiry, the more profoundly I felt my connection with the trees, birds, and people I saw, and the more open I felt to our shared kinship. "What is this 'me' exactly, that wants always to be protected and fulfilled?" I kept asking, "and that sees itself as separate?"

In Buffalo, we decided to head south and not look for any car rides at all, simply walking fifteen to twenty miles a day, from one little town to the next, entrusting ourselves as completely as possible into the care of the universe. We had no money and stayed mostly on the floors of churches in the towns we passed through, yet food always somehow presented itself to us. I became increasingly convinced of the truth of the teaching to *seek first the Kingdom of God, for then all else shall be added unto you*, as minor miracles unfolded practically every day in the form of fortuitous coincidences and meetings with people who seemed to us to be angels. Ironically, they often thought *we* were angels. Our security seemed to be our total vulnerability and, perhaps, the force field of the inquiry on which we focused.

I found my heart opening to others and wanting to help them. Sometimes that help was in learning to receive, and other times it was in being generous with our time and energy to help and counsel people who would naturally confide in us and seek our advice. We spent several hours every day sitting quietly, contemplating and inquiring into this seemingly infinite and impossible question, "Who am I?" The question still filled my mind as we walked for hours on end. Why do I think I am in this body only, and not in the body of that person or dog? Like me, they each have self-interest and strive to get what they like and avoid what they dislike. I found myself loosening an old tight grip on an idea that I am fundamentally separate, and began to see the same "I" in others. I could look through their eyes, understand their perspective, and feel their feelings. This began to have consequences.

At one point a friendly man directed us to a quaint little summer cabin on a stream where he said we could spend a few quiet days if we wanted to. We walked there and settled in, but there was no food so we started foraging. We found lots of wild carrots and some cattail roots, neither of which were appetizing, and since there were fishing poles there and I had learned to fish at Camp Challenge, I decided to catch a few fish.

It was drizzling, and I put the first fish I caught into my raincoat pocket, confident he would die before too long. When I caught a second fish, I put her into the other pocket. I went back to the cabin to cook supper, quite proud of myself. The cattail roots and wild carrots were cooking and I went to clean the fish, but to my dismay they were both still alive and flipping about convulsively. I realized that I was killing them, but they were not dead yet, so the old patterns kicked in and I grabbed one and slammed him down hard against the floor. Like waking from a nightmare, I could not believe what I was doing. Yet I did not think I could stop. The fish was still alive! Two more times I had to slam him against the floor, and then the other fish as well, before I could clean them, cook them, and we could eat them for dinner.

I could feel their terror and pain, and the violence I was committing against these unfortunate creatures, and I vowed never to fish again. The self-inquiry worked relentlessly to expose my conditioned behavior and hypocrisy. The old programming that they were "just fish" completely fell away, and I saw with fresh eyes what was actually happening, and how I had entered their world violently and deceitfully with intent to harm. Here I was on a spiritual pilgrimage, trying with all my heart to directly understand the deeper truths of being, yet I was acting contrary to this by first tricking the fish with a lure hiding a cruel barbed hook, and then killing them.

The next day Ed and I walked on, and though I still knew little about being a vegetarian, I began to think it would be a better—even a necessary—way to live. Walking on the small backcountry roads, we wended our way south through New York and into Pennsylvania, then across Pennsylvania into West Virginia. Most every evening we would look up a local minister and stay in a church, and sometimes be offered a meal as well. We also stayed in rescue missions, jails, homes, communes, fields, and forests. Thanks to Johnny Appleseed, our little packs were almost always filled with apples, and we would occasionally see abandoned gardens with ripe zucchini. I found myself beginning to minimize eating meat when it was offered, though I worried I might not get enough protein if I refused it completely.

Dogs were an occasional threat as we walked along the backcountry roads, I suppose because they would perceive us as strangers invading their territory. One morning as we walked by a house in rural West Virginia, a large German shepherd emerged without barking and walked behind us. I shivered when I suddenly felt his nose touch the back of my leg. We walked many miles and he stayed right with us, a beautiful animal, friendly and energetic, always running before us and acting like our protector. We stopped for lunch on a little hill above the road and ate a few apples and then meditated for about a half hour as we usually did. The dog sat quietly with us, looking alertly into the distance and radiating a profound sense of peace and power. We were quite in awe of this dog! He was clearly an accomplished meditator. We continued walking and, coming around a bend in the road, we saw a house on a hill above us—and a large dog who immediately rushed down the hill right at us, looking like he meant business. Our German shepherd friend was at the moment a few hundred yards behind us, and what a thrill it was to see him streaking from behind us across the hill and bowling the other charging dog over before he could reach us! After receiving some stern growls, the other dog ran back up to his house and we three continued on together, enjoying each other's company enormously, until the great dog eventually looked at us, turned, and trotted back toward his home. I wondered how anyone could fail to be touched by the spirit of this being—yet if he was kept in a cage or, as in China, seen only as a piece of meat to be eaten or, like a coyote or wolf, as a nuisance to be shot, his presence and individuality would be completely invisible.

Our long walk south continued through the hills of West Virginia and into eastern Kentucky, and then into Tennessee. People thought we were on an adventure to see the world, but for us it was an inner journey. Meditation and self-inquiry were the focus of every day, always coming back to the present moment and striving to approach cosmic consciousness. I felt certain that more elevated levels of consciousness than the ones I had experienced and saw displayed in people must be potentially available. Spiritual teachers and certain poets spoke clearly and passionately of their existence.

As the weeks went on, we gave up one thing after another. Extra shoes and spare clothes were all donated one by one, gradually lightening the load in our backpacks. It felt wonderfully liberating to let go of less physically bulky attachments as well, like the little address book with some friends around the country I thought we could visit on our journey. I discarded it early on in upstate New York, and soon after we gave away a $200 emergency fund we had in the form of four $50 bills hidden in our packs. I took my glasses off as well and put them away, which was quite a challenge, since my prescription was strong, with 20/400 vision in my better eye! The world was blurry for a few weeks but began clearing up noticeably as my eyes and mind gradually began to recover their natural ability to see again. I began realizing that it was my habit of wearing glasses and contacts that had caused my vision to deteriorate and would have made me a lifelong customer of the optometry industry. Though it was a bit frightening at first to remove those artificial barriers between the world and myself, it became increasingly liberating, and today I haven't worn corrective lenses for over twenty-five years.

As the golden autumn days rolled by and we continued walking south, I began to feel more alive than I ever had before. It was as if layers of armor were peeling away. Waves of pure joy would suddenly sweep over me and I would feel as if my heart were absolutely bursting with gladness. It was a joy that seemed to have little relation to what I had always thought would bring happiness. We had no money, virtually no possessions, and no idea where the next meal or lodging was coming from, and so why would these unexplainable waves bubble up from within so vividly? One thing was certain: we were living *our* life, not the life that had been dictated by media images or by parents, teachers, relatives, and authority figures. It was perhaps the essential joy of being that arises spontaneously when we are true to our inner calling to evolve. It seemed to create a field of freedom and blessing around us that was protective and almost palpable.

The quest for understanding was everything. We somehow knew

not to try to hang on to anything. I remember one Sunday in a small West Virginia town, when we were asked to give the morning lesson to the Sunday School children and we told them that we had found the truth of what Jesus taught us: *Seek first the Kingdom of God and everything else shall be added unto you.* Afterward, the church took up a special collection and gave us a surprise gift of $30 as we walked on to the next little town. The following day, after we bought two $5 lunches in a restaurant with the $30 windfall, we gave the waitress the remaining $20 as a tip and walked on again, pockets empty and hearts free. Once, when we had not eaten for quite a while and had nothing at all in our packs, I saw a plastic package up ahead by the side of the road. It was a fresh sandwich! We ate every bite as slowly and thankfully as we could. In all the months of walking, we never went seriously hungry.

Seeds of Community

Eventually we were somehow guided to a newly formed commune of about a dozen people in central Kentucky. They greeted us warmly, and we learned they were all vegetarians and were affiliated with The Farm in Tennessee! We learned how to cook soybeans and first heard of something called "tofu." Our hosts told us they wore vegetarian shoes and tried to minimize the suffering they caused to animals. I had been dimly aware of chickens pecking each other's eyes out in overcrowded factory farm cages, of calves being branded and castrated and pigs screaming in slaughterhouses, and I had seen the transport trucks filled with cattle, but I knew little of the details, or how to prepare healthy plant-based meals. In an atmosphere of openness and caring we talked of all these things. We worked and ate together, and played and meditated together, and it began to seem absurd and almost barbaric to even consider dining on the flesh of animals. I vowed within myself to be a vegetarian.

Soon we were heading south toward The Farm in Tennessee, continuing our pilgrimage and our practice. We eventually reached The Farm and stayed there several weeks. The experience absolutely sealed my vegetarianism and was worth the months of walking that it took to get there. Close to a thousand people, mostly living as married couples with kids in self-built homes, had created a community on a large piece of beautifully rolling farm and forest land. People wore their hair long as a statement for naturalness and against the military mindset that had been ravaging Vietnam. It was set up legally as a monastery, and it was strictly vegan to avoid harming animals, people, and the environment. The Farm had its own school, telephone system, soy dairy, publishing and printing company, rock band, Sunday morning church service, and Plenty, a blossoming outreach program that provided vegan food and health-care services both in Central America and in the ghettos of North America. Stephen Gaskin, the spiritual leader, was a student of Zen master Suzuki Roshi, founder of the San Francisco Zen Center.

The food was delicious, the atmosphere unlike anything I had ever experienced. People were friendly, energetic, bright, and there was a powerful sense of purpose: of working to create a better world, of sharing together and honoring each other and the local community. The soy dairy made tofu, soy milk, soy burgers, and "Ice Bean," the first soy ice cream, and the schoolhouse for the children served all vegan meals. The kids, vegan from birth, grew tall, strong, and healthy. Gardens, fields, and greenhouses provided food for everyone, and people worked on different crews, building, repairing, cooking, teaching, farming, and together making The Farm remarkably self-reliant. I worked in the book printing house, taking copies of The Farm's extremely popular *Spiritual Midwifery Guide* off the press. Women came from all over the country to The Farm's spiritual birthing center to have their babies delivered by The Farm's experienced and loving midwives. Women who were thinking of having abortions were told that if they had the baby at The Farm and decided not to keep the child, then he or she would be adopted by one of the couples on The Farm. Though many women came with this option in mind, never did a woman decide not to keep a baby after having gone through the birth process with The Farm's caring midwives.

I was deeply touched by the loving attentiveness people showed each other, and by the courage the whole community displayed in running almost completely contrary to the values of the larger society. The people there, like myself, had all been raised in a culture of domination that killed and abused animals for food, clothing, entertainment, and research, and that emphasized competition, private property, consumerism, and limited liability for large corporations. We had been raised to view the earth, animals, and even people as commodities to be used by the market for self-centered profit. The Farm was a living example of veganism, emphasizing gentleness, compassion, and respect for all creatures, a life of voluntary simplicity and appropriate technology, sharing resources, and finding happiness through strong, healthy family and social relationships, helping others, spiritual growth, and creative expression, rather than through personal aggrandizement. To me, it seemed these people were going much farther toward actually living the teachings espoused by Jesus than mainstream religions were. The lived ideal was that all life is sacred, and the attempt was to consciously create a community and lifestyle that reflected this ideal and would be an inspiration to others and a model for sustainable living. Needless to say, banking, corporate, and governmental institutions were all extremely hostile to The Farm. Though it is still going strong, it's smaller and somewhat less radical than it was in its heyday in the 1970s and early '80s.

Though we seriously considered joining The Farm, we eventually received intuitive guidance to walk farther south to Huntsville, Alabama. When we got there, we discovered the local Zen center, where we could devote our energy to meditation practice, sitting about eight hours daily and helping with the upkeep of the center. This was a perfect situation for us, and we were able to focus on our meditation practice and receive excellent instruction and guidance. Over the next several years, I continued living in Buddhist meditation centers in Atlanta and then in San Francisco, but loosened up somewhat on my vegan diet, since most people at these centers ate eggs and dairy products, and I was, at that point, unaware of the extent of the cruelty involved in these foods.

In 1980, while I was living at Kagyu Droden Kunchab, a Vajrayana (Tibetan Buddhist) meditation center in San Francisco, I had the auspicious opportunity to meet the Dalai Lama and present to him a translation of an ancient Tibetan practice text I had worked on and helped our center publish. Earlier in the day the Dalai Lama had conducted a ceremony with us in which we all took the Bodhisattva Vow, which is considered the foundation of Vajrayana meditation practice: the vow to attain complete spiritual enlightenment in order to be of maximum benefit to living beings. A difficult inconsistency for me and for many others was that while we were vegetarians, many of the Tibetan lamas we sought instruction from ate meat regularly. Even the Dalai Lama himself, while strongly condemning hunting and all forms of animal abuse and encouraging vegetarianism among both the Tibetan people and Western Buddhist practitioners, was eating animal flesh every other day, purportedly on the advice of physicians. Perhaps the reasons may have been political as well, because as the highest and most visible religious authority in the Tibetan tradition, it would take considerable courage to depart from the practice of most of the lamas and follow the ethical vegetarianism enjoined by the original Buddhist teachings. Fortunately, in April 2005, he displayed this remarkable political courage, and news services reported, "Saying he has recently turned to a vegetarian diet, the Dalai Lama called on people to stop killing and destroying animals."[1] Because of the Dalai Lama's eminence as an exemplar of peace, this is good news for all of us and there are encouraging signs that young Tibetans in India are moving in the same direction also.[2]

SonggwangSa Temple

In 1984 I had my second opportunity to live in a vegan community. This time it was an ancient Zen monastery in South Korea. I traveled there and participated as a monk in the summer's three-month intensive retreat. We rose at 2:40 A.M. to begin the day of meditation, practicing silence and simplicity, and eating vegan meals of rice, soup, vegetables, and occasional tofu, and retiring after the evening meditation at 9:00 P.M. The meals were eaten in silence with each of us using a set of four bowls: three for the rice, soup, and vegetables and the fourth for tea, which we used to clean our bowls and then drink, so that not even a single grain of rice would go to waste.

The community consisted of about seventy monks, with some lay people who helped with certain tasks, and the vegan roots there were old and deep. For many centuries in that temple, people had lived the same way, meditating and living a life of nonviolence. There was no silk or leather in any clothing, and though I was there in the summer mosquito season, it was absolutely not an option to kill a mosquito or any creature. We simply used a mosquito net in the meditation hall. Through the months of silence and meditation, sitting still for seemingly endless hours, a deep and joyful feeling emerged within, a sense of solidarity with all life and of becoming more sensitive to the energy of situations.

When after four months I returned to the bustle of American life, I felt a profound shift had occurred, and the vegetarianism I'd been practicing for about nine years transformed spontaneously and naturally into veganism with roots that felt as if they extended to the center of my heart. Until then, I had mistakenly thought that my daily vegan purchases of food, clothing, and so forth were my personal choices, simply options. Now I could clearly see that not treating animals as commodities was not an option or a choice, for animals simply are *not* commodities. It would be as unthinkable to eat or wear or justify abusing an animal as it would be to eat or wear or justify abusing a human. The profound relief and empowerment of completely realizing and understanding this in my heart has been enriching beyond words.

When I returned from Korea I was able to begin teaching humanities and philosophy courses at a college in the San Francisco Bay Area, through connections I'd made when getting a masters degree at San Francisco State University just prior to going to Korea. After about six months of teaching I decided to apply for entrance into a Ph.D. program in the U.C. Berkeley Graduate School of Education. For this I was required to take an aptitude test, the Graduate Record Examination, and it was interesting that when the results came back they were very high. Mensa told me that the scores corresponded to an I.Q. that was in the top one-quarter of one percent of the population. In my younger years as an omnivore and non-meditator I had never scored particularly high on such tests, but it's quite understandable. A vegan way of eating not only allows our system to run much cleaner, but more essentially, it frees us mentally to make connections. This ability is the foundation of intelligence. Regular meditative silence allows our mind to relax and connect with wellsprings of intuitive potential that also seem to increase our ability to make connections. Following a vegan diet and practicing inner silence is a powerful combination! I found, for example, that I was able to teach a full load of courses at the college and simultaneously take a full course load at Berkeley, so that I was typically juggling eight to ten courses at once. Not only did the teaching go wonderfully well, but I had only As and a couple of A-plusses in over sixty units of doctoral coursework, and my dissertation, *The Role of Intuition in Education*, was nominated for the Best Dissertation Award. There is nothing for me personally to be proud of or take credit for in this, because it's just one of countless human illustrations of the underlying principle that all of us have an enormous potential that can be fulfilled as we understand and live in accordance with our intrinsic nature. The main hindrance to this is the inherited food-enforced mentality of competition and exclusion that keeps us distracted, paralyzed, and unable to make meaningful connections.

After teaching college for about six years and enjoying it immensely, I felt guided to take up an itinerant lifestyle giving concerts of original piano music and seminars on developing intuition. Though the college offered me a salary increase to stay on, I felt a strong calling to return to the open road. I had found that in the years since embarking on my pilgrimage from New England, uplifting and swirling new music had begun pouring through me on the piano, and as I focused more on the music and played publicly, it got stronger and was received with enthusiasm. Through the music, I felt my heart and inner vision opening to an inspiring spiritual energy that connected me with the earth and with the plight of both animals and our human family. The music, emerging from the mystery of inner stillness, has always seemed to be a vehicle for carrying elevating and healing energy and intuitive understanding.

Although I hadn't been consciously aware of it at the time, while I was switching to a plant-based diet at The Farm in 1975, thousands of miles away in Switzerland, a young painter named Madeleine was simultaneously making a similar change. In 1990, while playing concerts in Europe, I met Madeleine fortuitously in a small Swiss village, and since then I have been wonderfully blessed with her presence as my life partner and loving companion.

The Power of Community

The communities we grow up in and call home affect us all profoundly. Understanding this, we can see why we view animals as commodities and often find it difficult to switch to a vegan diet and lifestyle. Our culture is completely saturated and defined by the exploitation of animals for food.

While cultures tend naturally to replicate themselves, they can and do evolve, or may be forced to change by outside pressure. The spread of the herding culture from central Asia into the Mediterranean and the Middle East and from there to Europe took several millennia and was accomplished by physical force, domination of women, and indoctrination of children, as Eisler documents in *The Chalice and the Blade*.[3] Jeremy Rifkin's *Beyond Beef* documents how the cattle culture came to North America from Europe and how European (especially British) demand for beef and its enormous financial investment in American cattle ranching supplied the capital that propelled our young country and its economy. Lynn Jacobs' *Waste of the West* documents the virtually complete decimation of western grazing lands and the near eradication of Indians, bison, prairie dogs, wolves, and all non-livestock "nuisance" animals. To this day, federal and state agencies like the USDA's "Wildlife Services" still poison, shoot, den, and trap millions of animals every year, including coyotes, bobcats, mustangs, prairie dogs, bison, beaver, raccoons, blackbirds, badgers, and bears. It is a tragedy involving unspeakable suffering.

When I was in Korea I marveled at beautiful terraced rice paddies nestled in valleys and climbing up hillsides, efficiently raising enough rice to feed the Korean people who, unlike in the U.S., could actually be seen every day in the paddies tending the crops. With U.S. and European capital investment, however, Korean culture was changing, and American food corporations and U.S. television programs and advertising were invading, creating demand for Western luxury foods, especially beef. Texas cattlemen were traveling to Korea, taking the opportunity to show investors how to convert rice paddies to cattle feedlots. Instead of feeding many people with rice, an area of land would now feed only a few rich people with beef and raise the price of rice beyond what poor people could afford, while creating the environmental nightmare of waste and pollution that modern animal agriculture always brings. The spread of the herding culture into Korea has received a strong boost from the Christian missionaries who have established a considerable presence there. It may be slowed down by the Buddhist monasteries and their teachings and example of compassion and veganism, but only to the degree they remain respected and relevant to the lives of an increasingly pressured population.

The spread of the herding culture has been going on for centuries and continues unabated today. Its wealth and willingness to use both financial pressure and physical violence make it difficult to resist, and as it spreads, so do oppression, inequality, violence, competition, and struggle. It is a culture of exploitation and predation that reinforces in all its members its core practice of herding and eating commodified animals.

To exist within the hostile environment of the herding culture, vegan communities must be strong and committed. Most, like The Farm and SonggwangSa Zen Temple, are essentially spiritual communities. Their practice of vegan living is part of a larger orientation of spiritual practice emphasizing compassionate living, cultivation of inner peace and harmony, and contributing to the moral regeneration of humanity. However, vegan community can also be experienced in many other places today, making the switch to veganism easier and more natural. The number of vegetarian and vegan communities is growing as a result of the proliferation of non-Western spiritual traditions here. There are a growing number of healing centers and religious retreat centers as well, emphasizing vegetarianism or veganism for reasons of both health and spiritual purification. There are also temporary communities, like animal rights and vegetarian conferences, as well as local vegetarian societies that provide knowledge and inspiration. Community support of some kind is vital, for it provides the context, examples, and practical guidance that are particularly essential in the beginning stages of switching to a more cruelty-free diet and lifestyle.

Seeds bear fruit after their kind. Both The Farm and SonggwangSa Temple are the blossoming of seeds planted by wise and compassionate people at least 2,500 years ago, and nurtured and replanted by countless dedicated people for centuries, often in the face of great adversity. The future generations of both humans and animals are depending on us to do what we can to nurture the seeds of nonviolence, intelligence, and compassion in our shared cultural garden so that they can inherit an earth that is healthy and a way of living that is based on freedom and caring. We can each be a field of freedom, and by the force of our example and intention we make it easier for those around us to do the same. The field will grow, spreading through our culture as a benevolent revolution.

While the journey I've been relating here is obviously unique, as all our individual journeys are, I believe the underlying pattern is universal. We have all been born into a herding culture that commodifies animals, and we have all been affected by the cruelty, violence, and predatory competitiveness that our meals require and that our culture embodies. We've also been taught to be loyal to our culture and relatively uncritical of it, to disconnect from the monumental horror we needlessly perpetuate, and to be oblivious to the disastrous effects this has on every level of our shared and private lives. We are all presented with the same evidence and hear the same call for mercy and justice.

Within us lie seeds of awakening and compassion that may be already sprouting. Our individual journeys of transformation and spiritual evolution call us to question who and what we've been told we and others are, to discover and cultivate the seeds of insight and clarity within us, and to realize the connections we've been taught to ignore. As we do this and as our web of journeys interweaves within our culture, cross-fertilizing and planting seeds, we can continue the transformation that is now well underway, and transcend the obsolete old paradigm that generates cycles of violence. When we uproot exclusion and domination from our plates, seeds of compassion can finally freely blossom, and this process depends primarily on us watering the seeds and fully contributing our unique journey. We depend on each other, and as we free the beings we call animals, we will regain our freedom. Loving them, we will learn to love each other and be fully loved.

CHAPTER FIFTEEN

LIVING THE REVOLUTION

◦ ◦

"My aim is not modest. I see that nothing short of the transformation of
humanity is necessary at this point in time."
—Jill Purce

"Every day forty thousand children die in the world for lack of food. We
who overeat in the West, who are feeding grains to animals to make
meat, are eating the flesh of these children."
—Thich Nhat Hanh[1]

"True human goodness, in all its purity and freedom, can come to the
fore only when its recipient has no power. Humanity's true moral test, its
fundamental test, consists of its attitude towards those who are at its
mercy: animals. And in this respect humankind has suffered a fundamental debacle, a debacle so fundamental that all others stem from it."
—Milan Kundera, author, *The Unbearable Lightness of Being*

The Holograph

The ripples that radiate from our choices to eat foods from animal
sources are incredibly far-reaching and complex. They extend deeply
into our essential orientation and belief system, and into our relationships with each other and the created order. From every perspective we

can possibly take, we discover that our culturally imposed eating habits are numbing, blinding, and confining us. Enslaving and eating animals is relentlessly polluting our mental and bodily environments, hardening our hearts and blocking feelings and awareness, instigating fear, violence, and repression in our relationships, laying waste our precious planet, gruesomely torturing and killing billions of terrorized beings, deadening us spiritually, and profoundly disempowering us by impeding our innate intelligence and our ability to make essential connections.

To come to terms with our multifaceted human dilemma is to come to terms with the mentality of oppression that our meals demand. Looking away, as we chronically do, our existence and our projects become ironic, self-deceptive, destructive, and suicidal. Seeing our eating habits for what they are, though, and answering the call of our spirit to understand the consequences of our actions, we become open to compassion, intelligence, freedom, and to living the truth of our interconnectedness with all life. There is an enormously positive revolution implicit in this, a spiritual transformation that can potentially launch our culture into a quantum evolutionary leap, from emphasizing consumption, domination, and self-preoccupation to nurturing creativity, liberation, inclusion, and cooperation. Are we ready for such a spiritual revolution? If we refuse, the strife, stress, and destruction will almost certainly intensify due to our ascending numbers and exploitive technology. When is a caterpillar ready to transform? The most obvious sign is the passing of its voracious appetite because an inner urge turns its attention to new directions.

The spiritual and cultural revolution that calls us must begin with our food. Food is our primary connection with the earth and her mysteries, and with our culture. It is the foundation of economy and is the central inner spiritual metaphor of our lives. There is no way to overstate the magnitude of the collective spiritual transformation that will occur when we shift from food of violent oppression to food of gentleness and compassion. The key to veganism is that it is lived. No one can be a vegetarian in theory only! Unlike many religious teachings that are primarily theoretical and internal, veganism is solidly practical. The motivation of veganism is compassion. It is not at all about personal purity or individual health or salvation, except as these bless others. It is a concrete, visible way of living that flows from, and reinforces, a sense of caring and connectedness.

Even if we are benumbed to the degree that we are not concerned about the suffering of animals, and we are only able to care about other humans, we soon realize that the human anguish caused by eating foods of animal origin requires us to choose a plant-based diet. Human starvation, the emotional devastation required to kill and confine animals, the pollution and waste of water, land, petroleum, and other vital resources, and the injustice and violence underlying our animal food production complex all compel us to abandon our acculturated eating habits. As we make connections and become open to feedback, it will be increasingly obvious that one of the greatest gifts any of us can give to the world, to the human family, to future generations, to animals, to ourselves, and to our loved ones is to go vegan and dedicate our lives to encouraging others to do the same.

This requires questioning the underlying assumptions and attitudes of our culture and freeing ourselves from them not just in theory, but in practice. This inner action of leaving home necessitates in many ways a spiritual breakthrough. The essential action is to stop turning away and disconnecting from the suffering we impose on others by our food choices. Being willing to look, see, respond, and reconnect with all our neighbors and live this interconnectedness inspires us naturally to choose food, entertainment, clothing, and products that cause a minimum of unnecessary cruelty to vulnerable living beings. As we do this, we become more mindful of the ripples our actions cause in the world. Our spiritual transformation deepens, and as our sensitivity increases we yearn to bless others more and to be a voice for the voiceless. Once a vegan, we are always so, because our motivation is not personal and self-oriented, but is based on concern for others and on our undeniable interconnectedness with other living beings.

This urge to show mercy and to protect those who are vulnerable is rooted deeply in us, and though it has been repressed by our herding culture, there is enormous evidence that it longs to be expressed by virtually all of us. We will collectively donate millions of dollars, for example, to help just one animal if we know the animal's story and our intelligence and compassion have been awakened by our connecting with this animal. The more we connect, the more we understand and the more we love, and this love propels us not only to leave home, questioning our culture's attitude of domination and exclusion, but also to return home, speaking on behalf of those who are vulnerable.

The opposite of love is not hate but indifference. When we lift the veil and see the suffering our food habits cause, when we connect with the reality of the defenseless beings who suffer so terribly because of our food choices, our indifference dissolves and compassion—its opposite—arises, urging us to act on behalf of those who are suffering. A primary danger is that we might leave home but not return; that is, we could awaken to the harmfulness inherent in our culture's commodification of living beings but fail to bring this awakening to our culture by becoming a voice for these beings. If our understanding isn't articulated in ways that are meaningful for us, it can become imprisoned within us and turn sour, becoming cynicism, anger, despair, and disease. This doesn't serve us or anyone else.

We all have unique gifts we can bring to the most urgent task we face at this point in our human evolution: transforming our inherited dominator mentality by liberating those we have enslaved for food. The crucial elements are adopting a vegan lifestyle, educating ourselves, cultivating our spiritual potential, and plugging in to help educate others. The spiritual revolution needs all of us, whatever our religious beliefs, ethnicity, class, or other variables may be. Every one of us has a piece of the puzzle to contribute, and our overall success depends on each of us discovering our talents and passion and persistently contributing them.

Victims, Perpetrators, and Bystanders

As we go vegan and begin to live much more lightly on the earth, we may also start to realize how powerfully we're affected by the omnivorous eating habits of the vast majority of our fellow citizens. Our freedom as omnivores to eat almost any non-human being we'd like limits others' freedom in many ways. For example, we find rivers and lakes polluted by animal agriculture so we can no longer enjoy or swim in them. We discover our air and groundwater needlessly polluted by animal abusing industries. We have to endure seeing our friends hunted and tortured by hunters and fishers, or view billboards with disgusting images of cooked animal flesh. Our money is taken from us by the government to support ranchers and dairy, factory farm, and feedlot operators, as well as predator control operations that needlessly kill more of our friends, and forests we could enjoy are destroyed to provide the immense desolate monocultures of livestock feed grains. The prices of the products and services we buy are higher than necessary because they have to include not just the government taxes that subsidize animal foods and make them artificially cheaper than they should be, but also the enormous medical insurance costs borne by corporations for their omnivore employees that are passed on to all consumers in higher prices for everything. The expensive medical procedures required by omnivores for heart disease, cancer, kidney disease, obesity, and so forth raise health insurance rates beyond the reach of many with lower incomes. The U.S. war machine is also forced upon us all; we must not only help pay for it but also see it destroy the lives of impoverished people to supply the cheap oil that wasting so much grain and energy on animal foods requires. When, as vegans, we become sensitized to the violence of the food system, we can also see that omnivores are victims of this food system as well.

There are many ways we can be part of the solution rather than part of the problem. When we buy or eat animal foods, we ourselves become the agents of our cultural perpetration of unnecessary and gruesome violence. (If we have any lingering doubt about this, we can view some of the videos listed in the resource section of this book and behold just the smallest tip of an iceberg of ongoing horror so vast and ghastly it overwhelms the mind.)

In violent crimes committed publicly, there are three roles acted out: that of the perpetrator, that of the victim, and that of the bystander or witness. It is well known that perpetrators hope bystanders will be silent and look the other way so they can successfully continue their hurtful actions, and that victims hope the bystanders will speak up, act, get involved, and do something to stop or discourage perpetrators from their harmful actions. With regard to eating animal foods, there are many perpetrators and victims and just a few bystanders. The perpetrators always encourage each other and regard the bystanders with suspicion and hostility, and the victims' voices cannot be heard.

Looking deeply, we see that the perpetrators are themselves victims of violence—that's why they've become perpetrators—and their violence hurts not only the animals but themselves and the bystanders as well. All three are locked in a painful embrace, and it is the bystanders who have the real power. They can either turn and look away, thus giving their tacit approval, or they can witness and bring a third dimension of consciousness and awareness to the cycle of violence that has the victims and perpetrators hopelessly enmeshed. The bystander offers an example of nonviolence and speaks on behalf of the victims who have no voice (and, on a subtler level, on behalf of the perpetrators who are also victimized by their own actions). Perpetrators may condemn bystanders for judging them and making them feel bad or guilty, but the bystanders are merely acting as the perpetrators' conscience, asking them to please become more aware and stop their violence, for everyone's sake. The guilt and shame perpetrators feel for their violent actions stem from their natural sense of kindness and caring, which they have blocked and are violating. Their attitude toward bystanders may even be indignation: "If you want to be a vegetarian, that's fine, but don't tell us what to do." While at first blush this seems reasonable, we quickly see that it is only because of the disconnections and bias inherent in our culture. Perpetrators wouldn't dare say, "If you don't want to beat and stab your pet dog, that's fine, but don't tell me not to beat and stab mine." We all recognize that we aren't entitled to treat others, especially those who are defenseless, however we like, and that if we are responsible for doing harm, people have every right to ask us to stop.

As perpetrators, we are thus profoundly challenged by the truth-field established by attentive and articulate bystanders. Eventually, we may respond to the challenge, examine our attitudes and, recognizing our behavior as morally indefensible, cease it and join the ranks of the bystanders. As bystanders, we are also deeply challenged to respond creatively to the situation with love, understanding, and skillful means, and to strive to live in ever more complete alignment with the values of com-passion, honesty, and integrity. The more we live in alignment with our values, the stronger the truth-field we emanate will be, and the more our words, gestures, and actions will carry weight with perpetrators. None of us is completely innocent, because to some degree we all are, and have been, in all three roles. As non-vegans, we are challenged by our spiritual and ethical disconnection to slow down, stop, pay attention, reconnect, embrace our disowned shadow, and begin the healing process. As vegans, we are challenged by our inconsistencies and fear of reprisal to pay attention and deepen our healing and awakening process by making the effort to align our thoughts, words, and actions with our understanding of interbeing and to ever more fully embody peace and courageous love. Cultivating awareness is essential to realizing happiness, peace, and freedom.

What about the victims, the animals? Who are these beings, so defenseless and unable to retaliate, so punished by a heartless, mechanized system developed for self-gratification and profit?

Our Connection with Animals

Though we are born into a culture that emphasizes our differences from other animals, our actual experience tells us differently. We are only comfortable eating animals when we exclude them from the categories we use to define ourselves, but our differences from animals are far less than our eating habits force us to believe they are. Those of us with companion animals, for example, know without doubt that they have distinct personalities and preferences, emotions and drives, and that they feel and avoid psychological and physical pain. Besides the enormous amount of anecdotal evidence that animals behave altruistically, both toward members of their own species and also to animals outside their species, there is clinical evidence as well, such as the typically cruel experiments in which monkeys were given food if they administered painful shocks to other monkeys. Researchers found that the monkeys would rather go hungry than shock other monkeys, especially if they had received shocks earlier themselves. The researchers were surprised (and perhaps somewhat ashamed?) by the monkeys' altruism. Though it is our true nature, one wonders if we humans would be so noble.

In addition to having the capacity for empathy, animals have the capacity to suffer psychologically, and often exhibit stereotypic behavior when they are forced into mental illness by our cruel treatment of them. The extreme confinement of animals used for food, fur, research, and entertainment causes such deep damage to their emotional and physical health that they repeat the same behaviors continuously, something they never do in the wild. Chimpanzees and pigs will bang their heads for hours against the metal bars of their cages, elephants will constantly sway their heads and lift their feet, and foxes confined in cramped cages in fur farms will circle manically and sway pathetically, driven insane by the impossibility of fulfilling their natural purposes. Like these animals, we humans may repeat stereotypic behaviors when we become deranged and lose our connection with the purpose we were born to fulfill.

It's illustrative to watch how the attributes we have proclaimed make us unique, such as using tools, making art, experiencing "higher" emotions, having a sense of the ludicrous, using language, and so forth, have all collapsed under the evidence as we get to know animals better. Of course, we have certain unique attributes and abilities. *Every* species has certain unique attributes and abilities. Eating animals makes us so subconsciously nervous that we neurotically overemphasize our uniqueness and our separateness from them. This allows us to exclude them from our circle of concern.

Besides sharing a common home on this beautiful planet here in outer space, animals share with us the vulnerability of mortality and all that entails. It is problematic to determine whether our lives as humans have actually improved over the centuries and millennia, for all our valiant efforts. Although we have comforts and possibilities undreamt of by our forebears, we also have stresses, diseases, and frustrations that they could not possibly have imagined. For animals, however, the situation has plainly deteriorated, especially over the more recent human generations. As food production industries brought their herds and flocks indoors into concentration camps, the extreme form of herding known as factory farming emerged. A new extreme form of factory farming is now emerging through genetic engineering, in which the animals are being tampered with at the genetic level, thus losing their biological integrity and identity. This is coupled with unparalleled destruction of habitat for wild animals and decimation of their populations for bush meat, pharmaceuticals, research, entertainment, and other human uses. Animals have thus gone from being free from human interference to being occasionally hunted, to being herded, to being imprisoned, and finally to being either forced into extinction or genetically mutated and confined as mere patentable property objects for human use.

It seems we're still so benighted as a culture that we'll refrain from committing violence only if we fear punishment or retaliation—and since animals are incapable of either, they have no protection from us at all. The new extremes to which animals are now subjected without remorse or awareness require that we adopt a more radically conscientious orientation that addresses the roots of our violent mentality. While it may seem extreme to our mainstream culture to advocate for a vegan revolution that utterly rejects our commodification of animals, it is only such an apparently extreme position that can be an antidote to the extreme abuse we now force upon animals. In fact, veganism is not extreme from the point of view of our innate nature, which longs for love, creativity, and spiritual evolution.

Heavens and hells are of our own sowing. We live in a culture that mindlessly exploits animals and encourages the domination of those who are vulnerable by the strong, the male, the wealthy, and the privileged. This culture has naturally created political, economic, legal, religious, educational, and other institutional vehicles to shield those in power from the effects of their actions, and to legitimize the violence and inequities required to maintain the system. Over the centuries it has developed an elaborate scientific and religious framework that in its reductionism and materialism denies the continuity of consequences in many ways. One of the many manifestations of this is its refusal to acknowledge the idea that we as consciousness may experience multiple dimensions and lifetimes, and especially the idea that human consciousness can be reborn as the consciousness of animals. These ideas are strenuously blocked for obvious reasons by our herding culture, but they are held as logical and true by many cultures that don't abuse animals as viciously and systematically as ours has for the past eight to ten thousand years. Perpetrators and victims are known to exchange roles over and over again in countless subtle and obvious ways. The cycle of violence may span larger dimensions than we in our herding culture would like to admit, and there are many wisdom traditions that affirm that it does. Until we see from the highest level, we had best heed the counsel of every enlightened spiritual teacher from every time: be ye kind to one another.

Paths Away from and Back to Sanity

The underlying assumptions of the culture into which we have been born are faulty and obsolete. If not questioned and changed, they will continue to drive us into deeper cultural insanity, just as they do the animals we mercilessly dominate. Recognizing the insanity of our actions and beliefs is the first and essential step to healing and awakening. The signs are evident: producing and using weapons of mass destruction while millions of people starve to death, attacking our living earth so savagely that within the space of just twenty-five years more species are forced into extinction than in the previous sixty-five million years combined, and genetically scrambling organisms with reckless disregard for the consequences these artificial creatures will have on the delicately interconnected living strands of our planet's biocommunities.

The powerful financial and media forces that block us from seeing any of this are continuing the spread of the herding culture and its obsolete and oppressive assumptions throughout the world. The transnational corporations that profit from abused animals are one example, and include gigantic retailers as well as the huge animal agriculture conglomerates that relentlessly push to expand their factory farm and slaughterhouse operations into the less industrialized cultures. In typically eating far fewer animals per person, these less wealthy societies represent markets with enormous potential for lucrative growth. The chemical, pesticide, and pharmaceutical corporations all profit from and encourage this same expansion. Charitable organizations like the

Heifer Project, which introduces animal agriculture into developing countries, often contribute directly to the same inhumane mentality that teaches people to see animals merely in terms of what the Heifer Project terms "the four Ms": meat, milk, manure, and money. The Heifer Project is simply another front for the iron fist of cruelty, indoctrinating the herding culture's regime of domination and abuse as far and wide as possible and hardening the hearts of indigenous children as it does so. Like the World Bank and the International Monetary Fund, the U.S. government in its foreign aid programs serves as an agent for our nation's powerful animal agriculture industry, buying their products for foreign distribution and concocting loans and programs that force impoverished countries to embrace the American model of petroleum-based industrial agriculture (which profits U.S. banking and petroleum companies and provides markets for the U.S. meat, dairy, egg, chemical, pharmaceutical, and medical industries). Two thirds of U.S. grain exports go to feed livestock rather than to feed hungry people.[2]

There are numerous uplifting and noble movements, organizations, and efforts that work to promote peace, social justice, equality, environmental protection, and to relieve the suffering of people who are disadvantaged, vulnerable, or marginalized. Unfortunately, virtually all of these efforts fail to address the underlying source of these problems in our domination of animals for food. As people learn more about the consequences of eating animal foods, however, we see increasing numbers of individuals and groups acting creatively to raise consciousness about this, thus helping to eliminate the roots of hunger, cruelty, pollution, and exploitation.

Food Not Bombs, for example, organizes volunteers and food donations to feed disadvantaged hungry people organic vegan food in over 175 cities throughout the Americas, Europe, and Australia. It is intentionally decentralized and web-like in its approach, with autonomous local units organizing their own compassionate operations.[3]

The worldwide followers of Ching Hai, a noted Vietnamese spiritual teacher with students numbering in the hundreds of thousands, have set up vegan restaurants in many cities and contribute vegan food, clothing, shelter, and aid to disaster victims, prisoners, children, and the elderly in countries around the world.[4] Though she requires students to meditate two and a half hours per day, vow to eat no flesh or egg products, refrain from alcohol and non-prescription drugs, and not work in jobs that promote the exploitation of animals or people, her movement continues to spread. It shows the effectiveness of a spiritual approach, because in less than twenty years she has been the proximate cause of hundreds of thousands of people's transition to veganism. Rather than impede her movement, her insistence that her students reduce the cruelty in their meals may paradoxically promote it. People who are serious about spiritual growth are apparently capable of embracing fundamental change in their lives, and may even welcome the opportunity.

These are but two encouraging examples of the vegan revolution of compassion, justice and equality taking firmer root in our culture and in the world. A positive momentum is unquestionably building in spite of the established forces of domination and violent control that would suppress it. Like a birth or metamorphosis, a new mythos is struggling through us to arise and replace the obsolete herding mythos, and the changes occurring may be far larger and more significant than they appear to be. They are ignored and discounted by the mass media, but what may seem to be small changes can suddenly mushroom when critical mass is reached. It is vital that we all contribute to the positive revolution for which our future is calling.

Implications for Further Research and Conversation

More thorough and open research and discussion of the implications of our food choices would increase our cultural awareness of the negative health, economic, environmental, psychological, and social consequences of eating animal foods, and illuminate the multiple benefits for everyone of a natural plant-based way of eating. There are virtually unending opportunities for further research and public discussion to deepen our understanding of our practice of commodifying and eating animals, and to explore more positive alternatives. Some examples include further research on the benefits of plant-based diets for individual health, and, on a larger scale, what moving to plant-based diets would mean in terms of improved air and water quality, increased food for hungry people, reduced demand for petroleum, antibiotics, drugs, chemicals, resources, and the implications of freeing up millions of acres of land currently being enslaved to graze livestock or grow their feed. The potential for enormous ecosystem healing and wildlife regeneration could be researched and discussed, as well as the economic, social, political, medical, psychological, and spiritual dimensions of these changes.

The psychological connections between abusing and killing animals and doing the same to human beings are already being explored and publicized, and this could certainly be taken further by researching the linkages between eating animal foods and obesity, teen pregnancy, collapse of family structures, disease, stress, emotional numbing, anxiety, suicide, and so forth. One particularly glaring inconsistency that should be further investigated is the underlying assumption of vivisection, that we can become healthier by destroying the health of other living beings. Our welfare is tied to the welfare of all beings; we cannot reap health in ourselves by sowing seeds of disease and death in others. We exhibit not only hubris but remarkable obtuseness in caging, torturing, and infecting animals in the name of improving our health. We can see the outcome of our actions already, as new diseases continue to arise and old ones spread, often becoming impervious to our increasingly devastating drugs. Another example of such research would be to investigate the connection between eating animal foods and the escalating use and abuse of damaging drugs like alcohol, narcotics, and pharmaceuticals. In 1915, during the temperance movement that led eventually to the prohibition era, Charles Fillmore wrote,

> The assertion has been made, and we have not heard it disproved, that there never was a vegetarian drunkard. Here then, is a remedy for intemperance far more effective than all the drug cures that men take. That the discontinuance of flesh eating will also carry off the craving for strong liquids, like beer, whiskey, wine, tea and coffee, anyone can test for himself. Stop eating meat for even one month and that unnatural thirst which accompanies and follows a diet of flesh will disappear. There is a physiological reason for this. Meat is always in a certain degree of putrefaction, and the decay is increased

when it is introduced into the stomach. The juicy steak which lovers of flesh smack their lips over is saturated with salty urea, which in the stomach calls for liquid. Physiologists say that this juice in the steak is the urine of the animal arrested on its way to the kidneys. In eating this mess man not only makes his system a sewer for the corrupting animal flesh, but he also puts into his stomach an irritant that demands a cooling solvent at once.

With this constant fever of rotting flesh in the stomach calling for a cooling draught, it is marvelous that any escape drunkenness. Blot out flesh eating and men will soon become temperate without the enactment of a single law. No one who eats the food that Nature prepared will have any desire for strong drink, not even tea or coffee. Then the sure cure for the drink habit is to stop eating meat and all animal products. This includes butter and eggs. Cereals, vegetables, nuts and oils have all the elements necessary to the body's sustenance.[5]

In addition to the physiological connection Fillmore describes between eating animal foods and craving strong drink, there are several other possible links that could be explored and discussed more broadly in our culture's battle against the horrendous effects of addiction to drugs and alcohol. There are the rather obvious psychological connections that were discussed earlier. Our herding culture is by its very nature abusive to its children, forcing them to disconnect from whom they're eating and to distance themselves from their natural feelings of empathy. This abuse, with its attendant hardening and disconnectedness, must certainly be a powerful contributing factor to substance abuse and to other pathologies as well. The drugs, hormones, artificial colors, preservatives, and toxic chemicals contained in animal foods may contribute to alcohol and drug addiction, as well as the fact that animal foods are filled with the vibrations of grief, misery, hopelessness, and despair—vibrations that would tend to push sensitive people who eat them into substance abuse and addiction. And, since we inevitably reap what we sow in others, we will unavoidably find ourselves reaping the consequences of our misguided "research" experiments on animals, which is more human addiction. Finally, there is also the macrobiotic perspective that animal foods are extremely yang in their energetic impact on the body, contracting the energy field, and that the body will then naturally and inevitably crave foods and substances that are extremely yin and expansive. These extreme yin foods are alcohol, white sugar, drugs of most every kind, tobacco, and caffeine. Grains, legumes, and vegetables tend to be neither excessively yin nor yang, but are more balanced, and so create few cravings. Eating extreme foods forces the body to gyrate continuously between the two poles, alternatively craving contracting foods like meat, cheese, eggs, and salt, and then expansive substances like sweets, coffee, alcohol, drugs, and tobacco, ad nauseam.

How can these connections be brought to attention in public forums? Perhaps, for example, the popular Twelve-Step programs could be made more effective by recognizing the insidious power of eating animal foods in driving the mental, emotional, and physical urge to consume alcohol and other harmful substances. The twelve steps of Alcoholics Anonymous, Narcotics Anonymous, Overeaters Anonymous, and similar programs are all grounded in the timeless principles of relying on support from others with similar aspirations by creating ongoing support groups and relying on "a Power greater than ourselves to restore us to sanity." Twelve-Step programs are effective because they take a basically spiritual approach, urging people to rise mentally and spiritually to a higher level of consciousness than the level at which they created the problem. They encourage introspection, humbly recognizing the harmful effects of past actions on other people and making amends to them, and improving conscious contact with the higher Power, and relying not on self-will but on the desire to fulfill the will of the higher Power.

Unfortunately, animals are not included in the moral inventory of those harmed by former actions, and eating and using animals isn't questioned. This helps explain perhaps why people in AA groups are taught they will always be alcoholics and can never take just a small drink, because in continuing to eat animals, the underlying pressures remain. The body and mind naturally still crave alcohol, drugs, sweets, extreme yin, and distraction from the horror that is being consumed every day at meals. By including animals within the circle of relevant beings that we harm with our actions, we can get to the root of the destructive addictions that plague people in our culture. This is not to imply that all patterns of addictive behavior will necessarily disappear with the adoption of a vegan orientation to living, but it is a powerful start; inner weeding, mindfulness, and cultivating inner silence, patience, generosity, and gratitude are also essential dimensions of spiritual health.

If we decrease our practice of exploiting animals for food, we will find our levels of disease, mental illness, conflict, and environmental and social devastation likewise decreasing. Rather than ravaging the earth's body and decimating and incarcerating her creatures, we can join with the earth and be a force for creating beauty and spreading love, compassion, joy, peace, and celebration. When we look with a relaxed eye at nature, we see an absolutely irrepressible celebration of living beauty. Animals in nature are both celebratory and inscrutable. They play, sing, run, soar, leap, call, dance, swim, hang out together, and relate in endlessly mysterious ways.

Freeing animals, we humans will be able to rejoin the celebration and contribute to it with our love and creativity. Competition and exploitation of other people can melt away as we regain our natural sensitivity. Our earth will naturally heal when we stop killing fish and sea life and polluting and wasting water in such unsustainable ways. Forests and wildlife will return because we'll need far less farmland to feed everyone a plant-based diet, and the whole earth will be relieved of the unbearable pressure exerted by omnivorous humans. We will be released from the paralysis that prevents us from creatively addressing the looming depletion of fossil fuels and the other challenges we face.

This change in our consciousness would usher in the first revolution since the herding revolution began with the domestication of sheep and goats ten thousand years ago. That revolution propelled us out of the garden into an existential sense of separateness, promoting competition and the cultivation of disconnected reductionism and materialistic technology. The evolutionary thrust is obviously now in a completely different direction, toward integration, cooperation, compassion, inclusiveness, and discovering our basic unity with all life. As we research, discuss, and deepen our understanding of the mind-body connection, of the human-animal connection, and of our connection with all the larger wholes in which we are embedded, our spiritual purpose will become manifest.

Privilege and Slavery

The message ritually injected into us by our culturally mandated meals is, at a fundamental level, the message of privilege. As humans, we see ourselves as superior to animals, whom we view as objects to be enslaved and killed for our use and pleasure, and with this herder mentality of our special and privileged position over animals, we inevitably create other categories of privilege. Wealth, gender, and race determine the extent of our privilege in a human hierarchy between rich white men on one end and impoverished non-white women and children on the other. Even poor humans have some privilege compared to animals, however, and it is this hierarchical, authoritarian social structure—pervasive, transparent, and taken for granted—that is the unavoidable outcome of commodifying animals and eating them.

The wealthy elite exerts its privilege and authority through all our social institutions, using food as a method of maintaining control. Because the quality of our food is directly connected to our mental and physiological health and to our quality of life, diminishing the quality of our food can make us sicker, weaker, and more distracted, violent, stressed, drugged, confused, and disempowered. This is perhaps the real agenda behind the vicious efforts to weaken the standards for organic foods and to introduce highly toxic foods through irradiation, genetic engineering, addition of artificial dyes, noxious flavor-enhancers like MSG, chemical preservatives, known carcinogens like aspartame, and dangerous genetically engineered hormones like rBGH and carcinogenic growth hormones. This is in addition to promoting animal-based meals, which concentrate the largest variety and intensity of toxins and are inherently confusing and disempowering. By controlling food and disseminating junk food and food sourced from animals, those with the most privilege can confuse and sicken our entire population, especially those who are most vulnerable and uninformed. There are well-documented connections, for example, between the deterioration of our food supply and certain newly invented pathologies like attention deficit disorder.[6]

We must explore these connections further and discuss them, and also take a hard look at our own abuse of privilege. As a culture, we regularly fail to make the connections between the suffering directly imposed on others and our privileged status. Those others may be fishes, chickens, pigs, or slaves on chocolate plantations. By refusing to dominate animals, we make the essential connections and open inner doorways to understanding and deconstructing the abuse of privilege in our lives. Justice, equality, veganism, freedom, spiritual evolution, and universal compassion are inextricably connected.

As long as we dominate others, we will be dominated. Even those at the top of pyramid, the rich white men who have the most privilege, are ironically enslaved. Planting seeds of fear and domination, they cannot reap inner peace, joy, love, and happiness. The misery, drug addiction, suicide, and insanity rampant among the wealthiest families illustrate the obvious and inescapable truth that we are all related, and spiritual health, our source of happiness, requires us to live this truth in our daily lives. As we bless others, we are blessed, and seeing beings rather than things, our own being is liberated and enriched.

The Last Days of Eating Animals

Is there adequate time for us as a human family to make the transition to compassionate vegan living? It's a matter of education and reaching critical mass. Every one of us has an essential part to play in this greatest of all tasks. The resistance from the dominant culture is understandably intense and manifests in a seemingly endless profusion of ways. Besides the ubiquity of the practice of eating enslaved animals, and all the media and cultural support that inevitably accrues to such a universal practice, and the justifications obediently fabricated by the religious and scientific institutions of our culture, there are predictable attempts to use governmental and legal means to protect the animal foods complex from any questioning. Many states have already passed "food disparagement" laws at the insistence of powerful meat, dairy, and egg interests, which actually disallow and criminalize public criticism of foods! The states with the strongest animal agriculture industries are also pushing to pass laws making it a felony to take pictures or videos inside farms, dairy operations, stockyards, fishing operations, and slaughterhouses without the permission of the industries and owners. There's obviously a lot to hide, and the fact that we live in a supposedly open society is a potent threat to the forces that would continue our omnivorism and block all discussion, questioning, and understanding of its consequences. There are also laws being passed making it illegal for people to talk about food publicly unless they are certified dieticians! An educator in Columbus, for example, was recently notified by the State Investigator of the Ohio Board of Dietetics that she couldn't show the video *Diet for a New America* publicly because "that could be construed as the practice of Dietetics because somebody might change their lifestyle habits as a result of seeing that movie."[7]

In addition to these strong-arm tactics, there are more subtle methods emerging. The National Eating Disorders Association has now listed a new type of eating disorder, which it calls "orthorexia nervosa":

Orthorexia Nervosa. Though not clinically recognized as an eating disorder, some health professionals are coming to believe that a pathological fixation on eating proper food, and obsession with "righteous eating" may eventually be considered a condition requiring treatment.[8]

Obviously, anyone unquestioningly eating the cruel and toxic Standard American Diet of fast-food burgers and hot dogs will be considered by mental health professionals to be psychologically healthy and normal, while those who refuse to do so may be considered to have a "pathological fixation on eating proper food" and an "obsession with 'righteous eating' " and may be obliged to undergo some kind of "treatment." It's hard to overestimate how subversive switching to a plant-based way of eating is to the established mentality of domination and exclusion, and to what lengths our culture will go to block and suppress open discussion and questioning of its defining rituals!

While it's easy to become discouraged in the face of the immense cultural inertia that propels the continued practice of eating animal foods, it's helpful to realize that it carries within it the seeds of its own destruction. At the rate it's ravaging our planet's ecosystems and resources—and our sanity and intelligence—it cannot last much longer. These may very well turn out to be humanity's last days of eating animals.

The Movie of Life on Earth

To awaken from the cultural trance of omnivorism we need only remember who we are. We have neither the psychology nor the physiology for predation and killing, but due to the culturally indoctrinated mentality required by our daily meals, we eat like predators. We become desensitized, exclusivist and materialistic, forgetting that we are essentially consciousness manifesting in time and space. As consciousness, we are eternal, free, and benevolent. We are interconnected with all other manifestations of consciousness, and at a deep level we are all united because we share the same source. This source is the infinite intelligence and consciousness that permeates and manifests as phenomenal reality. *To free the animals we are abusing, we must free ourselves from the delusion of essential separateness,* doing both the outer work of educating, sharing, and helping others, and the inner work of uncovering our true nature.

Metaphorically, we are all part of the movie of life on earth, and while we may appear to be the images on the screen, at a deeper level we share a common heritage—we are all also the light that makes the movie possible. This light is consciousness, and it is our fundamental nature, emanating from an infinite and inconceivable source. Glimpsing this essential nature that we share with all beings not only deepens our yearning to relieve their suffering but also strengthens our ability to work effectively to do so. Seeing victims and perpetrators not merely in these roles but in their spiritual perfection and completeness is profoundly healing. We see that there are no enemies—no essentially evil people or completely hopeless or destructive situations. There are, rather, opportunities to grow, learn, serve, and work together to raise consciousness and bring compassion and understanding to the painful and unjust situations we may see unfolding around us. Recognizing that we are all profoundly related, the greatest blessing we can give others, both animal and human, is to see their beauty, innocence, and upright-ness, and address that in them.

The world we see is a product of our thoughts and way of seeing. Looking deeply into the animal-derived food on our plates, we see enor-mous suffering, abusive hands, and hardened hearts. Looking more deeply, we see that these hands and hearts have themselves been abused and wounded but yearn to be comforted and loved, and to comfort and love. As we see that abusers have always been abused themselves, we seek less to judge and more to understand, and to protect the vulnera-ble from abuse. As we heal our wounds and stop eating animal foods we become better able to contribute to the healing of our culture. We see that we need less to be the hands of judgment and punishment—for pain willfully inflicted is unavoidably received again in the fullness of time—but rather to be the hands of mercy, help, and healing.

As we realize our interconnectedness with all living beings, our pur-pose naturally becomes to help and bless others, and it is a role we can carry without burnout or anger. The terrible suffering we see may cer-tainly disturb and outrage us, but the outrage turns to compassion and creativity rather than to anger, despair, or vindictiveness. Rising above anger and despair while still keeping our hearts open to the ocean of cruelty, indifference, and suffering on this earth is not easy. It requires cultivating wisdom and compassion—both the inner silent receptivity that links us to the eternal truth of our being and the outer actions of serving and helping others that give meaning to our life. By creating an inner field of peace, kindness, joy, and unity, we contribute to building a planetary field of compassion that reflects this consciousness.[9]

As we hold steadfastly to the truth of being, knowing that compas-sion is irresistible and that it encircles the earth through us and many others, and as we live this understanding in our daily lives and share it with others, we create a field of kindness and sow seeds of cultural transformation. There are no enemies because we are all related. The spiritual connection between animals and humans grows out of understanding that we are all expressions of eternal benevolent consciousness, and as we acknowledge this interconnection and live in harmony with it, our lives become prayers of compassion and healing. A positive approach is essential because it mobilizes our spiritual resources, generates enthusiasm, and brings more joy and love into our world.

Just as waves are manifestations of the ocean and inseparable from it, we are both the light that makes the movie possible and the images on the screen illuminated by that light, each of us unique and contributing our voice, passion, and spirit to the unfolding story. With this understanding, we can live to help and bless others with both a sense of urgency, which is required and appropriate, and a sense of spaciousness that doesn't blame others or fight with them. Blaming and fighting only generate resistance and reinforce the delusion of separateness. Our human spiritual evolution is a calling to liberate ourselves and the animals we hold in bondage. It's founded upon recognizing the unity of cause and effect: whatever seeds we sow in our consciousness we will reap in our lives. The ancient teaching holds true: "Hatred ceases not by hatred, but by love. This is the everlasting law."[10] In the end, as Mahatma Gandhi emphasized, we must be the change we want to see in the world.

The Elk's Message

One August night in 1991, high in the Olympic mountains of western Washington, I was climbing up a seemingly endless and steep series of switchbacks, trying to get back to my van parked at the trailhead. I had gone too far to reach an alpine lake, and now returning many miles in steep terrain, without food or water, I was as physically exhausted as I'd ever been in my life. Every step took enormous effort, and in the dim moonlight I prayed for the strength and energy to continue the arduous climb back up to the top of the ridge. Feeling almost completely spent, I thought I might have to bivouac on the cold barren slope when I felt a presence beside me. Plodding along in the eerie light, dragging each foot with all my strength, I looked to my right and saw, only four or five yards away, a magnificent elk walking slowly along beside me. In the somewhat surreal mental state I was already in from being exhausted and alone on the mountain in the moonlight, it somehow wasn't surprising. We continued along together for several minutes, and just having this powerful animal walking so close to me gave me an enormous boost. Mentally thanking him as we walked for caring and for helping me, I felt a profound sense of kinship, beyond the usual concept of that term. I felt our utter relatedness as a basic fact. With him beside me, it was natural to feel my energy increasing, and soon I was able to walk faster and with more confidence. Before long, the elk picked up his pace and crossed over in front of me, disappearing into the night. Within another ten minutes, I made it to the top of the ridge and could descend to the parking lot.

Though I was enormously thirsty and hungry, and my little van was well stocked with food and water, I waited and silently thanked the elk and the benevolent mystery of this universe. My heart was filled with gratitude for the overwhelming presence of love and compassion I felt shining on me through the elk. I saw I didn't need to thank the elk, my brother, with thoughts or words, for he understood our connection. Any thanks I could give him could only be through my actions to protect him and all my brothers and sisters of this earth, sacred expressions of an infinite love that smiled at me that evening from the elk, the stars, the moon, and the night mountain air.

The elk taught me to take time every day to be grateful, to feel my connection with the great Mystery, and to open to the inner wellsprings of joy and peace. The most powerful antidotes to cruelty, abuse, and indifference are not anger and sadness, but love, peace, joy, and open-hearted creative enthusiasm for this precious gift of a human life. Just as Thich Nhat Hanh has wisely said that without inner peace, we cannot contribute to the peace movement, so it is also that without inner freedom, we cannot contribute to the liberation of animals, which is the essential prerequisite to meaningful human freedom.

The experience with the elk is one of many blessings I have found that being vegan brings. Veganism kindles a deep sense of peace in nature and of kinship, fellowship, and harmony with all life. It encourages a sense of inner richness that keeps growing and deepening as years go by, a sense of gentleness and of purpose. Becoming vegan is not so much a decision made with our intellect as it is a natural consequence of inner ripening. While it's certainly helpful to comprehend intellectually the vast mandala of negative consequences of eating animal foods, we find that we are propelled into veganism by our intuition. As our intuitive heart opens, it opens to understanding our connection with others and to including them within the sphere of our concern.

In our culture, which is so permeated by the mentality of domination and exclusion, veganism requires a spiritual breakthrough. This breakthrough cannot be forced in any way by others, but it can definitely be encouraged. Looking behind the curtain to the horrific suffering inherent in animal foods, asking questions, contemplating spiritual teachings, cultivating the higher knowing of intuition, and observing the example of other vegans all contribute to the ripening process. Once we can clearly see the universal law or principle underlying veganism, we can experience a spiritual transformation that allows greater possibilities of freedom and happiness. Once we see and understand, we become a voice for the voiceless, a note in the glorious chord of healing and awakening that is unfolding in our shared consciousness.

From Obsolete Exclusivity to All of Us

Our inherited meal traditions require a mentality of violence and denial that silently radiates into every aspect of our private and public lives, permeating our institutions and generating the crises, dilemmas, inequities, and suffering that we seek in vain to understand and effectively address. A new way of eating no longer based on privilege, commodification, and exploitation is not only possible but essential and inevitable. Our innate intelligence demands it.

Vegan congressman Dennis Kucinich said in a speech in 2002,

> I have seen groups of people overcome incredible odds as they became aware they are participating in a cause beyond self and sense the movement of the inexorable which comes from unity.
>
> Violence is not inevitable. War is not inevitable. Nonviolence and peace are inevitable. We can make of this world a gift of peace which

will confirm the presence of universal spirit in our lives. We can send into the future the gift which will protect our children from fear, from harm, from destruction.[11]

As our hearts open to deeper understanding, our circle of compassion naturally enlarges and spontaneously begins to include more and more "others"—not just our own tribe, sect, nation, or race, but all human beings, and not just humans, but other mammals, and birds, fish, forests, and the whole beautifully interwoven tapestry of living, pulsing creation. All beings. All of Us.

When we are then drawn toward a plant-based way of eating, it is in no way a limitation on us; rather it is the harmonious fulfillment of our inner seeing. At first we think it's an option we can choose, but with time we realize that it's not a choice at all but the free expression of the truth that we are. It is not an ethic that we have to police from outside, but our own radiant love spontaneously expressing, both for ourselves and for our world. Caring is born on this earth and lives through us, as us, and it's not anything for which we can personally take credit. It is nothing to be proud of. Refraining from eating and using animals is the natural result of seeing that is no longer chained within the dark and rigid dungeon of narrow self-interest. From the outside, it may look like and be called "veganism," but it is simply awareness and the expression of our sense of interconnectedness. It manifests naturally as inclusiveness and caring. It's no big deal because it's the normal functioning of our original nature, which unfailingly sees beings rather than things when it looks at our neighbors on this earth.

We owe the animals our profoundest apologies. Defenseless and unable to retaliate, they have suffered immense agonies under our domination that most of us have never witnessed or acknowledged. Now knowing better, we can act better, and acting better, we can live better, and give the animals, our children, and ourselves a true reason for hope and celebration.

NOTES

Chapter 1—Food's Power

1. To name just a few: Weber, Durkheim, Veblen, Mumford, Riesman, Fromm, Wirth, Marcuse, and Bellah in sociology and social theory, James, Freud, Adler, Reich, Jung, Maslow, Skinner, Sheldon, Rogers, and Allport in psychology, Heidegger, Husserl, Sartre, Whitehead, Camus, Buber, Wittgenstein, Popper, Kuhn, Polanyi, Gebser, and Jaspers in philosophy, Bateson, Churchman, Varela, Mitroff, Fuller, and Prigogine in systems theory, and countless others.

2. Some of these contemporary radical voices include Noam Chomsky, Mary Daly, Helen Caldicott, Daniel Berrigan, David Icke, Michael Parenti, Howard Zinn, E.F. Schumacher, Theodore Roszak, Jim Hightower, and Adrienne Rich. Just a few of those who are writing today about holistic health, spirituality, and peace are Matthew Fox, John Shelby Spong, Ken Wilber, Jean Houston, Gary Zukav, Andrew Harvey, Eckhart Tolle, Deepak Chopra, Pema Chödrön, Andrew Cohen, Ram Dass, Joan Borysenko, Wayne Dyer, Stanislav Grof, George Leonard, Neale Donald Walsh, Larry Dossey, Caroline Myss, Dan Millman, David Hawkins, Marianne Williamson, Robert Johnson, Sam Keen, James Twyman, and Peter Russell.

Chapter 2—Our Culture's Roots

1. Jim Mason, *An Unnatural Order: Why We Are Destroying the Planet and Each Other* (New York: Continuum, 1993), p. 143.
2. Ibid., p. 138.
3. Ibid., pp. 142–143.
4. *Merriam-Webster's Collegiate Dictionary*, Tenth Edition (Springfield, MA: Merriam-Webster, 1996), p. 308.
5. Cynthia Eller, *The Myth of Matriarchal Prehistory: Why an Invented Past Won't Give Women a Future* (Boston: Beacon Press, 2000), p. 41.
6. Riane Eisler, *The Chalice and the Blade: Our History, Our Future* (New York: HarperCollins, 1987), p. 44.
7. Riane Eisler, *Sacred Pleasure: Sex, Myth, and the Politics of the Body* (New York: HarperCollins, 1995), p. 92.
8. Ibid., pp. 95–96.
9. Ibid., p. 96.
10. Mason, p. 140.
11. Ibid.
12. Ibid., p. 146.
13. Cappeller dictionary: f. gavyaa. desire for cows, ardour of battle; see also Monier Williams: goSu + gam=>, to set out for a battle [to conquer cows] RV. ii, 25, 4; v, 45, 9; viii, 71, 5; from author's correspondence with Claude Setzer, Ph.D.

14. Mason, p. 137.
15. Leonardo da Vinci, *Notes*, cited in Andrea Wiebers and David Wiebers, *Souls Like Ourselves* (Rochester, MN: Sojourn Press, 2000), p. 62.
16. Joanne Stepaniak, *Being Vegan* (Los Angeles: Lowell House, 2000), p. 3.

Chapter 3—The Nature of Intelligence

1. See, for example, John Bradshaw, *Bradshaw on: The Family* (Deerfield Beach, FL: Health Communications, 1988, 1996).
2. Charles Fillmore, "Vegetarianism," *Unity Magazine*, June 1915.
3. Charles Fillmore, "The Vegetarian," *Unity Magazine*, May 1920.
4. Charles Fillmore, "The Unity Vegetarian Inn" (Unity Village, MO).
5. Keith Akers, *The Lost Religion of Jesus* (New York: Lantern Books, 2000), p. 157.
6. Gregory Bateson, *Mind and Nature* (New York: Bantam, 1979), p. 12.
7. For a discussion of some of the unexplained dimensions of intelligence in animals, see Rupert Sheldrake, *Dogs That Know When Their Owners Are Coming Home and Other Unexplained Powers of Animals* (New York: Three Rivers Press, 1999) and also his *Seven Experiments That Would Change the World* (New York: Inner Traditions, 2002), as well as Jean Houston, *Mystical Dogs: Animals as Guides to Our Inner Life* (Makawao, HI: Inner Ocean Publishing, 2002). These are only a small sampling of the books addressing this theme.
8. Dan Kindlon and Michael Thompson, *Raising Cain: Protecting the Emotional Life of Boys* (New York: Ballantine, 1999), p. 174.
9. *Rainforest Alliance Newsletter*, September 2001, p. 1.
10. Greg Critser, *Fat Land* (New York: Houghton Mifflin, 2003), p. 171.
11. Ronald Goodman, *Circumcision: The Hidden Trauma* (Boston: Vanguard Publications, 1997).
12. Paul M. Fleiss, "Protect Your Uncircumcised Son: Expert Medical Advice for Parents," *Mothering*, November–December 2000, p. 44.
13. John Robbins, *The Food Revolution: How Your Diet Can Save Your Life and the World* (Berkeley: Conari Press, 2001), p. 48.
14. John Robbins, *Diet for a New America* (Walpole, NH: StillPoint, 1987), p. 330.
15. The United States, for example, has one of the highest per capita rates of animal food consumption in the world and also has the highest incarceration rate. With only four percent of the world's population, the U.S. has twenty-five percent of the world's prisoners; the country with the most animal prisoners also has the most human prisoners.
16. Amnesty International, *Torture Worldwide: An Affront to Human Dignity* (New York: Amnesty International, 2000), p. 2. See also www.amnestyusa.org.
17. Ibid., pp. 112–113.
18. Jim Mason, "Inside a Turkey Breeding Factory: Of Rape and Pillage," *Farm Sanctuary News*, Fall 1997, pp. 5–7.
19. U.S. Bureau of Justice Statistics, *Criminal Victimization, 2003* (Washington DC: September 2004). See R.A.I.N.N. (Rape, Abuse, & Incest National Network), www.rainn.org/statistics.html. In 2003 there were 198,500 victims of rape or sexual assault (one every roughly two minutes), and 87,000 victims of completed rapes (one every six minutes).
20. Michael Greger, "SARS: Another Deadly Virus from the Meat Industry," *VegNews* May–June, 2003, p. 10.

Chapter 4—Inheriting Our Food Choices

1. Joseph Mercola and Rachael Droege, "Why Junk Food Is so Tempting, and How to Beat Your Temptation," Mercola-com e-newsletter, Issue 516, March 17, 2004.

2. Neal Barnard, *Turn Off the Fat Genes* (New York: Three Rivers Press, 2001), p. 108.
3. Neal Barnard, "Breaking the Food Seduction," in *Good Medicine from the Physicians Committee for Responsible Medicine,* Summer 2003, pp. 10–12.
4. According to Russell Blaylock, M.D., for example, fast-food restaurant chains add large amounts of monosodium glutamate (MSG), a toxic and addictive artificial flavor enhancer, to their meats. See Russell Blaylock, *Excitotoxins: The Taste that Kills* (Santa Fe, NM: Health Press).
5. See, for example, Carol Simontacchi, *The CrazyMakers: How the Food Industry is Destroying our Brains and Harming Our Children* (New York: Putnam, 2000), p. 99: "MSG or other flavor enhancers give food a greater-than-nature, "better-than-good" taste, blunting the taste for the natural flavors found in real food. By contrast, real food tastes bland, setting children up to permanently dislike natural food."

Chapter 5—The Intelligence of Human Physiology
1. John McDougall, "Vegan Diet Damages Baby's Brain—Sensationalism!" *VegNews* March–April 2003, p. 10.
2. E. A. Hooton, *Man's Poor Relations* (Garden City, NY: Doubleday, 1940), p. 412.
3. Carnivorous animals have over three times as much phosphate of magnesia in their teeth to harden them as we have: "Human teeth usually contain 1.5 percent phosphate of magnesia, whereas the teeth of carnivores are composed of nearly 5 percent phosphate of magnesia." Vasu Murti, *They Shall Not Hurt or Destroy: Animal Rights and Vegetarianism in the Western Religious Traditions* (Cleveland: Vegetarian Advocates Press, 2003), p. 122.
4. Carnivorous animals have digestive systems three times their body length while primates, classified as frugivores, have a digestive system twelve times their body length. Herbivores such as ungulates and ruminants have digestive systems roughly thirty times their body length. See Ibid., pp. 121–122.
5. Robert O. Young and Shelley R. Young, *The pH Miracle* (New York: Warner, 2002).
6. John McDougall, "Need Potassium? Take Vegetables, Not Pills," *McDougall Newsletter*, April 2004.
7. Riane Eisler, *Sacred Pleasure: Sex, Myth, and the Politics of the Body* (New York: HarperCollins, 1995), p. 38.
8. National Academy of Sciences Institute of Medicine Dietary Reference Intakes for Energy, Carbohydrate, Fiber, Fat, Fatty Acids, Cholesterol, Protein, and Amino Acids (Macronutrients) (2002), cited in Michael Greger, *Carbophobia* (New York: Lantern, 2005, p. 83). Dr. Greger continues, "In their report condemning trans fats they couldn't even assign a Tolerable Upper Daily Limit of intake because 'any incremental increase in trans fatty acid intake increases coronary heart disease risk.' "
9. In *Turn off the Fat Genes* (New York: Harmony, 2001, p. 132), Neil Barnard writes, "The old notion that you need to carefully combine or 'complement' various plant foods to get adequate protein has been set aside. Both the U.S. government and the American Dietetic Association hold that, so long as your diet includes a normal variety of plant foods, you will easily get enough protein, even without any special combining."
10. V. Messina and K. Burke, "Position of the American Dietetic Association: Vegetarian Diets," *Journal of the American Dietetic Association*, 97, 1997, pp. 1317–1321.
11. Colin Campbell, interview, 1994, cited in Andrea Wiebers and David Wiebers, *Souls Like Ourselves* (Rochester, MN: Sojourn Press, 2000), p. 51.
12. John Robbins, *Diet For A New America*, pp. 172–173.
13. Ibid., p. 177.

14. Andrew Weil, *Spontaneous Healing* (New York: Random House, 1995), pp. 145–147.
15. Andrew Weil, *Eight Weeks to Optimum Health* (New York: Random House, 1997), p. 70.
16. Young and Young, *The pH Miracle*, p. 23.
17. Cited in Greg Lawson, "The Broccoli Link," *Animal Rights Online* newsletter, June 5, 2003; see also http://biology.berkeley.edu/crl/index.shtml.
18. R. Mazess, "Bone Mineral Content of North Alaskan Eskimos," *Journal of Clinical Nutrition*, 27:916, 1974.
19. John McDougall, *McDougall's Medicine* (Piscataway, NJ: New Century Publishers, 1985), p. 67.
20. For a good overview of the research connecting animal food intake with disease, and list of primary sources, see John Robbins, *The Food Revolution*, Part 1, pp. 11–150.
21. "A Diet Rich in Profit," *Adbusters Journal*, November–December 2002.
22. For more details, see Felicia Drury Kliment, *The Acid Alkaline Balance Diet* (New York: Contemporary Books, 2002).
23. J. T. Dwyer, L. G. Miller, N. L. Arduino, et al. "Mental Age and I.Q. of Predominately Vegetarian Children." *Journal of the American Dietetic Association*, 76, 1980, pp. 142–147. In this study, pediatric developmental tests indicated that brain development in vegetarian children is normal. In fact, the mental age of the children advanced over a year beyond chronological age, and mean IQ was well above average (with an average of 116 points).
24. Plutarch, "On Eating Flesh," *Moralia*, William Watson Goodwin, ed. (London: S. Low, Son, and Marston, 1870), Vol. 5, Tract 1.
25. Greg Critser, *Fat Land* (New York: Houghton Mifflin, 2003), p. 170.
26. "A Diet Rich in Profit," *Adbusters Journal*, November–December 2002.
27. Neal Barnard, *Turn off the Fat Genes*, p. 134.
28. U.S. Department of Agriculture, "A Comparison of Low-Carbohydrate vs. High-Carbohydrate Diets," cited in Eve Hightower, "Pasta Preferred," *E Magazine*, January–February 2003, p. 42.
29. Andrew Weil, *Spontaneous Healing* (New York: Random House, 1995), pp. 145–147.
30. Sheldon Rampton and John Stauber, *Mad Cow U.S.A: Could the Nightmare Happen Here?* (Monroe, ME: Common Courage Press, 1997), pp. 39–51, 210–218.
31. Nicholas Fox, *Spoiled: The Dangerous Truth About a Food Chain Gone Haywire* (New York: Basic Books, 1997), pp. 178–179.
32. *45 Days: The Life and Death of a Broiler Chicken*, Compassion Over Killing, Washington, DC, DVD, 2004.
33. "Factsheet—January 2000," National Cattlemen's Beef Association.
34. Gail Eisnitz, *Slaughterhouse: The Shocking Story of Greed, Neglect, and Inhumane Treatment Inside the U.S. Meat Industry* (Amherst, NY: Prometheus Books, 1997), p. 219.
35. Ibid., p. 175.
36. Ibid., p. 177.
37. Julie Vorman, "US Groups Seek Food Safety Warning Label on Meat," Reuters News Service, January 13, 2000.
38. "Microbiologists Battle E. Coli," *Meat Industry Insights*, October 26, 1999.
39. Eisnitz, pp. 174–175.
40. Ibid., p. 173.
41. Ibid., p. 183.
42. Ibid., p. 167.
43. Ibid., p. 168.
44. Ibid., p. 287.

45. John McDougall, "Diet and Diabetes: The Meat of the Matter," *EarthSave Magazine*, November 2002, p. 4.
46. Ibid., p. 22.
47. Dean Ornish, *Eat More, Weigh Less*, (New York: HarperCollins, 1993).
48. For an informative and eye-opening discussion of the placebo effect in a variety of medical and healing modalities, see Andrew Weil, *Health and Healing*, pp. 199–274. See also Lolette Kuby, *Faith and the Placebo Effect* (Novato, CA: Origin Press, 2001).
49. Jeffrey Hildner, "Destination: Healing," *The Christian Science Journal*, November 2003, pp. 6–7.
50. "Subway: The New King of Fast Food," Organic Consumers Association, July 2004. See www.organicconsumers.org/corp/subway071504.cfm.
51. Weil, *Eight Weeks to Optimum Health*, p. 104.
52. Brenda Davis and Vesanto Melina, *Becoming Vegan* (Summertown, TN: Book Publishing Company, 2000).
53. World Health Organization Technical Report Series 916. *Diet, Nutrition and the Prevention of Chronic Diseases* (Geneva, 2003).
54. *European Journal of Clinical Nutrition*, 57, August 2003, p. 947. Also, USDA, *Food and Nutrient Intakes by Individuals in the United States, by Region, 1994–1996.* Cited in Michael Greger, "Latest in Human Nutrition," *Dr. Michael Greger's Monthly Newsletter*, September 2003. (www.drgreger.org/september2003.html).
55. Howard Lyman points out in *Mad Cowboy* (New York: Scribner, 1998, p. 126), that not only does it take enormous amounts of pesticide-laden grain to make the animal foods we consume, but also that " . . . governmental limitations, lax though they are, on the use of pesticides for human consumption do not apply to crops destined for livestock. The lion's share of the agrochemical poisons sprayed into the air and falling onto the ground are dedicated to the production of meat."
56. Howard Lyman, author of *Mad Cowboy*, occasionally offers this metaphor in his public addresses.

Chapter 6—Hunting and Herding Sea Life
1. Farley Mowat, *Sea of Slaughter* (New York: Atlantic Monthly Press, 1984), p. 404.
2. Minority Staff of the U.S. Senate Committee on Agriculture, Nutrition, and Forestry, "Animal Waste Pollution in America: An Emerging National Problem," December 1997.
3. Michael Satchel, "The Cell from Hell," *U.S. News and World Report*, July 28, 1997, pp. 26–28.
4. Tim Beardsley, "Death in the Deep: 'Dead Zone' in the Gulf of Mexico Challenges Regulators," *Scientific American*, November 1997, pp. 17–18.
5. Lewis Regenstein, *How to Survive in America the Poisoned* (New York: Acropolis, 1982), p. 103.
6. K. Noren, "Levels of organochloride contaminants in human milk in relation to the dietary habits of the mothers," *Acta Paediatrica Scandinavica*, 72(6), November 1983, pp. 811–816.
7. Michael Klaper, *Vegan Nutrition: Pure and Simple* (Paia, HI: Gentle World, 1998), pp. 26–27. This passage from the book is slightly modified and updated by Dr. Klaper through his correspondence with the author of February 2004.
8. Brenda Davis and Vesanto Melina, *Becoming Vegan* (Summertown, TN: Book Publishing Company, 2000), pp. 60–76.
9. Office of Pollution Prevention and Toxics, EPA, "Management of Polychlorinated Biphenyls in the United States" (Washington, DC: Government Printing Office, 1997).

10. See www.fao.org/docrep/005/y7300e/y7300e00.htm for an overview of world fisheries.
11. christie Aschwanden, "Is Salmon Good for You?" *Alternative Medicine*, June 2005, p. 71. See also www.fishinghurts.com.
12. Canthaxanthan, the pink salmon pigment marketed by pharmaceutical giant Hoffman-LaRoche, has been linked to retinal damage, though its use is still allowed in the commercial aquaculture industry. It is also fed to hens in the egg industry to make their egg yolks more yellow. See "Fish Farms Become Feedlots of the Sea," *Los Angeles Times*, December 9, 2002.
13. "Fishy Business" *New Internationalist*, July 2000, p. 11.
14. Ann P. McGinn, "Blue Revolution—The Promises and Pitfalls of Fish Farming," *WorldWatch*, March/April 1988, p. 10.
15. Cornelia Dean, "Fish Farms Tied in Study to Imperiling Wild Salmon," *New York Times*, March 30, 2005; see also "The Fish Business," Animal Aid (U.K.) at www.animalaid.org.uk.
16. Mowat, p. 167.
17. S. Holt, "The Food Resources of the Ocean," *Scientific American*, 22, 1969, pp. 178–94.
18. See www.fishinghurts.com/HealthConcerns.asp.
19. "America's Fish: Fair or Foul?" *Consumer Reports*, February 2001.
20. See www.fishinghurts.com/EnvironmentalConcerns.asp.
21. See www.environmentaldefense.org/seafood/oceansinperil.cfm.
22. Paul Watson, "Consider the Fishes," *VegNews*, March–April 2003, p. 27.
23. Ibid.
24. Paul Watson, *Sea Shepherd Log* #58, 2002, p. 20.
25. Ibid.
26. Ibid., p. 10.
27. Ibid.
28. Rod Fujita, *Heal the Ocean: Solutions for Saving Our Seas* (Gabriola Island, BC: New Society Publishers, 2003), p. 125.
29. Barry Kent MacKay, "Catch and Release," *Animal Issues*, Spring 2003, p. 20.
30. Richard H. Schwartz, "Troubled Waters: The Case Against Eating Fish," *Vegetarian Voice*, Spring 2004, p. 7.
31. Ibid., pp. 22–23.
32. Joan Dunayer, *Animal Equality* (Derwood, MD: Ryce Publishing, 2001), p. 69.
33. Barry Kent MacKay, p. 20.
34. BBC News, "Scientists Highlight Fish 'Intelligence,' " reprinted in Animal Rights Online, September 7, 2003. See http://news.bbc.co.uk/1/hi/england/west_yorkshire/3189941.stm.
35. Ibid.
36. Cited in Dawn Carr, "They Die Slowly . . ." *PETA's Animal Times*, Summer 2003, p. 9.
37. Paul Watson and Joseph Connelly, "The VN Interview: Captain Paul Watson," *VegNews*, March–April 2003, p. 25.

Chapter 7—The Domination of the Feminine

1. Karen Davis, *Prisoned Chickens, Poisoned Eggs: An Inside Look at the Modern Poultry Industry* (Summertown, TN: Book Publishing, 1996), p. 50.
2. Mary Baker Eddy, *Science and Health with Key to the Scriptures* (Boston: The First Church of Christ, Scientist, 1903), p. 449.
3. Thomas Lynn Rodgers, forty-year dairy farmer, in a recorded and transcribed interview in August 1997 in Salt Lake City.

4. Jim Mason and Peter Singer, *Animal Factories* (New York: Harmony Books, 1990), p. 92.
5. See www.organicconsumers.org/monlink.html.
6. Rodgers interview.
7. Mason and Singer, *Animal Factories*, p. 129.
8. Rodgers interview.
9. Ibid.
10. Frank Oski, *Don't Drink Your Milk: Frightening Medical Facts About the World's Most Overrated Nutrient* (Brushtown, NY: Teach Services, 1983), pp. 15–45.
11. *Practical Techniques for Dairy Farmers*, 3rd Edition, University of Minnesota, 2000. See http://www.ansci.umn.edu/practical-techniques/book.htm.
12. Ibid.
13. Shirley Roenfeldt, "Stop BLV," *Dairy Herd Management*, December 1998.
14. *Journal of Infectious Diseases* 161 (1990): 467–472. Cited in Michael Greger, "Latest Meat and Dairy Infection Risks: Have Millions of Americans Been Infected with a Cow Cancer Virus?" *Dr. Michael Greger's Monthly Newsletter*, January 2004.
15. Mason and Singer, *Animal Factories*, p. 14.
16. Jeramia Trotter, "Hogwashed," *Waterkeeper Magazine*, Summer 2004, p. 23. Trotter adds in the article, "That's twenty-five million pounds of antibiotics for uses other than fighting illness, compared to the roughly three million pounds humans consume."
17. J. M. Tanner, "Trend Towards Earlier Menarche in London, Oslo, Copenhagen, the Netherlands, and Hungary," *Nature*, 243 (1973), pp. 75–76. Cited in Kerrie Saunders, *The Vegan Diet as Chronic Disease Prevention* (New York: Lantern Books, 2003), p. 137. Saunders writes, "The World Health Organization has been gathering statistics on the age of puberty worldwide for many years. In 1840, the average age of puberty in female humans was 17 years of age. Today, it is 12.5 years. The age of puberty is also dropping in England, Norway, Denmark, and Finland— other countries that eat the 'western' diet."
18. Kagawa, Y., "Impact of Westernization on the Nutrition of Japanese: Changes in Physique, Cancer, Longevity, and Centenarians," *Preventive Medicine*, 7 (1978), pp. 205–217. Cited in Saunders, *The Vegan Diet as Chronic Disease Prevention*, p. 137.
19. Saunders, *The Vegan Diet as Chronic Disease Prevention*, p.137.
20. Vicki Griffin, Diane Griffin, and Virgil Hulse, *Moooove Over Milk*, foreword by Attwood and Campbell (Hot Springs, NC: Let's Eat!, 1997), p. vii.
21. See www.lifesave.org for more information on the low numbers of pathogens in grains, vegetables, fruits, legumes, and nuts.
22. Oski, *Don't Drink Your Milk*, p. 54. The U.S. Public Health Service allows 20,000 bacteria per milliliter of pasteurized milk, which is 4,800,000 bacteria per cup.
23. "Milk: Why is the Quality so Low?" *Consumer Reports*, January 1974, p. 70.
24. Oski, *Don't Drink Your Milk*, pp. 64–65.
25. Ibid., pp. 17–59.
26. T. Colin Campbell, "New York Times: Reality Check Needed," www.vegsource.com/articles/campbell_nyt_brody2.htm, November 28, 2000.
27. Cited in Griffin, Griffin, and Hulse, *Moooove Over Milk*, p. 102.
28. Davis, *Prisoned Chickens, Poisoned Eggs*, p. 54.
29. Ibid., pp. 56–64.
30. USDA NASS, Agricultural Statistics 2001.
31. Page Smith and Charles Daniel, *The Chicken Book: Being an Inquiry into the Rise and Fall, Use and Abuse, Triumph and Tragedy of Gallus Domesticus* (Boston:

Little, Brown, 1975), p. 180, cited in Davis, *Prisoned Chickens, Poisoned Eggs*, p. 39.

32. C. David Coats, *Old McDonald's Factory Farm: The Myth of the Traditional Farm and the Shocking Truth about Animal Suffering in Today's Agribusiness* (New York: Continuum, 1989), pp. 93–94, cited in Davis, *Prisoned Chickens, Poisoned Eggs*, pp. 39–40.

33. For more information on "free-range" practices, see www.upc-online.org/freerange.html.

Chapter 8—The Metaphysics of Food

1. Ken Wilber, *A Brief History of Everything* (Boston: Shambhala, 1966), p. 4.

2. D. Olwens, et al. "Circulating Testosterone Levels and Aggression in Adolescent Males: A Causal Analysis," *Psychosomatic Medicine*, 50, 1988, pp. 261–272.

3. Neal Barnard, *Eat Right, Live Longer* (New York: Crown Books, 1993).

4. Ibid.

5. Jianghong Liu, et al., "Early Nutrition and Antisocial Behavior," *American Journal of Psychiatry*, November 2004. See www.newstarget.com/006194.html, also www.usc.edu/uscnews/stories/10773.html.

6. The Heisenberg uncertainty principle is based on the realization in the 1920s that light manifests as a nonlocal continuous wave or as discrete particles depending on the choice and will of the observer. There is inherent uncertainty in observation of small particles because it is impossible to discern simultaneously and with high accuracy both the position and the momentum of a particle such as an electron or photon. The very act of observing and measuring inherently changes the nature of the particle wave. The observer effect is based on the realization by researchers (not just in the "hard" sciences such as physics, but also in anthropology and other social sciences) that the act of observation necessarily influences whatever is being observed. The apparent subject/object split is increasingly seen to be illusory. For more information on these ideas, see Fritjof Capra, *The Tao of Physics* and *The Turning Point*; Gary Zukav, *The Dancing Wu Li Masters*; Ishtak Bentov, *Stalking the Wild Pendulum*; Fred Alan Wolf, *Mind Into Matter*; Amit Goswami, *The Self-Aware Universe: How Consciousness Creates the Material World*; and others.

7. Cited in Gregg Braden, "Living in the Mind of God," *Horizons Magazine*, February 2003, p. 9.

8. Andrew Weil, *Health and Healing* (New York: Houghton Mifflin, 1998), pp. 199–254.

9. See J. Alan Boone, *Kinship With All Life* (New York: HarperCollins, 1954), as well as previously cited books by Rupert Sheldrake.

10. Thich Nhat Hanh, *Peace Is Every Step* (New York: Bantam, 1991), p. 24.

11. Thich Nhat Hanh, *Anger* (New York: Penguin Putnam, 2001), pp. 15–16.

12. Charles Fillmore, "As to Meat Eating," *Unity Magazine*, October 1903.

13. Charles Fillmore, "Flesh-Eating Metaphysically Considered," *Unity Magazine*, May 1910.

14. Wendy Melillo, "Doctor's Group Blasts Milk Ads," *Adweek*, May 7, 2001, p. 8.

15. "Reverence," *Albert Schweitzer Fellowship Quarterly*, Fall 1997, p. 27.

16. Shabkar, *Food of Bodhisattvas*, translated by the Padmakara Translation Group (Boston: Shambhala, 2004), p. 60.

17. Lobsang Lhalungpa, tr., *The Life of Milarepa* (New York: Penguin, 1977), p. 154.

18. Cited in Andrew Linzey, *Animal Theology* (Urbana and Chicago: University of Illinois Press, 1995), p. 56.

19. J. R. Hyland, *God's Covenant with Animals: A Biblical Basis for the Humane Treatment of All Creatures* (New York: Lantern, 2000), p. xii.

20. Misri, quoted in Ellen Kei Hua, ed., *Meditations of the Masters*, cited in Andrea Wiebers and David Wiebers, *Souls Like Ourselves* (Rochester, MN: Sojourn Press, 2000), p. 42.
21. Albert Einstein, letter dated 1950, quoted in H. Eves, *Mathematical Circles Adieu*, 1977.
22. Michael Dilbeck, et al., "Consciousness as Field: The Transcendental Meditation and TM-Siddhi Program and Changes in Social Indicators." *The Journal of Mind and Behavior*, Winter 1987.
23. See Larry Dossey, *Healing Words: The Power of Prayer and the Practice of Medicine* (New York: Harper, 1994); also *Reinventing Medicine* (New York: HarperCollins, 1999).

Chapter 9—Science and Religion
1. Vandana Shiva, interviewed in *A Cow at My Table*, produced by Jennifer Abbott, VHS, 1998.
2. For further information, see www.soaw.org.
3. Henryk Skolimowski, "Life, Entropy, and Education," *The American Theosophist*, October 1986, p. 306.
4. Carolyn Merchant, *The Death of Nature* (New York: Harper & Row, 1980).
5. See, for example, Rauni Kilde, M.D., "Microchip Implants, Mind Control & Cybernetics," *Spekula*, 3rd Quarter 1999. See http://www.mindcontrolforums.com-/implants-kilde.htm. Besides microchip implants, the U.S. government is developing Pulsed Energy Projectiles (PEPs) that "cause excruciating pain from up to two kilometers away." See David Hambling, "Maximum Pain Is Aim of New U.S. Weapon," *New Scientist*, March 5, 2005. These devices are tested extensively on animals.
6. David Streitfeld, "First Humans to Receive ID Chips," *Los Angeles Times*, May 9, 2002, p. A-1. See also Will Weissert, "Chip Implanted in Mexico Judicial Workers," Associated Press, July 14, 2004.
7. Ibid.
8. "Swine Producer Protein Sources LLP Implements Digital Angel's PigSMART System for Improved Herd Management and Data Collection," PR Newswire, June 8, 2004.
9. For example, Lynn McTaggart, *The Field: The Quest for the Secret Force of the Universe* (New York: HarperCollins, 2002), p. 227.
10. See, for example, McTaggart, *The Field*, for a recent documentation of the work being done by holistically oriented scientists.
11. Steven Rosen, *Diet for Transcendence* (Badger, CA: Torchlight, 1997), p. 23.
12. J. R. Hyland, *God's Covenant with Animals: A Biblical Basis for the Humane Treatment of All Creatures* (New York: Lantern Books, 2000).
13. Matthew Fox, *Original Blessing* (New York: Tarcher/Putnam, 1983/2000).
14. Joseph Campbell, *The Masks of God*, Volume 1 (New York: Penguin, 1978), p. 77.
15. Ibid., p. 129.

Chapter 10—The Dilemma of Work
1. Matthew Fox, *The Reinvention of Work* (New York: Harper, 1994), p. 128.
2. Ralph Waldo Emerson, "Fate," *The Conduct of Life*, 1860.
3. Laura Moretti, "Another Death in the Family," *The Animals' Voice: Of Animal Rights and Its Defenders*, www.animalsvoice.com/PAGES/home.html.
4. Gail Eisnitz, *Slaughterhouse: The Shocking Story of Greed, Neglect, and Inhumane Treatment Inside the U.S. Meat Industry* (Amherst, NY: Prometheus Books, 1997), p. 271.
5. John Byrnes, *Hog Farm Management*, September 1976.

6. People for the Ethical Treatment of Animals, *North Carolina Pig Farm Investigation*, narrated by James Cromwell, VHS, 2002.
7. Eisnitz, *Slaughterhouse*, p. 75.
8. *A Cow at My Table*, produced by Jennifer Abbott, VHS, 1998.
9. Joby Warrick, "Modern Meat: A Brutal Harvest. They Die Piece by Piece" *Washington Post*, April 11, 2001.
10. Lance Gompa, professor of industrial and labor relations at Cornell University, lead researcher in Human Rights Watch's report *Blood Sweat, and Fear: Workers' Rights in U.S. Meat and Poultry Plants*, January 2005. See also Steven Greenhouse, "Human Rights Watch Report Condemns U.S. Meat Packing Industry For Violating Basic Human And Worker Rights," *New York Times*, January 25, 2005. According to Gompa, "Dangerous conditions are cheaper for companies—and the government does next to nothing."
11. Eisnitz, *Slaughterhouse*, pp. 172, 174, 271, 274.
12. Ibid., p. 273.
13. Though neither the industry nor government keeps figures on the percentage of animals improperly stunned before being cut and bled and either skinned or scalded, and because they don't want anyone else to know about this, we have to rely mainly on the testimony of the workers themselves, as found, for example, in Eisnitz's *Slaughterhouse*. According to farmedanimal.net, a study in Germany found one third of chickens under-stunned, one third properly stunned, and one third overly stunned.
14. People for the Ethical Treatment of Animals, *Victims of Indulgence*, VHS.
15. Donald McNeil, "KFC Supplier Accused of Animal Cruelty," *New York Times*, July 20, 2004.
16. Eisnitz, *Slaughterhouse*, pp. 92–93.
17. Ibid., p. 87.
18. Fox, p. 95.

Chapter 11—Profiting From Destruction
1. The Fertilizer Institute, *U.S. Fertilizer Statistics*, http://www.tfi.org/Statistics/USfertuse2.asp.
2. Albert Gore, Introduction to Rachel Carson, *Silent Spring* (Boston: Houghton Mifflin, 1962, 1994), p. xix, cited in Howard Lyman, *Mad Cowboy* (New York: Scribner, 1998), p. 72.
3. Lee Hitchcox, *Long Life Now* (Berkeley: Celestial Hearts, 1996), p. 59.
4. Ron Eisenberg and Virgil Williams, "Cost of a Meat-based Diet—for Your Body and for the Planet," *The Argus: 4-Bay Area Living*, June 2, 2000.
5. Robin Hur and David Fields, "Are High-Fat Diets Killing Our Forests?" *Vegetarian Times*, February 1984; cited in John Robbins, *Diet for a New America*, pp. 360–361. Hur and Fields estimate 260 million acres, which is 406,000 square miles of deforested land, and a rate of one acre every 5 seconds. Conservatively reducing their estimate to one acre every 8.5 seconds, we arrive at the estimates in the text.
6. Ibid.
7. Mario Giampietro and David Pimentel, *Food, Land, Population and the U.S. Economy, Executive Summary*, Carrying Capacity Network, November 1994.
8. Eisenberg and Williams, "Cost of a Meat-based Diet."
9. Giampietro and Pimentel, *Food, Land, Population and the U.S. Economy.*
10. William Lagrone, "The Great Plains," in *Another Revolution in US Farming?*, Scherz, et al., USDA, ESCS, Agricultural Economic Report No. 441, December 1979, cited in John Robbins, *Diet for a New America* (Walpole, NH: StillPoint, 1987), p. 370.
11. John Robbins, *The Food Revolution*, p. 237.
12. Cited in Ibid., p. 237.
13. Ibid., p. 266.

14. For more on the relationship between increased food production and population growth, see Daniel Quinn, "Population: A Systems Approach." Center for Biotechnology Policy and Ethics, Texas A&M University, reprinted in Quinn, *The Story of B* (New York: Bantam, 1996).

15. Mario Giampietro and David Pimentel, "Land, Energy and Water: The Constraints Governing Ideal U.S. Population Size," *Focus*, Spring 1991.

16. Worldwatch Institute, *Vital Signs 1999* (Washington, DC: 1999), p. 114. "Today nearly 1,000 major agricultural pests—including some 550 insect and mite species, 230 plant diseases, and 220 weeds—are immune to pesticides, a development almost unheard of at mid-century."

17. Giampietro and Pimentel, *Food, Land, Population and the U.S. Economy.*

18. Ibid.

19. Richard Heinberg, *The Party's Over: Oil, War and the Fate of Industrial Societies* (Gabriola Island, BC: New Society Publishers, 2003).

20. Colin J. Campbell, *Peak Oil*, Presentation at the Technical University of Clausthal, Germany, December 2000. See page 7 of http://energycrisis.org/de/lecture.html.

21. Ibid, p. 2.

22. *Adbusters Journal*, November–December 2002.

23. "Animal Waste Pollution in America: An Emerging National Problem," report of the Minority Staff of the U.S. Senate Committee on Agriculture, Nutrition, and Forestry, December 1997, p. 1.

24. John Robbins, *Diet for a New America*, p. 373.

25. "Scientists Fear Antibiotics Fed to Animals Pollute Streams," *Iowa Farmer Today Online*, March 29, 2001.

26. Elliot Diringer, "In Central Valley, Defiant Dairies Foul the Water," *San Francisco Chronicle*, July 7, 1997, p. A1.

27. According to The Sierra Club's 2002 "Rap Sheet on Animal Factories," a report compiled after nearly three years of reviewing state and federal regulatory agencies' records, "Millions of gallons of liquefied feces and urine seeped into the environment from collapsed, leaking, or overflowing storage lagoons, and flowed into rivers, streams, lakes, wetlands, and groundwater."

28. "U.S. Sets New Farm-Animal Pollution Curbs," *New York Times*, December 16, 2002.

29. "Concentrating on Clean Water: The Challenge of Concentrated Animal Feeding Operations," *Iowa Policy Project*, April 2005. See also "Report Says Factory Farms Cost Taxpayers," WOI-TV / Associated Press, April 6, 2005.

30. "Smogburgers Would Be Out Under Air-Quality Plan," *San Jose Mercury News*, September 6, 1994, p. 3B.

31. C. Spedding, "The Effect of Dietary Changes on Agriculture," in B. Lewis and G. Assmann, eds., *The Social and Economic Contexts of Coronary Prevention* (London: Current Medical Literature, 1990), cited in John Robbins, *The Food Revolution: How Your Diet Can Save Your Life and the World* (Berkeley: Conari Press, 2001), p. 294.

32. "Diverse Diets, with Meat and Milk, Endanger World Food Supply," *Hearst News Service*, March 8, 1997.

33. Robbins, *Diet for a New America*, p. 277.

34. Vasu Murti, *They Shall Not Hurt or Destroy: Animal Rights and Vegetarianism in the Western Religious Traditions* (Cleveland: Vegetarian Advocates Press, 2003), p. 127.

35. Marion Nestle, *Food Politics* (Berkeley: University of California Press, 2002), p. 3.

36. For an historical analysis of how corporations gradually became the powerful "persons" they are legally and economically today, see David Korten, *When Corporations Rule the World* (West Hartford, CT: Kumarian Press, 1995).

37. "Top Ten Drugs of 2001," *Pharmacy Times*, April 2002; 68(4), pp. 10–15.
38. Mickey Z., "Pills a Go-Go," *VegNews*, March–April 2003, p. 12.

Chapter 12—Some Objections Answered
1. Peter Kropotkin, *Mutual Aid: A Factor in Evolution* (New York: Penguin, 1939).
2. Jim Mason, *An Unnatural Order: Why We Are Destroying the Planet and Each Other* (New York: Continuum, 1993), p. 72. See also Donna Hart and Robert W. Sussman, *Man the Hunted: Primates, Predators, and Human Evolution* (New York: Pereseus, 2005), p. 10.
3. Hart and Sussman, p. 244. According to these anthropologists, early humans such as *Australopithecus* (2.5–7 million years ago) "depended mainly on fruits, herbs, grasses, and seeds, and gritty foods such as roots, rhizomes, and tubers. A very small proportion of [their] diet was made up of animal protein; mainly social insects (ants and termites) and, occasionally, small vertebrates captured opportunistically."
4. Mason, p. 70. According to fossil analysis carried out by M. Teaford and P. Ungar, "The early hominids were not dentally preadapted to meat—they simply did not have the sharp, reciprocally concave shearing blades necessary to retain and cut such foods." ("Diet and the Evolution of the Earliest Hominids," *Proceedings of the National Academy of Science* 97 (25): 13, p. 511.)
5. Ibid., p. 81.
6. Hart and Sussman, p. 190.
7. Plutarch, "On Eating Flesh," *Moralia*, William Watson Goodwin, ed. (London: S. Low, Son, and Marston, 1870), Volume 5, Tract 1.
8. Peter D'Adamo, *Eat Right for Your Type* (New York: Putnam, 1996).
9. For an overview of many of these, see Steven Rosen, *Diet for Transcendence: Vegetarianism and the World Religions* (Badger, CA: Torchlight, 1997).
10. Keith Akers, *The Lost Religion of Jesus* (New York: Lantern Books, 2000), p. 117.
11. See Matthew 15:11 through 15:20 for entire relevant passage.
12. Matthew 15:19.
13. Gary Zukav, *Seat of the Soul* (New York: Simon and Schuster, 1989), p. 276.
14. Ibid., p. 278.
15. See Marjorie Spiegel, *The Dreaded Comparison: Human and Animal Slavery* (New York: Mirror Books, 1999) for more on the treatment of black slaves as animal livestock in the standard practices of extreme confinement in transport, family destruction, branding, mutilation, and domination. See Sam Keen, *Faces of the Enemy: Reflections of the Hostile Imagination* (San Francisco: Harper & Row, 1986) as well as his PBS documentary of the same name for more on how we humans have dehumanized people we intended to systematically harm (such as slaves and enemies), seeing them as sub-human—as animals. Keen shows, for example, how Nazi propaganda films equated Jewish people with rats, and U.S. World War II propaganda films and posters portrayed Japanese people as hordes of beetles, among other instances.
16. Georgio Cerquetti, *The Vegetarian Revolution* (Badger, CA: Torchlight, 1997), p. 31.
17. Ibid., p. 30.
18. Howard Lyman, *Mad Cowboy* (New York: Scribner, 1998), p. 125.
19. See Lynn Jacobs, *Waste of the West*, for a thorough discussion and reporting of the disastrous effects of cattle ranching in the American West. See also Howard Lyman, "Bovine Planet," in *Mad Cowboy*, pp. 121–153.

Chapter 13—Evolve or Dissolve
1. Helen Caldicott, *The New Nuclear Danger* (New York: The New Press, 2002), p. 1.

2. Based on Department of Agriculture statistics for the slaughtering of over ten billion mammals and birds in the U.S. in 2002, and the 2004 U.S. military budget of $400 billion.

3. The World Game Institute, in "What the World Wants." Cited in Helen Caldicott, *The New Nuclear Danger.* See www.worldgame.org; also www.idealog.us/2004/02/ever_hear_of_th.html.

4. Ten billion land animals slaughtered per year works out to about three hundred animals being killed in the U.S. every second. One way to get a feel for this abstract number is to imagine a line the length of a football field, with animals standing on the line next to each other and each animal occupying an average of one foot of space. A new one-hundred-yard line filled with three hundred animals whizzes by every second around the clock.

5. Katsuki Sekida, *Zen Training* (New York: Weatherhill, 1975), p. 62.

6. Steven Rosen, *Diet for Transcendence* (Badger, CA: Torchlight, 1997), pp. 59–76. See also Vasu Murti, *They Shall Not Hurt or Destroy: Animal Rights and Vegetarianism in the Western Religious Traditions* (Cleveland: Vegetarian Advocates Press, 2003), pp. 101–106.

7. Norm Phelps, *The Dominion of Love* (New York: Lantern Books, 2002), p. 33.

8. Peter Walker, "Makah Whaling Also a Political Issue," *Whales Alive!*, Cetacean Society International, October 4, 1999; see http://csiwhalesalive.org/csi99409.html.

9. Dan Kindlon and Michael Thompson, *The Emotional Life of Boys* (New York: Ballantine, 1999), p. 250.

10. Ibid., p. 87.

11. Matthew Scully, *Dominion: The Power of Man, the Suffering of Animals, and the Call to Mercy* (New York: St. Martin's Press, 2002), pp. 199–226.

12. Cited in Beverly-Collene Galyean, *MindSight: Learning Through Imagery* (Long Beach: Center for Integrative Learning, 1983), p. 5.

Chapter 14—Journey of Transformation

1. "Dalai Lama Campaigns to End Wildlife Trade," Environmental News Service, April 8, 2005.

2. Though most Tibetan lamas eat meat, there is also a strong tradition in Tibetan Buddhism of abstaining from meat and showing great kindness and respect to animals. Tibet's cold, harsh climate is another factor. For more details, see Shabkar, *Food of Bodhisattvas*, translated by Padmakara Translation Group (Boston: Shambhala, 2004) and Norm Phelps, *The Great Compassion: Buddhism and Animal Rights* (New York: Lantern Books, 2004). Besides the Dalai Lama, there are other noted contemporary Buddhist spiritual leaders who have strongly taught and exemplified compassion for animals, particularly Thich Nhat Hanh, Bhiksuni Cheng Yen, S. N. Goenka, A. T. Ariyaratne, and the late Roshi Philip Kapleau and Tripitika Master Hsuan Hua.

3. Eisler, *The Chalice and the Blade: Our History, Our Future* (New York: HarperCollins, 1987), pp. 42–103.

Chapter 15—Living the Revolution

1. Thich Nhat Hanh, *Creating True Peace* (New York: Simon & Schuster, 2003), p. 77.

2. Jeremy Rifkin, "The World's Problems on a Plate: Meat Production Is Making the Rich Ill and the Poor Hungry," *The Guardian*, May 17, 2002.

3. See www.foodnotbombs.org for further information.

4. See www.godsdirectcontact.org for further information. Ching Hai has said, "If everyone practiced meditation and ate a wholesome diet without killing involved,

the world would long since have been in a peaceful state. There's no need to give up your property; just give up the meat-based diet. That would be enough to save the world."

5. Charles Fillmore, "The Twins: Eating and Drinking," *Unity Magazine*, June 1915.

6. See Carol Simontacchi, *The CrazyMakers: How the Food Industry Is Destroying Our Brains and Harming Our Children*. New York: Putnam, 2000.

7. For the complete story and interview with Dr. Pam Popper of the "Wellness Forum," see http://www.madcowboy.com/02?MCIview02.000.html.

8. Mary Spicuzza, "Eating on the Edge," *The Seattle Times*, September 3, 2003. See also http://www.nationaleatingdisorders.org.

9. There are many ways to cultivate this inner field of loving-kindness and compassion. One helpful resource is Judy Carman's book *Peace to All Beings* (New York: Lantern Books, 2003), which contains prayers, meditations, and stories that help readers deepen their spiritual connection with animals. Another is the *Four Viharas Guided Meditation* compact disc by the author of this book, which teaches a 2,500-year-old practice designed to help us reconnect with our inner spiritual abode of loving-kindness, compassion, joy, and equanimity. A third resource is the compact disc album *AnimalSongs*, also by the author, which contains original piano music blended with the voices of animals, with special attention to those species we use for food. See the Resources section for further information.

10. Thomas Byrom, tr., *The Dhammapada*, attributed to Gautama Buddha (New York: Bantam, 1976).

11. Dennis Kucinich, "Spirit and Stardust," address given at the Dubrovnik Conference on the Academy of Peacebuilding, June 4–11, 2002.

RESOURCES

AnimalSongs. Music CD by Will Tuttle. Original piano blended with voices of animals; special focus on animals used for food production. 61 mins.

Circles of Compassion: Essays Connecting Issues of Justice. Edited by Will Tuttle. Essays by internationally recognized authors on the intersectionality of justice issues. Vegan Publishers, 2014. 320 pages.

Conscious Eating: The Power of our Food Choices. DVD by Will Tuttle. Fully illustrated interview, plus three other programs, including a World Peace Diet keynote lecture. 110 mins.

Four Viharas Guided Meditation. CD by Will Tuttle. Meditation on loving-kindness, compassion, joy, and peace, for cultivating inner and outer harmony, with original piano music. 45 mins.

Living in Harmony with All Life. CD by Will Tuttle. In-depth monologue covering the main ideas presented in *The World Peace Diet*. 75 mins.

The World Peace Diet audio book. CD by Will Tuttle. Contains the entire *World Peace Diet* text in an unabridged reading by the author. 31 tracks. It is 13.5 hours long, in an MP3 format.

World Peace Meditations—Eightfold Path for Awakening Hearts. CD by Will Tuttle. Eight guided meditations with original piano and flute music, plus *World Peace Diet* passages for meditation. 79 min.

World Peace Diet Cookbook: Food for People Who Eat. Book by Mark Stroud (foreword by Will Tuttle). Cincinnati, Ohio: Heärt Books, 2016.

World Peace Yoga: Yogs for People Who Breathe. Book by Anna Ferguson (foreword by Will Tuttle). Cincinnati, Ohio: Heärt Books, 2016.

World Peace Diet Mastery and Facilitator Training Programs. Self-paced online training by Will Tuttle: worldpeacemastery.com.

YouTube video channel with Dr. Tuttle's lectures and interviews, as well as vegan kitchen and crafts videos by Madeleine Tuttle.

See worldpeacediet.com and/or willtuttle.com for more information and downloading. Audio recordings also available through online commercial sources.

INTUITIVE COOKING
Happy Dining for Body, Soul, and Spirit

BY MADELEINE TUTTLE

~~~~

Here are some basic recipes for one week (which can be repeated or mixed and matched in different ways) with a shopping list at the end. I kept the dishes pretty simple, but there is a lot of variety. Please use only organic ingredients if possible!

It can be convenient to cook pasta, potatoes, rice, and other grains in a large quantity and store them in the fridge to use later in stir fries, salads, and other meals. Some recipes call for leftover grains.

I purposefully don't mention measurements, just the different ingredients. So let your intuition create wildly and have fun!

I love to "paint" the meals. For example, add paprika if it lacks red, or herbs, baby leaves, or sprouts for green, and turmeric, curry, or peppers for yellow.

- **Favorite breakfast**—a Green Smoothie! Feel great 'til lunch! Blend fruits in season, bananas, citrus, apples, kale, ginger, flaxseeds (can be ground first in coffee grinder), cinnamon, clove, nuts, seeds, herbs, and water.
- **Favorite lunch**—Tortillas! Spread vegan mayo or tahini on tortilla, add lettuce, sprouts, tomatoes, carrots, cucumber, grated horseradish, herbs. Variations: walnuts, avocado, tofu, tempeh, "fakin bacon," etc.
- **Favorite dinners**—Mashed potatoes topped with veggie ragout. Boil cut-up potatoes in water. When soft, pour most of the water into a bowl and save. Add olive oil, nutmeg, celtic salt, and mash with potato masher. Add some water back if necessary. Steam seasonal veggies, and when al dente add olive oil, tamari, herbs, minced garlic, and mix. Add herbs and nutritional yeast to leftover potato water for a delicious soup. Save leftover mashed potatoes for Shepherd's Pie (below)!
- ❖ **Spaghetti**—Cook spaghetti with chunks of kabocha squash in water, and when nearly soft, put broccoli flowers on top. Cover and cook till al dente. Pour water off (as a soup) and serve with tomato sauce, or with a grated ginger-tahini sauce (add water to tahini and stir until smooth).
- ❖ **Salad**—Chop and mix greens, peppers, tomatoes, cucumbers, celery, onions, carrots, etc.; add olive oil, lemon, tamari, herbs, and spices (or tahini sauce above), and mix. Variations: add tofu, tempeh cubes, leftover rice, noodles, kasha, or cut-up boiled potatoes, or eat with bread or crackers.
- ❖ **Couscous**—Boil water and pour over couscous in a bowl with added cumin seeds. Sauté onions, squash, cabbage, and a few potato chunks and curry. When soft, add

olive oil, celtic salt, ground pepper, peppermint, and mix. Place in the middle of bed of couscous.

❖ **Polenta**—Boil water with rosemary; with whisker, stir in cornmeal. Steam seasonal veggies, add tofu. When soft, add olive oil, tamari, garlic, Italian herbs. Top cornmeal with nutritional yeast, add veggie mix.

❖ **Quinoa**—Boil quinoa in water (approximately 3:1) for 45 minutes. Add kale when two-thirds done. Sauté slices of tofu, then sauté mushrooms with onions. Top quinoa with sauté and fresh basil.

❖ **Carrot salad**—Mix greens with finely grated carrots, (raisins,) and pine nuts or walnuts. Mix tahini butter with water, lemon, tamari, and peppermint herbs until smooth, and pour over carrot salad.

❖ **Shepherd's Pie**—Sauté onions and zucchini in a wide shallow pan with lid. Spread peas and crumbled Sunburger or tempeh, top it with leftover mashed potatoes and cook until warm.

❖ **Rice**—Cook rice with wild rice. Mix raw sauce containing finely-cut peppers, celery, tomatoes, parsley, walnuts, olives, olive oil, lemon, herbs, and spices. Mix and pour over cooked rice.

❖ **Millet with roasted leek**—Cook millet (4:1) for 30 mins. Sauté leeks. When soft, add olive oil, minced garlic, and tamari. Serve over millet with a few drops of lemon. Adorn with baby spinach.

❖ **Pumpkin soup**—Boil Kabocha squash (or other winter squash) in water. When soft, pour into blender. Add tahini and blend. When served, add a little tamari or celtic salt.

❖ **Bean tortillas**—Spread fresh cooked or refried beans on tortillas. Cut up cilantro and/or other greens, tomatoes, cucumbers. Add tomato sauce or salsa, cayenne, pepper, and roll up.

❖ **Angel-hair noodles on kale bed**—Cook angel hair noodles or spaghettini. Steam kale (not too long). Serve pasta on a bed of kale with roasted sesame seeds, tamari, and toasted sesame oil and paprika.

❖ **Sablé cookies**—Mix spelt flour, Sucanat, vanilla, and a pinch of salt with liquefied coconut and/or canola oil and water. Shape into long bars 1½ inches in diameter. Put into refrigerator for half hour. When firm, cut into ¹/₃-inch cookie slices. Put onto baking pan and bake at 350 until light brown (ca. 20–30 mins). Variation: add hazelnuts or shredded almonds or raisins.

❖ **Chocolate cookies**—Mix spelt flour, chocolate powder, shredded coconut, crushed walnuts, and a pinch of salt. Add maple syrup or Sucanat and canola oil. Spread onto baking sheet and bake about 20–30 mins. When still warm, cut into squares or bars.

Instead of refined oils, try making nut butter/water/blended veggie/yeast sauces—delicious and healthy!

* * *

Shopping list

Allow yourself a good hour to explore and buy the following items, always *organic*, fair trade, and non-GMO. The more love you feel, the better the outcome. Remember: only the most evolved monks are allowed to cook in some Asian traditions.

Grains: rice, millet, spaghetti, angel-hair, couscous, quinoa, buckwheat/kasha, wild rice, cornmeal.

Veggies: in season, pumpkin/squash, leek, onions, garlic, kale, cabbage, ginger, horseradish, broccoli, peppers, mushrooms, carrots, lettuce/greens, sprouts, edamame, spinach, tomatoes, cucumbers, celery, avocado, cilantro, peas (fresh or frozen), green beans, yams, asparagus potatoes.

Proteins: Tofu, tempeh, "fakin bacon", Sunburgers, seitan. Lentils, split peas, beans, and other legumes.

Dried herbs: peppermint, Italian seasoning mix, basil, dill, cilantro, paprika, cayenne, curry, turmeric, pepper, nutmeg powder, cumin seeds, rosemary, nutritional yeast.

Fruits: citrus, apples, bananas, grapes, berries, avocado, etc.

Other: Almonds, walnuts, hazelnuts, pine nuts; raisins. Flax, sunflower and sesame seeds.

Tahini (sesame butter), organic Vegenaise, tomato sauce, olive oil, tamari or shoyu, refried beans.

Spelt flour, Sucanat, Celtic salt, vanilla, canola oil, coconut oil, chocolate powder, shredded coconut.

Also explore the plant-based cheeses, milks, butters, yogurts, meats, creams, and ice creams.

When you sit down to eat, look at what you've created. Enjoy the colors, smells, tastes, and the love that blesses the food. The Oneness of all beings!

Bon Appetit!

Stay in touch—feel free to copy!

For more details and ideas, see Madeleine's YouTube channel.

SELECTED BIBLIOGRAPHY

Adams, Carol J. *The Inner Art of Vegetarianism*. New York: Lantern Books, 2002.
_____. *Living among Meat Eaters*. New York: Three Rivers Press, 2001.
_____. *The Pornography of Meat*. New York: Continuum, 2003.
_____. *The Sexual Politics of Meat: A Feminist-Vegetarian Critical Theory*. New York: Continuum, 1998.
Adams, Carol J., and Josephine Donovan, eds. *Animals and Women: Feminist Theoretical Explorations*. Durham: Duke University Press, 1995.
Akers, Keith. *The Lost Religion of Jesus: Simple Living and Nonviolence in Early Christianity*. New York: Lantern Books, 2000.
Altman, Nathaniel. *Ahimsa: Dynamic Compassion*. Wheaton, IL: Quest Books, 1980.
Amory, Cleveland. *Man Kind? Our Incredible War on Wildlife*. New York: Harper and Row, 1974.
Badiner, Allen, ed. *Mindfulness in the Marketplace: Compassionate Responses to Consumerism*. Berkeley: Parallax Press, 2002.
Baker, Ron. *The American Hunting Myth*. New York: Vantage Press, 1985.
Barnard, Neal. *Breaking the Food Seduction*. New York: St. Martin's Press, 2003.
_____. *Turn Off the Fat Genes*. New York: Three Rivers Press, 2001.
Bateson, Gregory. *Mind and Nature*. New York: Bantam, 1979.
Bauston, Gene. *Battered Birds, Crated Herds*. Watkins Glen, NY: Farm Sanctuary, 1996.
Berman, Morris. *The Reenchantment of the World*. Ithaca: Cornell University Press, 1981.
Berry, Rynn. *Famous Vegetarians and Their Favorite Recipes*. New York: Pythagorean Publishers, 1999.
_____. *Food for the Gods: Vegetarianism and the World's Religions*. New York: Pythagorean Publishers, 1998.
Boone, J. Allen. *Kinship with All Life*. New York: HarperCollins, 1954.
Bowlby, Rex. *Plant Roots: 101 Reasons Why the Human Diet Is Rooted Exclusively in Plants*. Burbank, CA: Outside the Box Publishing, 2003.
Bradshaw, John. *Bradshaw on: The Family*. Deerfield Beach, FL: Health Communications, 1988, 1996.
Burwash, Peter. *Total Health*. Badger, CA: Torchlight Publishing, 1997.
Bucke, R. M. *Cosmic Consciousness*. New York: Dutton, 1901/1969.
Byrom, Thomas, tr. *The Dhammapada*. New York: Random House, 1976.
Caldicott, Helen. *The New Nuclear Danger*. New York: The New Press, 2002.
Campbell, Joseph. *The Masks of God*. New York: Penguin, 1978.
Campbell, T. Colin. *The China Study: The Most Comprehensive Study of Nutrition Ever Conducted and the Startling Implications for Diet, Weight Loss and Long-term Health*. Dallas: Benbella Books, 2004.

Campolo, Tony. *How to Rescue the Earth without Worshipping Nature: A Christian Call to Save Creation.* Nashville: Thomas Nelson Publishers, 1992.

Capra, Fritjof. *The Tao of Physics.* New York: Bantam, 1975.

_____. *The Turning Point.* New York: Simon & Schuster, 1982.

Carman, Judy. *Peace to All Beings: Veggie Soup for the Chicken's Soul.* New York: Lantern Books, 2003.

Carson, Rachel. *Silent Spring.* Boston: Houghton Mifflin, 1962, 1994.

Cerquetti, Giorgio. *The Vegetarian Revolution.* Badger, CA: Torchlight Publishing, CA, 1997.

Chang, Garma C. C. *The Buddhist Teaching of Totality.* University Park, PA: Pennsylvania State University Press, 1971.

Ching Hai, The Supreme Master. *I Have Come to Take You Home.* San Jose: ISMCH-MA, 1995.

Churchman, C. West. *The Systems Approach and Its Enemies.* New York: Basic Books, 1979.

Coats, C. David. *Old McDonald's Factory Farm: The Myth of the Traditional Farm and the Shocking Truth about Animal Suffering in Today's Agribusiness.* New York: Continuum, 1989.

Coe, Sue. *Dead Meat.* New York: Four Walls Eight Windows, 1996.

Cohen, Robert. *Milk: The Deadly Poison.* Englewood Cliffs, NJ: Argus Publishing, 1998.

_____. *Milk A–Z,* Englewood Cliffs, NJ: Argus Publishing, 2001.

Critser, Greg. *Fat Land.* New York: Houghton Mifflin, 2003.

Davis, Brenda and Vesanto Melina. *Becoming Vegan.* Summertown, TN: Book Publishing Company, 2000.

Davis, Gail. *Vegetarian Food for Thought.* Troutdale, OR: Sage Press, 1999.

Davis, Karen. *More Than a Meal: The Turkey in History, Myth, Ritual, and Reality.* New York: Lantern Books, 2001.

_____. *Prisoned Chickens, Poisoned Eggs.* Summertown, TN: Book Publishing Company, 1996.

Deval, Bill and George Sessions. *Deep Ecology.* New York: Peregrine Smith, 1985.

Diamond, Harvey and Marilyn. *Fit for Life.* New York: Warner Books, 1987.

Dossey, Larry. *Healing Words: The Power of Prayer and the Practice of Medicine.* San Francisco: HarperSanFrancisco, 1993.

_____. *Reinventing Medicine,* New York: HarperCollins, 1999.

Dunayer, Joan. *Animal Equality.* Derwood, MD: Ryce Publishing, 2001.

Eddy, Mary Baker. *Science and Health with Key to the Scriptures.* Boston: The First Church of Christ, Scientist, 1903.

Eisler, Riane. *The Chalice and the Blade: Our History, Our Future.* New York: Harper & Row, 1987.

_____. *Sacred Pleasure: Sex, Myth, and the Politics of the Body—New Paths to Power and Love.* New York: HarperCollins, 1995.

Eisnitz, Gail. *Slaughterhouse: The Shocking Story of Greed, Neglect, and Inhumane Treatment Inside the U.S. Meat Industry.* New York: Prometheus Books, 1997.

Fillmore, Charles. *The Twelve Powers of Man.* Unity Village, MO: Unity Books, 1930.

Fox, Matthew. *Original Blessing.* New York: Tarcher/Putnam, 1983/2000.

_____. *The Reinvention of Work: A New Vision of Livelihood for Our Time.* San Francisco: HarperSanFrancisco, 1994.

Fox, Michael W. *The Boundless Circle.* Wheaton, IL: Quest Books, 1996.

Fox, Nicholas. *Spoiled: The Dangerous Truth about a Food Chain Gone Haywire.* New York: Basic Books, 1997.

Francione, Gary. *Introduction to Animal Rights: Your Child or the Dog?* Philadelphia: Temple University Press, 2000.

Freire, Paulo. *Pedagogy of the Oppressed.* New York: Herder and Herder, 1970.

Fromm, Erich. *Escape from Freedom.* New York: Farrar and Rinehart, 1941.

Fujita, Rod. *Heal the Ocean: Solutions for Saving Our Seas.* Gabriola Island, BC: New Society Publishers, 2003.

Geertz, Clifford. *The Interpretation of Cultures.* New York: Basic Books, 1973.

Geldard, Richard. *The Spiritual Teachings of Ralph Waldo Emerson.* Great Barrington, MA: Lindisfarne Books, 2001.

Goodman, Ronald. *Circumcision, the Hidden Trauma: How an American Cultural Practice Affects Infants and Ultimately Us All.* Boston: Vanguard Publications, 1997.

Goswami, Amit. *The Self-Aware Universe: How Consciousness Creates the Material World.* New York: Tarcher/Putnam, 1993.

Govinda, Lama Anagarika. *Insights of a Himalayan Pilgrim.* Berkeley: Dharma Publishing, 1991.

Grandin, Temple. *Thinking in Pictures and Other Reports of My Life with Autism.* New York: Doubleday, 1995.

Griffin, Vicki, Diane Griffin, and Virgil Hulse. *Moooove Over Milk.* Hot Springs, NC: Let's Eat! Books, 1997.

Hall, Edward T. *The Hidden Dimension.* New York: Doubleday, 1966.

Hammitzsch, Horst. *Zen in the Art of the Tea Ceremony.* New York: Avon, 1982.

Harris, William. *The Scientific Basis of Vegetarianism.* Honolulu: Hawaii Health Publishers, 1995.

Hart, Donna, and Robert W. Sussman. *Man the Hunted: Primates, Predators, and Human Evolution.* New York: Perseus, 2005.

Heinberg, Richard. *The Party's Over: Oil, War and the Fate of Industrial Societies.* Gabriola Island, BC: New Society Publishers, 2003.

Houston, Jean. *Mystical Dogs: Animals as Guides to Our Inner Life.* Makawao, HI: Inner Ocean Publishing, 2002.

Hubbard, Barbara Marx. *The Revelation: Our Crisis Is a Birth.* Novato, CA: Nataraj Publishing, 1993.

Hyland, J. R. *God's Covenant with Animals: A Biblical Basis for the Humane Treatment of All Creatures.* New York: Lantern Books, 2000.

Icke, David. *Alice in Wonderland and the World Trade Center Disaster.* Wildwood, MO: Bridge of Love Publishers, 2002.

Jacobs, Lynn. *Waste of the West.* Tucson: Lynn Jacobs, 1991.

Kaufman, Stephen R., and Nathan Braun. *Good News for All Creation: Vegetarianism as Christian Stewardship.* Cleveland: Vegetarian Advocates Press, 2002.

Kapleau, Philip. *To Cherish All Life: A Buddhist Case for Becoming Vegetarian.* Rochester, NY: The Zen Center, 1986.

Kindlon, Dan, and Michael Thompson. *Raising Cain: Protecting the Emotional Life of Boys.* New York: Ballantine, 1999.

Klaper, Michael. *Pregnancy, Children, and the Vegan Diet.* Paia, HI: Gentle World, 1994.

_____. *Vegan Nutrition: Pure and Simple.* Paia, HI: Gentle World, 1998.

Kliment, Felicia Drury. *The Acid-Alkaline Balance Diet.* New York: Contemporary Books, 2002.

Korten, David. *When Corporations Rule the World.* West Hartford, CT: Kumarian Press, 1995.

Kowalski, Gary. *The Souls of Animals.* Walpole, NH: Stillpoint Publishing, 1991.

Krishnamurti, J. *Beyond Violence.* New York: Harper & Row, 1973.

Kropotkin, Peter. *Mutual Aid: A Factor in Evolution.* New York: Penguin, 1939.

Kuby, Lolette. *Faith and the Placebo Effect: An Argument for Self-Healing.* Novato, CA: Origin Press, 2001.

Kuhn, Thomas. *The Structure of Scientific Revolutions.* 2nd ed. Chicago: University of Chicago Press, 1962, 1970.

Lappé, Frances Moore. *Diet for a Small Planet.* 2nd rev. ed. New York: Ballantine, 1987.

Lappé, Frances Moore and Joseph Collins. *Food First: Beyond the Myth of Scarcity.* Boston: Houghton Mifflin, 1977.

Lappé, Frances Moore and Anna Lappé. *Hope's Edge: The Next Diet for a Small Planet.* New York: Penguin Putnam, 2002.
Lhalungpa, Lobsang, tr. *The Life of Milarepa.* New York: Penguin, 1977.
Linzey, Andrew. *Animal Gospel.* Louisville: Westminster John Knox Press, 2000.
_____. *Animal Theology.* Urbana: University of Illinois Press, 1995.
Luk, Charles, tr. *The Surangama Sutra.* London: Rider, 1966.
Macy, Joanna. *Dharma and Development: Religion as Resource in the Sarvodaya Self-Help Movement.* West Hartford, CT: Kumarian Press, 1983.
Marcus, Erik. *Vegan: The New Ethics of Eating.* Ithaca, NY: McBooks Press, 1998.
Mason, Jim, and Peter Singer. *Animal Factories: What Agribusiness Is Doing to the Family Farm, the Environment, and Your Health.* New York: Harmony Books, 1990.
Mason, Jim. *An Unnatural Order: Why We Are Destroying the Planet and Each Other.* New York: Continuum, 1993.
Masson, Jeffrey Moussaieff. *The Pig Who Sang to the Moon: The Emotional World of Farm Animals.* New York: Ballantine, 2003.
Masson, Jeffrey Moussaieff and Susan McCarthy. *When Elephants Weep: The Emotional Lives of Animals.* New York: Delacorte Press, 1995.
McDougall, John. *McDougall's Medicine.* Piscataway, NJ: New Century Publishers, 1985.
_____. *The McDougall Plan.* Piscataway, NJ: New Century Publishers, 1983.
McElroy, Susan. *Animals as Teachers and Healers: True Stories and Reflections.* New York: Ballantine, 1996.
Merchant, Carolyn. *The Death of Nature.* New York: Harper & Row, 1980.
Mitroff, Ian and F. Sagasti. "Epistemology as General Systems Theory: An Approach to the Design of Complex Decision-Making Experiments." In *Philosophy of the Social Sciences,* 3:1973.
Moran, Victoria. *Compassion: The Ultimate Ethic, An Exploration of Veganism.* Wellingborough, UK: Thorsons Publishers Limited, 1985.
Moretti, Laura A., ed. *All Heaven in a Rage: Essays on the Eating of Animals.* Chico, CA: MBK Publishing, 1999.
Mowat, Farley. *Sea of Slaughter.* New York: Atlantic Monthly Press, 1984.
Murti, Vasu. *They Shall Not Hurt or Destroy: Moral and Theological Objections to the Human Exploitation of Nonhuman Animals.* Cleveland: Vegetarian Advocates Press, 2003.
Nestle, Marion. *Food Politics.* Berkeley: University of California Press, 2002.
Newkirk, Ingrid. *Free the Animals.* New York: Lantern Books, 2000.
Nhat Hanh, Thich. *Anger.* New York: Penguin Putnam, 2001.
_____. *Creating True Peace.* New York: Simon & Schuster, 2003.
_____. *Peace is Every Step.* New York: Bantam, 1991.
Noddings, Nell. *Caring: A Feminine Approach to Ethics and Moral Education.* Berkeley: University of California Press, 1984.
O'Barry, Richard. *To Free a Dolphin.* Los Angeles: Renaissance Books, 2000.
Oski, Frank. *Don't Drink Your Milk.* Brushtown, NY: Teach Services, 1983.
Page, Tony. *Buddhism and Animals: A Buddhist Vision of Humanity's Rightful Relationship with the Animal Kingdom.* London: UKAVIS Publications, 1999.
Patterson, Charles. *Eternal Treblinka: Our Treatment of Animals and the Holocaust.* New York: Lantern Books, 2002.
Phelps, Norm. *The Dominion of Love.* New York: Lantern Books, 2002.
_____. *The Great Compassion: Buddhism and Animal Rights.* New York: Lantern Books, 2004.
Pipher, Mary. *Reviving Ophelia: Saving the Selves of Adolescent Girls.* New York: Ballantine, 1994.
Quinn, Daniel. *The Story of B.* New York: Bantam, 1996.

Rampton, Sheldon and John Stauber. *Mad Cow U.S.A.* Monroe, ME: Common Courage Press, 1997.

Randour, Mary Lou, Ph.D. *Animal Grace: Entering a Spiritual Relationship with Our Fellow Creatures.* Novato, CA: New World Library, 2000.

Regan, Tom. *The Case for Animal Rights.* Berkeley: University of California Press, 1983.

Regenstein, Lewis. *How to Survive in America the Poisoned.* New York: Acropolis, 1982.

Reinhardt, Mark Warren. *The Perfectly Contented Meat-Eater's Guide to Vegetarianism.* New York: Continuum, 1999.

Rifkin, Jeremy. *Beyond Beef: The Rise and Fall of the Cattle Culture.* New York: Dutton, 1992.

Robbins, John. *Diet for a New America.* Walpole, NH: StillPoint, 1987.

_____. *The Food Revolution: How Your Diet Can Save Your Life and the World.* Berkeley: Conari Press, 2001.

_____. *Reclaiming Our Health.* Tiburon, CA: H. J. Kramer, 1996.

Rosen, Steven. *Diet for Transcendence: Vegetarianism and the World Religions.* Badger, CA: Torchlight Publishing, 1997.

Ruesch, Hans. *Slaughter of the Innocent: Animals in Medical Research.* New York: Bantam, 1978.

Russell, Peter. *The Global Brain.* Los Angeles: Tarcher, 1983.

Schoen, Allen M. *Kindred Spirits: How the Remarkable Bond between Humans and Animals Can Change the Way We Live.* New York: Broadway Books, 2001.

Schumacher, E. F. *A Guide for the Perplexed.* New York: Harper & Row, 1977

Scully, Matthew. *Dominion: The Power of Man, the Suffering of Animals, and the Call to Mercy.* New York: St. Martin's Press, 2002.

Sekida, Katsuki. *Zen Training.* New York: Weatherhill, 1975.

Shabkar. *Food of Bodhisattvas.* Translated by the Padmakara Translation Group, Boston: Shambhala Publications, 2004.

Sheldrake, Rupert. *Dogs That Know When Their Owners Are Coming Home and Other Unexplained Powers of Animals.* New York: Three Rivers Press, 1999.

_____. *Seven Experiments That Would Change the World.* New York: Inner Traditions, 2002.

Simontacchi, Carol. *The CrazyMakers: How the Food Industry Is Destroying Our Brains and Harming Our Children.* New York: Putnam, 2000.

Sinclair, Upton. *The Jungle.* New York: Bantam, 1906, 1981.

Singer, Peter. *Animal Liberation.* New York: Random House, 1990.

Skolimowski, Henryk. *The Theatre of the Mind.* Wheaton, IL, Quest Books, 1984.

Sorokin, Pitirim. *The Reconstruction of Humanity.* Boston: Beacon Press, 1948.

Spiegel, Marjorie. *The Dreaded Comparison: Human and Animal Slavery.* New York: Mirror Books, 1999.

Stepaniak, Joanne. *Being Vegan: Living with Conscience, Conviction, and Compassion.* Los Angeles: Lowell House, 2000.

Suzuki, D. T. *Essays in Zen Buddhism.* Series 1–3. New York: Samuel Weiser, 1971.

_____, tr. *The Lankavatara Sutra.* Boulder: Prajna, 1978.

Thoreau, Henry David. *Walden and Other Writings.* New York: Bantam, 1854, 1981.

Watson, Paul. *Ocean Warrior.* Key Porter Books, Toronto, 1994.

Webb, Stephen H. *Good Eating.* Grand Rapids, MI: Brazos Press, 2001.

Weil, Andrew. *Eight Weeks to Optimum Health.* New York: Random House, 1997.

_____. *Health and Healing.* New York, Houghton Mifflin, 1998.

_____. *Spontaneous Healing.* New York: Random House, 1995.

Weil, Simone. "The Iliad or the Poem of Force." In *Politics*, November 1945.

Wiebers, Andrea and David Wiebers. *Souls Like Ourselves.* Rochester, MN: Sojourn Press, 2000.

Wilber, Ken. *A Brief History of Everything.* Boston: Shambhala Publications, 1996.

_____. *Up from Eden.* Boston: Shambhala Publications, 1984.

Wolf, Fred Alan. *Mind into Matter: A New Alchemy of Science and Spirit*. Portsmouth, NH: Moment Point Press, 2001.
Young, Richard Alan. *Is God a Vegetarian? Christianity, Vegetarianism, and Animal Rights*. Peru, IL: Open Court, 1999.
Young, Robert O. and Shelley R. Young. *The pH Miracle*. Warner, New York, 2002.
Zukav, Gary. *The Dancing Wu Li Masters*. New York: Bantam, 1979.
_____. *Seat of the Soul*. New York: Simon & Schuster, 1989.

INDEX

absurdities, belief in, 213, 215
abuse of animals, suppression of aware-
    ness of, 30, 31, 33–34
acid, 72, 73
Adams, Carol J., 47
addiction, 61, 281–284
advertising, 57
agribusiness. *See* agriculture industry
agricultural revolution, effects on forager
    cultures, 21
agriculture
    plant *vs.* animal, 21
    See also animal agriculture
agriculture, animal. *See* animal agricul-
    ture; animal food industry
Agriculture, Department of, 112
agriculture, industrial. *See* animal agricul-
    ture; animal food industry
agriculture industry
    protection of, 112
    spread of American model, 279
    See also animal agriculture
ahimsa, 231
Akers, Keith, 210–211
alcoholism, 281–284
Alcott, Bronson, 248
Alcott, Louisa May, 249
All Heaven in a Rage (Moretti), 167–168
altruism, animals', 275–276
American Cancer Society, 89
American Heart Association, 89
American Indian cultures, 235
Amnesty International, 46
analysis, 227
animal agriculture
    government support of, 190, 194
    as men's work, 21
    petroleum required for, 187
    pollution from, 96, 187, 190–191
    toxins in, 189–191
    See also animal food industry

animal-derived foods
    acid in, 72
    and addiction, 61, 281–284
    beginnings of eating of, 204
    blood in, 60
    considered natural, 202–206
    descriptions of, 7–8
    disguising of, 60
    effects of choosing to eat, 269–270,
        272–273
    effects on humans, 271
    effects on intelligence, 75
    and environment, 185, 216
    fat in, 61, 70, 76, 78
    and health, 74–76, 93
    as hindrance to fulfilling potential,
        265
    and incarceration rate, 296n15
    inefficiency of, 189
    lack of carbohydrates in, 70
    lack of fiber in, 70
    lack of need for, 94
    and limitations on freedom, 272–273
    petroleum needed to produce, 187
    raw, 59–60
    and suffering, 8, 9
    taste of, 60–61
    toxins in, 76, 78–84, 135
    as unnecessary, 67
    vibrations in, 139
    waste products in, 60
    See also beef; dairy; eggs; fish; omni-
        vores
animal feed, 79, 80, 112–113, 185–187,
    190
animal food industry
    destructiveness of, 184
    inhumanity of, 183
    marketing pressure by, 56–57
    omnivores as victims of, 273
    propaganda by, 74

STUDY QUESTIONS

(These are just a few suggestions. Please feel free to create more.)

~~~

Chapter 1—Food's Power

1. What do you think is meant by "the power of food?" What is the source of this power?
2. Why might it be that the more forcefully we ignore something, the more power it has over us? What are the effects of this ignoring and denial? Can you think of any examples of this?
3. In what ways have we inherited abusiveness? Are we responsible for this?
4. What is compassion? How does the dictionary definition of compassion relate to our food choices?
5. In what ways do we practice I–Thou and I–It relations with others during our day? How does the I–It sense of self compare with the I–Thou sense of self?
6. What is the shadow archetype as articulated by Carl Jung? Why is it significant?

Chapter 2—Our Culture's Roots

1. What is the core mentality of our culture, according to *The World Peace Diet*?
2. How did this mentality arise and develop?
3. How is it still reinforced today, do you think?
4. What is the relationship between herding animals, war, the domination of women, elitism/privilege, social injustice, and the establishment of a wealthy ruling class?
5. What is the Pythagorean Principle?
6. What is veganism? What are its roots? What is its defining motivation?

Chapter 3—The Nature of Intelligence

1. How might consumerism be connected to omnivorism?
2. Why are the "secrets" of dysfunctional families so damaging? How is this related to our treatment of animals for food?
3. What is intelligence? What are the cognitive and affective components of intelligence?
4. "We are what we practice." How does this relate to our culture's loss of real intelligence?
5. What is the purpose of non-human animals? Of humans?
6. What are some examples of the "boomerang effect"—of reaping the seeds we sow in our mistreatment of animals? Can you think of other boomerang effects that are not in the book?
7. How do we increase joy and peace in our lives?

Chapter 4—Inheriting Our Food Choices
1. Why is it difficult to contemplate or question indoctrinated beliefs?
2. What is "leaving home?" Why is it important, do you think?
3. What are the three main reasons people eat animal-derived foods, according to the book? Are there others?
4. What are the types of social pressure we are subjected to that push us to eat animal foods? Which types do you think are strongest?
5. What factors influence taste?
6. Is taste a good reason to eat foods derived from animals? Why or why not?
7. Does anyone in this culture freely choose to eat the flesh and secretions of animals? Explain.

Chapter 5—The Intelligence of Human Physiology
1. What types of foods are we humans physiologically designed to eat? What is the evidence for this?
2. What are the effects of eating animal protein?
3. What is the relationship between carbohydrates and obesity?
4. Which foods contain the highest levels of toxins? What are some examples of these toxins?
5. What is the relationship between the proliferation of CAFOs (factory farms) and what the author refers to as the meat-medical complex?
6. What is the placebo effect? How may the placebo effect operate in those who stop eating animal foods?
7. Why is buying organic produce and grains important?

Chapter 6—Hunting and Herding Sea Life
1. Why is the flesh and oil of fish so extremely high in concentrated toxins?
2. What is "herding fish" and what are the effects of this practice on animals and the environment?
3. What is "bycatch" and why is this so devastating to our oceans?
4. What are some of the effects of "sport" fishing?
5. Can fish feel pain? Are they intelligent?

Chapter 7—The Domination of the Feminine
1. How are dairy cows pushed to produce more milk than they naturally would? What are the effects of this?
2. What are some of the toxins in milk? Is cow's milk designed for humans?
3. What are the four pathways a calf born on a dairy might take?
4. What is the effect of drinking milk on the age of menarche?
5. What happens to males born on egg production facilities, "free-range" or not? What are some of the types of suffering caused to hens by battery cages? Are "free-range" egg operations much better?
6. What is Sophia? Discuss her significance for us today, and her oppression by our culture's food institutions.

Chapter 8—The Metaphysics of Food
1. What are metaphysical toxins?

2. What is the emerging understanding of the relationship between matter, energy, and consciousness? Why is this significant?
3. What is materialism, and why is a culture with violent food likely to be materialistic?
4. What is *prana*? Why do many mothers in India consider it important in preparing food?
5. What might be the relationship between eating violence and violence in movies, music, art, and the media?
6. What is *ahimsa*? Why is it important?
7. What is "the Maharishi effect?"

Chapter 9 – Reductionist Science and Religion
1. What are "the two bickering brothers?" They are the sons of what?
2. How do they reinforce one another? Who do they both join in attacking? Why is this ironic?
3. What is reductionist science? How is it damaging to the world and us? What are some examples of holistic science?
4. What is reductionist religion? How is it damaging?
5. How is our violence toward animals for food related to our sense of evil?

Chapter 10—The Dilemma of Work
1. What types of work do slaughterhouse and animal farm workers actually do?
2. What are some of the effects of doing this work on the workers?
3. What is the significance of effect? How does it affect everyone?
4. What should work be, ideally?
5. What does "resurrecting work" mean?

Chapter 11—Profiting from Destruction
1. "The foundation of agriculture has switched from soil to oil." Discuss this and its significance.
2. Why is eating animal-derived foods extremely wasteful of water, land, energy, and fossil fuels?
3. What is monocropping? What are the consequences of this practice?
4. Why do diets high in animal foods decimate wildlife and destroy habitat?
5. What types of pollution are caused by animal agriculture?
6. What are some ways trans-national corporations profit from people eating animal-based diets?
7. Why do gene theories of disease have appeal to corporations?

Chapter 12—Some Objections Answered
1. Discuss the first objection—that our mistreatment of animals is ethically trivial.
2. Are humans naturally predatory? What types of evidence are there?
3. Why has the blood-type diet been popular?
4. How does science often support violence toward animals? How could it change?
5. How does religion often support violence toward animals? How could it change?
6. "Imagining our culture as a vegan culture is truly imagining an almost completely different culture." Discuss.

Chapter 13—Evolve or Dissolve
1. What are "the two limited perspectives" regarding our abuse of animals?
2. Discuss the cycle of violence as it relates to abusing animals routinely for food. How does this generate "The Shadow" and what are the effects of this?
3. "All sentient beings have interests." Discuss.
4. What is "the intuitive imperative?"
5. What are *shojin* and *samadhi* and how are they related?
6. What is "the emotional miseducation of boys" and its significance?

Chapter 14—Journey of Transformation
1. Discuss the jeweled web metaphor. How are all journeys interconnected?
2. Why is community important in influencing human consciousness and behavior? Examples?
3. What are some types of vegan communities? How can we best spread the vegan message?
4. What seeds of compassion are unfolding in your life journey now?

Chapter 15—Living the Revolution
1. "The opposite of love is not hate but indifference." Discuss.
2. Discuss the roles of victim, perpetrator, and bystander, and their significance for us today as vegans.
3. What are "the four M's?" How does this mentality affect us and our institutions?
4. Discuss some of the implications for further research and conversation.
5. What is "orthorexia nervosa" and what is its significance?
6. "Veganism requires a spiritual breakthrough." Discuss.
7. How can we best be the change we would like to see in the world?